SFCR Experts Series

Volume 1

Spinal surgery has evolved considerably in recent years, making it particularly challenging for the spine surgeon to have the latest and most relevant knowledge in the field of spinal diseases at his disposal. French spine surgeons have always been innovative in the field of spinal treatment, introducing new concepts and breakthrough theories for many years, and some of them, such as Doctor Pierre Stagnara, Professor Raymond Roy-Camille and Professor Jean Dubousset, are considered masters in the field and recognised pioneers throughout the world. This series has been conceived by a group of experts from the French Spine Society with an 'encyclopaedic spirit', and the aim of bringing together the best knowledge, scientific literature, personal experience and expert opinion in all areas of spinal pathologies. It will cover a wide range of topics (trauma/degenerative/tumours), from decision-making and artificial intelligence to surgical strategy, new technologies and complications, as well as specific conditions such as spinal deformities, spinal infections, cranio-vertebral junction, osteoporotic spine or paediatric spine. A unique panel of French experts and of international contributors with extensive experience in the field are involved, ensuring a high quality scientific level of content. The friendly format, with illustrations and tables and concise chapters, undoubtedly makes the books easy and enjoyable to read.

Cédric Y. Barrey
Editor

Spine Surgery

General Considerations and Fundamental Concepts Vol. 1

Springer

SFCR

Editor
Cédric Y. Barrey
Department of Spine and Spinal Cord Surgery
Hôpital P. Wertheimer, GHE, Hospices Civils de Lyon (HCL),
and University Claude Bernard of Lyon 1
Lyon, France

ISSN 3004-8850 ISSN 3004-8869 (electronic)
SFCR Experts Series
ISBN 978-3-031-85445-3 ISBN 978-3-031-85446-0 (eBook)
https://doi.org/10.1007/978-3-031-85446-0

This Springer imprint is published by the registered company Springer Nature Switzerland AG
The registered company address is: Gewerbestrasse 11, 6330 Cham, Switzerland

I dedicate this book to my wife, Hélène, for its unfailing daily support, and to our two great sons, Corentin and Maximilien, for their unlimited love; to my mentor, Professor Gilles Perrin for his transmission of knowledge and sharing his huge experience; to my patients for their unshakeable confidence; and finally, to my colleagues, residents, and fellows, and all the team, for their insatiable curiosity and for giving me the force to always do better.

Also, I would like to thank all the chapter authors for their invaluable work and for their complete engagement into the project; the editorial committee for their constant inspiration; as well the SFCR and Springer team for supporting the book collection series.

SFCR Foreword

The French Spine Surgery Society (SFCR) was created in 2004 under the initiative of an orthopedic group (Daniel Chopin, Arnaud Blamoutier, Pierre Guigui). From 2011, after several joint meetings, French spine neurosurgeons were unified to the SFCR representing so far, all the spine surgeons in France. Over the years, the society has considerably grown organizing many activities not only in scientific and academic fields but also regarding socio-professional and medico-economic aspects. Each year, the members have the opportunity to present their scientific works, learn from the most recent advances in the field, and share their opinions through interactive discussion sessions during the Annual Meeting of the society. SFCR is also strongly connected with other spinal societies, especially in Europe, being regularly involved in international conferences and symposiums.

France has a tradition of innovative concepts in spine surgery and Professor Raymond Roy-Camille and Professor Jean Dubousset, both from Paris, represent undoubtfully the most world recognized French pioneer surgeons who have revolutionized the spine surgery in the 1960s and the 1980s, respectively. More recently, under the impulsion of Madame Duval-Beaupère, the French spine school considerably contributed to a better understanding of sagittal balance concepts introducing new parameters and developing modern ideas.

To perpetuate the tradition of French school in the field of spine surgery, the SFCR desired to establish a collaboration with Springer in order to edit a book collection series around spinal concepts with an encyclopedic spirit. The finality is to address all the features of spinal pathologies through the book collection editing 1 to 2 volumes per year. The first volume is dedicated to the fundamentals and basic concepts. Volumes 2 and 3 will treat about lumbar and cervical degenerative diseases, and Volumes 4 and 5 will be focused on thoraco-lumbar and cervical traumas, respectively.

At the end, it is our great pleasure to contribute to the diffusion of knowledge in spinal disorders, for the next spine surgeon's generation. We assume that the "SFCR Experts Series" collection will provide to them useful tools and decision-making for their daily practice.

SFCR presidents:

2004/2005: D. Chopin	2010: P. Guigui	2015: J. Beaurain	2020: J. Allain
2006: JP. Lemaire (†)	2011: R. Assaker	2016: H. Parent	2021: JL. Barat
2007: JM. Vital	2012: A. Blamoutier	2017: J. Huppert	2022: P. Tropiano
2008: P. Roussouly	2013: J. Destandau	2018: JC. Le Huec	2023: C.Y. Barrey
2009: T. David	2014: JP. Steib	2019: S. Litrico	2024: V. Fiere

For the SFCR,
Prof. Cédric Y. Barrey (SFCR President 2023)

Preface

Spine surgery has considerably evolved over the last years by challenging the spine surgeons to have available the most recent and relevant knowledge in the field of spinal diseases.

A group of experts from the French Spine Surgery Society (SFCR) aimed to edit a book series, with an "encyclopedic spirit," regrouping the best knowledge, scientific literature, personal experience, and expert opinion in all the domains of spinal pathologies. This book represents the first volume of the collection "SFCR Experts Series." The aim of this volume is to regroup all the fundamental concepts around spine surgery thus offering to the spine surgeon a unique overview in the field. The volume will concentrate the basic concepts that all spine specialist should be informed about.

To understand the present and anticipate the future, it is essential to know the past. The volume will thus start with the history of spine surgery describing the most significant key steps of the discipline.

The present of spine surgery will then be discussed through the epidemiology of spine practice and spinal pathologies nowadays.

The fundamentals, including surgical anatomy, biomechanics, spinal instrumentation and biomaterials, bone fusion biology and bone substitutes, spinal cord injury and regeneration, represent "the heart" of the volume and will be successively depicted and illustrated within the pages by well-renowned experts. The authors will make efforts to present the most relevant concepts and synthetize the most useful knowledge.

Finally, the section on data management, artificial intelligence, innovations, and emerging technologies will give to the reader the perspectives and future of spine surgery.

At the end, the content of this "SFCR Experts Series" Volume 1 should doubtless be appreciated by spine surgeons, both orthopedists and neurosurgeons!

Lyon, France Cédric Y. Barrey

Contents

History of Spine Surgery

Vincent Challier and Jean Meyblum

1 Introduction

From the ancient civilizations of Egypt and India to the modern era of advanced medical technology, the field of spinal surgery has undergone a remarkable evolution shaped by centuries of innovation, discovery, and perseverance. This chapter delves into the rich tapestry of history, tracing the foundational principles and pivotal inventions that have shaped the practice of spinal surgery as it is known today. As we journey through the annals of history, uncovering the ingenuity and perseverance of those who dared to explore the complexities of the spine, their contributions have transformed spinal surgery from a rudimentary art to a sophisticated science, offering hope and healing to countless individuals afflicted by spinal disorders. Embark on a voyage through time with this exploration of the evolution of spinal surgery and the indelible mark, it has left on the landscape of medicine.

V. Challier (✉)
Hôpital Privé du Dos Francheville, Hôpital Privé Francheville 4, Francheville, Périgueux, France
e-mail: drchallier@hpdf.fr

J. Meyblum
Pôle Rachis Eure-et-Loire, Hôpital Privé d'Eure-et-Loire, Mainvilliers, France

2 Part I: The Founding Principles of Spinal Surgery

2.1 Antiquity (−3500 to 476)

2.1.1 Ancient Egypt

It was not until the papyrus discovered by Edwin Smith (1822–1906) in Ancient Egypt that the first observations on the spine were made [1–3]. The exact author is not known, but archaeologist James Henry Breasted (1865–1935) speculates that the papyrus may be attributed to the work of the architect, priest, and physician Imhotep (−3000). The papyrus contains a precise description of spinal lesions, including a case of fracture–luxation with a full description of tetraplegia. On the subject of a comminuted fracture of the vertebral body, the author has few solutions to offer: "*It's a medical problem that can't be cured.*" Thus, this work on spinal pathology and its management is the first known treatise on the subject, and thus the birth of our specialty. Despite anatomical dissections, no direct connection was initially established between the anatomy and functionality of the spinal cord.

2.1.2 The Hindu Origin of Axial Traction

The first description of scoliosis and the concept of axial traction is reported in "*Srimad Bhagivat Mahapuranam*," an Indian legend [4]. This legend (−3500/−1800) describes the feat of Lord

C. Y. Barrey (ed.), *Spine Surgery*, SFCR Experts Series 1,
https://doi.org/10.1007/978-3-031-85446-0_1

Krishna, correcting the deformity of one of his next Kubja two fingers under the chin, one foot on her foot. This passage is the earliest known reference to the concept of axial traction, predating Hippocrates (−460/−370) by over a millennium.

2.1.3 Greco-Roman Influence

Hippocrates (−460/−370) classified spinal pathologies into five groups: kyphosis, scoliosis, "seisis" (medullary contusions), vertebral dislocation, and spinous process fractures [5].

He established and codified the basis for orthopedic treatment of spinal fractures using external maneuvers, aided by his Hippocratic board. Although his writings suggest that real surgery on the spinal column was a rarity, he advocated open-focus reduction of fractures, in particular using an anterior approach. However, he warned patients to beware of charlatans who used treatment methods more to impress their audience than to heal, even if it meant doing harm. "*Primum non nocere*" [6].

Herophilus of Chalcedon (335–280 BC), who settled in Alexandria and benefited from the goodwill of the authorities who freely allowed him to perform autopsies, traced the anatomical origin of the nerves to the spinal cord [7]. However, there is no mention of the anatomy of the spine or the biomechanics of the spine in his work, which comprises nine treatises, all of which tragically disappeared in the library fire.

Claude Galien of Pergamon or Galen (129–216 AD), born in Asia Minor to a wealthy family, set out on a journey through the Greco-Roman world to meet the most renowned physicians. He drew his knowledge from the observation of cadavers, but above all from his dissections of animals, extrapolating his discoveries to human anatomy, particularly the study of the spinal cord and peripheral nerves [8]. He described the various vertebral segments and observed metameric correlation. His anatomical doctrines would remain the standard for over 14 centuries.

2.2 The Middle Ages (476–1492)

The tragic burning of the Library of Alexandria and the decline of the Roman Empire marked a troubled period in the West, leading to a relative loss of the knowledge accumulated during Antiquity. Fortunately, the expansion of Islam led to the migration of knowledge to the Byzantine Empire and the development of an Arabic medicine based on principles inherited from the Greco-Roman period.

Paulus Aegina (625–690 AD) is credited with the first described surgical approaches to the spine, involving debridement and removal of bone debris, mainly in traumatized patients with neurological complications [9–12]. Born in Aegina, Greece, he studied medicine in Alexandria, immersing himself in the knowledge inherited from Hippocrates and Galen. He then traveled to the Middle East, where he was inspired by Arab scientific thought. He published the seven-volume *Epitome of Medicine (Pléiade)*, incorporating Greco-Roman theories and adding his own personal innovations. Endowed with great surgical skill and a keen sense of observation, he described his experiments, including several surgical approaches. His volume on the art of surgery was masterfully translated in 1855 by René Briau (1810–1886) [13], a French physician and librarian at the Académie de Médecine, and constitutes a compendium considered, along with the writings of Celsus (first century), to be the first treatises on surgery. The paragraph on fractures reads as follows:

> *The contours of the vertebrae are sometimes affected by contusion, but rarely by fracture. In such cases, if the vertebral meninges or the medulla itself are compressed, nerve sympathies are aroused and rapid death ensues; especially if the condition occurs on the cervical vertebrae. It is therefore necessary, after warning of the danger, to dare, if possible, to remove the compressing bone by means of an incision.*

Abulcasis (Abul-Qasim Al Zahrawi) (936–1013), born in Cordoba, produced a 30-volume medical treatise, the last of which contains three books on general, orthopedic, and traumatological surgery [14, 15]. Inventor of numerous surgical instruments, including the forerunner of the suction cannula, he insisted on the need for clean surgery and described procedures for reducing and stabilizing the spinal column.

Avicenna (980–1037 AD), a Persian physician, is considered one of the most important scientists of the ancient world. He perfected Galen's writings by proposing the *Canons of Medicine*, the medical reference text until 1650 and one of the most widely printed works after the Bible. Chapters 6, 7, 8, 9, 10, 11, 12, and 13 contain an unprecedented description of the functional and biomechanical anatomy of the spine, with particular reference to the cranio-spinal junction, and the coupling phenomenon of the thoracolumbar spine [16].

It would be inaccurate to describe the Middle Ages as a period of medical obscurantism. From the twelfth century onward, the term surgery (from the Greek keir: hand and ergon: activity) was used to designate a practice that gradually became distinct from the medical art and developed despite its condemnation by the Christian Church at the Council of Tours in 1163 with the famous maxim "ecclesia abhorret a sanguine" [17]. Jean Pitard (1248–1328) is credited with asking Saint Louis (1214–1270) to create the *Confrérie de Saint-Côme*, which defined and organized the profession of surgeon for the first time around 1260 [18]. The same period saw the founding of the first faculties of medicine in Montpellier (1220) and Paris (1253). The first surgical treatises by Henri de Mondeville (1260–1320) and his pupil Guy de Chauliac (1300–1368) set the standard for the treatment of battlefield wounds, introducing notions of antisepsis inspired by Theodoric Borgognoni (1205–1298) [19–21]. It was in the fifteenth and sixteenth centuries that the French scientific approach to surgery clearly took shape, with the flowering of anatomical studies in the artistic and scientific effervescence of the Renaissance, of which Leonardo da Vinci (1452–1519) and André Vésale (1514–1564) remain the undisputed benchmarks [22].

3 Part II: The Development of Spinal Surgery Through Various Inventions

3.1 The Birth of "Modern" Spine Surgery: Laminectomy

The evolution of medical techniques inevitably accompanies those of death. On the battlefield, Ambroise Paré (1509–1590) revolutionized traumatic surgery, inventing a number of new instruments, notably cranial drill bits, favoring vascular suturing over cauterization, developing a device for spinal traction in cases of dislocation, and evoking the possibility of incising and decompressing neurological structures, without publishing any cases of vertebral surgery [23, 24]. Fabricius Hildanus (1560–1634) proposed a bloody reduction of cervical dislocation, which the famous figure of the *seton* or *setaceum* in his famous posthumous *Opera Omnia* of 1646 misrepresented for decades [25]. Geraud was perhaps the first surgeon to accurately describe a direct approach to the spine during the Battle of Fontenoi in 1753 [26, 27]. He extracted a bullet and compressive bone fragments from the third lumbar vertebra of an Irish soldier who, despite an infection, seemed to recover the use of his legs. "*After this operation, the paralysis of the extremities gradually disappeared, and the diseased was happily over.*"

Published in 1836, Antoine Louis (1723–1792) memoir of vertebral fractures and dislocations at the public session of the Académie Royale de Chirurgie on April 18, 1774, remains a classic that describes the spinal cord as follows [28]: "*It is clearly the continuation of the brain, enclosed in the canal of the vertebrae, where it is protected from external insults, like the brain in the skull. The importance of the functions of the spinal cord is no less than that of this viscera, which has hitherto been considered the primary motive of the animal economy.*"

The text contains a series of 14 cases of spinal cord or radicular trauma, including the story of Captain de Villedon, shot in Amöneburg in 1762, with several extraction and decompression procedures inspired by treatments for head injuries, resulting in long-term recovery.

The early nineteenth century saw the emergence of one of the most formidable controversies concerning the surgical treatment of traumatic neurological compression, accurately described in Donald Armour's (1869–1933) esteemed "Lettsomian lecture" of 1927 [29]. The debate raged between proponents and detractors of spinal surgical decompression in cases of trauma accompanied by neurological disorders [30, 31]. Indeed, in 1815, the young George

Hayward (1791–1863) described a procedure to remove the posterior arch from T7 to T9 in a traumatized patient, carried out on June 15, 1814 by Henry Cline (1750–1827), unfortunately without success, resulting in death on the 19th day [32]. The affair caused quite a stir and divided the community violently to the point of pitting two great figures of the time and long-time friends against each other: Charles Bell (1774–1842), a fierce critic [33], and Astley Cooper (1768–1841) [34], a radical defender who did not hesitate to call his detractors "blockheads" [35]. The battle intensified as subsequent attempts failed, notably those by Tyrell in 1822 and Barton in 1824, until the international recognition of a successful operation by Edwards in 1838 [36]. In fact, posterity overlooked the case of Alban Gilpin Smith (1788–1869), a Kentucky surgeon who performed a laminectomy in 1829 with long-term success [37]. It was not until advances in surgical antisepsis by the illustrious Joseph Lister (1827–1912), inspired by the work of Louis Pasteur (1822–1895), in general anesthesia by William Morton (1819–1868) [38] and in neurophysiology by the phenomenon Charles Brown-Sequard (1817–1894) [39] that a gradual change of opinion took place around 1860. In 1861, Hutchison presented a review of the 20 cases published to date, demonstrating that surgery was not inevitably fatal [40]. Other successful surgical indications, infectious by William Mac Ewen (1848–1924) [41] and tumoral by Victor Horsley (1857–1916) [42–44], were described. In 1869, the fifth edition of John Erichsen (1818–1896) surgical bible was finally published, changing his opinion in favor of Cline's procedure [45]. The name laminectomy appeared later, in 1893, in an article by Arbuthnot Lane (1856–1943) on a case of lumbar spondylolisthesis [46, 47]. The laminectomy technique evolved toward a less and less invasive procedure, and it was Alfred Taylor (1860–1942), an illustrious New York surgeon and inventor of numerous instruments including the famous retractor, who in 1908 proposed the first unilateral procedure, the hemilaminectomy [48, 49]. His brilliant pupil Byron Stookey (1887–1966) perfected the technique, and in 1928 published the seminal article on degenerative cervical myelopathy, using extensive laminectomies and a transdural approach to extract what were considered chondromas [50, 51]. Hiyoshi Hirabayashi modified hemilaminectomy in the 1970s for the posterior cervical approach with his famous laminoplasty, popularized in Japan, the land of multilevel cervical spinal compression by ossification of the posterior vertebral common ligament [52–54]. In 1986, Jacques Sénégas (1938–2025) invented lumbar recalibration, which frees stenosis by clamping the adjacent hemi-laminae, respecting as far as possible the articular joints and the stability of the posterior intervertebral mobile segment [55].

3.2 Radiology

The development of modern spinal surgery is closely linked to advances in scientific technology, and to the birth and development of imaging techniques that enable precise lesion diagnosis, informed prognosis, and surgical planning.

The history of radiology began with the discovery and medical use of the X-ray by Wilhelm Roentgen (1845–1923) in 1895 [56, 57]. The first medical imaging departments opened in early 1896, and he was awarded the Nobel Prize for Physics in 1901. In the interests of medicine, he did not patent his discovery, but donated his Nobel Prize money to the University of Würzbürg. In 1921, Jean-Athanase Sicard (1872–1929), neurologist and radiologist, head of department at Necker Hospital, suggested to his intern Jacques Forestier (1890–1978) to work on the radiological properties of lipiodol, synthesized 20 years earlier by Marcel Guerbet (1861–1938) [58–60]. Forestier observed the opacification of the rabbit's spinal canal and invented myelography, a term left to posterity by the Germans.

In 1970, the scanner was developed by English engineer Godefrey Hounsfield (1919–2004), and American physicist Allan MC. Cormack (1924–1998), who were awarded the Nobel Prize in 1979, even though the latter had no doctorate [61, 62]. Their work was inspired by the seminal paper on tomographic reconstruction published in 1961 by the American neurologist William

Oldendorf (1925–1992), combining X-rays with computerized image processing [63].

In 1974, American Raymond Damadian (1936–2022) patented an imaging device based on the principles of nuclear magnetic resonance, first described by Swiss physicist and Nobel Prize winner Félix Bloch (1905–1983) in 1946 [64].

Modern software techniques for three-dimensional image splicing in the early 2000s represented a significant advance in lesion recognition and surgical planning.

The advent of whole-body imaging using EOS technology, an application of the work of Georges Charpak (1924–2010), winner of the 1992 Nobel Prize in Physics [65], by Biospace and the ENSAM team led by Wafa Skalli, marks a turning point in the diagnosis and management of spinal deformities [66].

3.3 The Discovery of the Anatomo-clinical Correlation: The Herniated Disc

Sciatica as a clinical entity was first described by Domenico Cotugno (1736–1822) in 1764 [67] and amusingly enough, the famous sign of Ernest-Charles Lasègue (1816–1883) is not mentioned in his 1864 princeps article describing sciatic pain [68], but rather in the thesis of one of his students, Jean Joseph Forst (1851–?), published in 1881 [69]. In fact, the sign had been discovered and published a year earlier [70] by Lazar Lazarevic (1851–1891), physician to the King of Serbia, and its pathophysiological mechanism elegantly demonstrated on cadavers by Lucien De Beurmann (1851–1923) [71–73]. In 1857, Rudolph Virchow (1821–1902) considered disc rupture to be tumoral in origin [74]. Emil Kocher (1841–1917), Nobel prize Laureate, observed a traumatic rupture of a disc during the autopsy of a man who had fallen [75]. The etiopathogenetic link between annulus tear, sciatica, and neurologic sign was suggested in 1911 by Joel Goldthwait (1866–1961) [76]. In 1908, Fedor Krause (1857–1937) and Hermann Oppenheim (1858–1919) described lumbar laminectomy combined with a transdural approach to remove a "cartilage mass" [77]. In 1922, Alfred Adson (1887–1951) made the first description of surgical removal of herniated nucleus pulposus, by extradural approach [78]. At the time, the pathophysiology of herniated discs was not fully understood, and they were considered to be enchondromas. In 1929, Walter Dandy (1886–1946) noted that these lesions were related to disc material and stressed that their origin was traumatic rather than tumoral [79], in accordance with the conclusion of Otto Veraguth (1870–1944) and Christian Schmorl (1861–1932) [80], followed in 1930 by the French Théophile Alajouanine (1890–1980) and Daniel Petit-Dutaillis (1889–1968), for whom the origin was malformative [81]. Despite the above-mentioned numerous publications on disc herniation, the concept of disc herniation and its relationship to radiculopathy was finally defined by William Mixter (1880–1958) and Joseph Barr (1901–1963) in 1934, in the *New England Journal of Medicine* after initially being banned from publication by their hierarchy, considered too polemical to be presented in congress [82, 83]. For more than two decades, almost all of herniated discs were cured by durotomy until the outstanding work of Grafton Love (1903–1987) [84, 85], describing the extradural interlaminar approach. In 1967, Gazi Yasargil introduced the microscope for discectomy [86], quickly followed by Wolfhard Caspar (1938–2019), who added a tubular medial facetectomy to the procedure [87–89]. In 1973, Parviz Kambin (1931–2020) introduced the idea of endoscopic lumbar discectomy, leaving his famous triangle to posterity [90].

3.4 Degenerative Stenosis

Unlike herniated discs, narrowed spinal canals were described relatively early as the nineteenth century. Sir William Arbuthnot Lane (1856–1943) described a case of laminectomy on spondylolisthesis in 1893 [46, 47]. Bernard Sachs (1858–1944) and Joseph Fraenkel (1867–1920) entrusted Arpad Gester (1848–1923) with a

48-year-old Russian patient presenting with rapid neurological decompensation due to T11–T12 stenosis and demonstrated the efficacy of laminectomy for spinal stenosis [91]. Recognition of the degenerative nature of the clinical entity of narrowed lumbar canal was established by Pearce Bailey (1865–1922) and Louis Casamajor (1881–1962), neuropsychiatrists at *New York City Hospital* in 1911 [92]. They described a series of five patients with signs of spinal cord and radicular compression. Two patients in the series suffered from paraparesis and benefited from the laminectomy successfully performed by the founding father of spinal cord surgery, the legendary Charles Elsberg (1871–1948) [93, 94], the first describer of cervical laminectomy in 1926, who along with Harvey Cushing (1869–1939) and Charles Frazier (1870–1936) had convinced the venerable *American College of Surgeons* to designate neurosurgery as a specialty in its own right. In 1948, Dutch neurologist Christopher Van Gelderen (1872–1945) published the first description of neurogenic claudication associated with lumbar spinal stenosis, based on two cases, one of which was successfully operated on. He observed that cycling was painless and ruled out an ischemic cause but concluded that lordosis aggravated the symptoms [95]. In 1954, Henk Verbiest (1909–1997) published the first series of seven cases of symptomatic lumbar spinal stenosis with myelography, a classic in the literature [96].

3.5 Posterior Instrumentation

The bone grafting process differentiates between the concepts of instrumented stabilization (device without graft), fusion (graft without device), and instrumented fusion (device and graft), which have evolved over the last 130 years. In 1887, Walter Wilkins (1848–1935) performed the first internal fixation of a T12–L1 dislocation with spina bifida in a newborn, using a silk thread mounted in a figure-of-8 on the spinous processes. This case, published in 1891 by Berthold Hadra (1842–1903), a Russian immigrant to Texas, inspired the author to describe a similar technique of C6–C7 interspinous lacing in a young patient suffering from cervical trauma with neurological damage [97]. In 1895, the famous François Calot (1861–1944), who gave his name to the Berck-sur-mer center, used periosteal suturing between the laminae and transversalis in combination with his plastered corset for the treatment of tubercular deformities, which he soon abandoned [98]. In 1909, German surgeon Fritz Lange (1864–1952) proposed the first multistage internal fixation of the spine, using steel rods on either side of the spinous processes with silk and then silver wire [99]. In 1910, Samuel Mixter (1855–1926) and Robert Osgood (1873–1956) published a brilliant review of the literature on high cervical spine trauma, including a case of laminectomy, but also the invention of C1–C2 stabilization, an interspinous lacing in a 15-year-old trauma patient, with great success [100]. These early trials cannot be considered as fusion procedures, as by definition they do not involve bone grafting. Posterolateral vertebral fusion was initiated in tuberculosis patients by Russel Hibbs (1869–1932) and Fred Albee (1876–1945), two New York orthopedists, completely independently, in 1911 [100, 101]. The former described an autologous bone graft extracted from the product of decortication of the laminae and spinous processes. The second deconstructed the cartilage of the intervertebral joints and fixed tibia rods between the bisected spinous processes. In 1939, Canadian William Gallie (1882–1959) reported on a stabilization–fusion technique using posterior cervical interspinous lacing in cervical dislocations [102]. He also published a fascinating retrospective of the evolution of orthopedic surgery in the first half of the twentieth century [103]. In 1948, Mather Cleveland (1889–1979) was the first to describe a surprisingly unilateral intertransverse graft [104], followed in 1961 by Keith Mc Elroy (1915–2005), who published the bilateral technique universally used to this day [105]. These spinal arthrodesis procedures do not involve instrumented stabilization and require postoperative immobilization, but bone grafting will be associated with the stabilization techniques subsequently described, modified by the addition of iliac cancellous bone.

In 1948, Donald King (1903–1987) first described the use of transfacet screws to avoid postoperative immobilization and preserve healthy spinal segments [106]. He observed solid fusion in 90% of cases in his series of 44 patients at 2 and 7 years, a success rapidly tempered by the results published by Walter Thompson (1911–?), who found over 55% pseudarthrodesis with this technique in 1949 [107]. In 1959, HH Boucher further developed trans-articular fixation by inventing transarticulo-pedicular targeting in a series of 175 patients with degenerative lesions, including 49 spondylolisthesis patients with laminectomies without postoperative immobilization, with encouraging results [108]. In addition to screw fixation, some patients tried plate fixation, as had already been done for limb lesions. Philip Wilson (1886–1969), a surgeon who played an active part in the postwar restoration of the venerable Hospital for Special Surgery in New York City [109], proposed interspinous plate fixation in 1945. He operated on the celestial artist Frida Kahlo (1907–1954) using this technique, and counted other celebrities among his patients, including Marlene Dietrich (1901–1992). These interspinous plates were used in traumatology by Frank Holdsworth (1904–1969), who proposed the first definition of spinal stability introducing the two-column model of the spine [110], a model adjusted by Francis Denis (1946–2020) in 1983 [111] and René Louis in 1985 [112], thus forming the three-column complex still in use today. This led to a classification of vertebral fractures, the forerunner of today's AO-MAGERL classification [113].

In April 1963, Raymond Roy-Camille (1927–1994) was an orthopedic surgeon at the Garches hospital in the Paris region. Its proximity to the dreaded Saint-Cloud tunnel, which handles hundreds of road injuries every year, makes it one of France's leading trauma centers. The disappointing results of the immobilization techniques of Jörg Böhler (1918–2005) and Ludwig Guttman (1899–1980) in patients with unstable fractures prompted him, under the guidance of Robert Judet (1909–1980), to propose posterior internal fixation, initially using plates screwed into the posterior articular joints but above all into the pedicles, a source of remarkable stability [114]. The anatomical work of Gérard Saillant and Christian Mazel subsequently contributed to the codification of pedicle targeting [115]. The pedicle screw and its technique were not patented, as the inventor's main aim was to disseminate knowledge. This team was also behind Friedrich Magerl (1931–2020) [116] modified technique for screwing cervical articular masses. The period of litigation concerning the use of pedicle screws in the United States, from 1994 to 1999, was a difficult one for the *Scoliosis Research Society* (SRS), accused of providing training on a product considered dangerous and even threatening its existence. Despite their widespread and safe use in other countries, the FDA had classified them as an unapproved device, leading to a series of lawsuits, notably against its promoter in the United States, the eminent Art Steffee. SRS faced significant legal challenges but was ultimately released from any financial liability. This litigation led to the creation of the *International Meeting for Advanced Spinal Techniques* (IMAST), which became an essential component of the SRS educational program. Plate fixation methods rapidly evolved toward the screw–rod couple, thanks in particular to Randy Puno, Robert Winter, and Abbot Byrd, whose PWB system in 1984 prefigured the polyaxial screw concept [117, 118], also developed by Thomas Errico in New York. In the 1980s, posterior pedicle fusion systems and associated complications, pseudarthrodesis and adjacent syndromes, inspired the flexible stabilization movement, firstly interspinous [119] by Jacques Sénégas (1938–2025) and then interpedicular by Henri Graf [120]. A multitude of devices and techniques have followed this evolution.

Technological advances in posterior lumbar interbody fusion took off in the second half of the twentieth century. In 1944, Henry Briggs and Paul Milligan proposed the first posterior lumbar interbody fusion (PLIF) procedure with bone chips in their series of 70 patients [121], modified in 1953 by Ralph Cloward (1908–2000), a great mentor from Honolulu, who used bone plugs from the iliac crest to increase stability in a series of 321 patients, a technique little appreciated by surgeons, probably because of the apprehension of neurological complications [122]. This, at least, was the opinion of Paul Lin (1927–2017) of Philadelphia, who in 1977 published a variant of PLIF, less aggressive on the posterior articular joints, insisting on hemostasis of the epidural vessels, with fusion observed at 4 months in 94% of his series of 75 patients. The article is followed by a long, lapidary commentary by the master of Hawaii [123]. Despite his efforts, stand-alone PLIF did not gain in popularity, and in 1988, the genius Art Steffee published the first series of patients to benefit from posterior circumferential fusion by PLIF and combined pedicle screwing [124], then joined John Brantigan and engineer Carl Mc Millin in the adventure of PEEK-type polymer cages in 1993 [125]. In 1982, Jürgen Harms introduced a new method of interbody fusion using a bone graft-filled cage via the TLIF transforaminal approach, supplemented by screw fixation in 1998, which paved the way for current techniques [126].

3.6 Anterior Approach

The anterior approach to the spine is closely linked to the treatment of *Mycobacterium tuberculosis*, described by Percival Pott (1714–1788), who observed an improvement in neurological symptoms in patients with spontaneous evacuation of paravertebral abscesses, and recommended drainage [127]. Victor Ménard (1854–1934), a tireless worker and head of department at the Berck Maritime Hospital from 1891 to 1914, appointed after a fierce battle with François Calot, proposed the first anterior approach to the spine by costo-transversectomy in order to preserve the spinal column's means of stability, which was rapidly abandoned due to the high risk of infection. In 1906, Wilhelm Müller (1855–1937), a German surgeon based in Rostock, performed the first transperitoneal approach to the lumbosacral spine, also for tuberculosis [128]. Despite the success of this first operation, subsequent attempts failed. In 1934, Hiromu Ito modified the approach, using an extraperitoneal approach with drainage associated with bone grafting [129]. This surgical option was rapidly abandoned owing to the advent of streptomycin in 1947. Sometime earlier, in 1932, Norman Capener (1898–1975) described a theoretical anterior fixation of spondylolisthesis in what appears to be the first brilliant biomechanical description of the disease [130]. In 1933, Bryan Burns (1896–1985), president of the orthopedic section of the Royal Society of Medicine and eccentric aristocrat, proposed transcorporeo-sacral L5–S1 drilling with an anterior tibial graft after a three-cadaver study in a 14-year-old male with spondylolisthesis due to isthmic lysis [131]. He concludes his article with: "*It is possible that the intervertebral disc is not the ideal situation for a graft.*"

In 1936, Scottish surgeon Walter Mercer (1890–1971) published the first series of discectomies associated with an interbody iliac graft in two cases of spondylolisthesis, one of whom died of mesenteric arterial thrombosis, the cause of which the author attributed to surgical trauma [132]. The surgical indication was extended to degenerative disc disease in 1948 by John Lane and Emory Moore, who published an arthrodesis discectomy technique with heterograft according to Svante Orell (1889–1968) [133]. Particular attention was paid to the preparation of the vertebral endplates to optimize fusion. The French school was not to be outdone, with Robert-Aimé Merle d'Aubigné (1900–1989) and Jean Cauchoix (1912–2009) published their transperitoneal fusion technique for lumbar spondylolisthesis in 1950 [134]. The retroperitoneal approach, whose authorship remains controversial (several works attribute it to Torao Iwahara in 1944, whose publication is absolutely untraceable), was described by Wayne Southwick (1923–2016) [135], director of the orthopedics program at Yale University and a great sculptor, and then in 1960 by Paul Harmon (1906–1988), head of department at the Hollywood Presbytarian Hospital in Los Angeles, in an article whose teachings are still relevant today and whose drawings are of fantastic pedagogical power [136]. He also proposed a set of dedicated instruments that would remain part of the ancillary equipment for decades to come. The year 1968 was also revolutionary in terms of the previous approach, with the discovery by Arthur "Hoddy" Hodgson (1915–1993), head of the Hong Kong orthopedics department, who, in addition to his legendary expertise in the surgical treatment of Pott's disease, demonstrated the indirect canal decompression enabled by the technique through comparative myelographic analysis [137]. The following year, Allan Dwyer (1920–1975), an Australian surgeon, proposed his famous anterior scoliotic reduction technique [138]. Between the end of the twentieth century and the beginning of the twenty-first century, implanted interbody material evolved rapidly. Initially made up of iliac or fibular grafts, then portions of frozen femur in the shape of cylindrical pins, the first interbody implant was invented by the legendary Georges Bagby and his *Bagby Basket*, initially proposed for equine cervical arthrodesis in *Wobble Syndrome*, and adapted by Stephen Kuslich (1943–2004) for human use with this threaded titanium profile for greater stability, the results of whose study published in 1998 are breathtaking [139–141]. Charles Ray (1928–2011), cofounder of the *North American Spine Society,* proposed a screw-in version in 1997 [142]. Fusion rates have always been a matter of debate in the community, and it was O'Brien who published the first double anterior and posterior time technique for circumferential fusion in 1985 [143]. In order to save posterior time, the anterior implant was instrumented with a plate in the early 2000s, followed by a *stand-alone* screw-retained version by Nicholas Boeree (1958–2012) and his *Hartshill Horseshoe cage* [144, 145] or incorporated wings. This was followed by modern cages in PEEK and then PEEK–Titanium hybrids, with the most recent models in pure titanium printed in three dimensions [146–149].

The anterior approach was also a fantastic laboratory in the quest for mobility in the second half of the twentieth century, which was contemplating the success of hip arthroplasty. In 1955, Ulf Fernstrom (1915–1985), a Swedish surgeon, proposed a technique of disc replacement with a ball, which was implanted in over 250 patients, most of whom used the posterior approach, attracting sharp criticism from some in the community [150]. His contemporary, Alf Nachemson (1931–2006), also Swedish, famous promoter of *Evidence Based Medicine* and editor of *Spine* for 20 years, had no hesitation in describing the procedure as a "*rape of the spine*" [151]. In the 1970s, Art Steffee worked on a prototype with a polyethylene core between two titanium plates, which was abandoned due to debris production [152]. Karin Büttner-Janz, Olympic gymnastics champion in Munich in 1972 and President of the *Spine Arthroplasty Society*, developed the first widely used *Charité* device with Kurt Schellnack (1932–2023) [153], which paved the way for the modern models invented in the 1990s–2000s by Thierry Marnay, Patrick Tropiano, Jean-charles Le Huec, and Jean-Yves Lazennec [154, 155].

For the cervical spine, the technique of anterior approach with discectomy and fusion by interbody graft was published almost simultaneously in 1958 by three teams: from Baltimore Georges Smith (1916–1964) and Robert Robinson (1914–1990), from Honolulu Ralph Cloward (1908–2000), and from Leuven, Belgium Albert Dereymaeker (1916–1988) and Joseph Mulier (1922–2017). The latter had already published their technique, in an article in French unfortunately forgotten by the authors, in 1956 and should today be appropriately honored [156–159]. The anterior graft was then stabilized with a screw plate by pioneers Jacques Senegas (1938–2025) or Streli, but also with a dedicated ancillary proposed by the mythical Wolfhard Caspar (1938–2019), who gave his name to the interbody retractor [160]. Cervical corpectomy, or more precisely stepped somatotomy, was described in 1984 by the vigorous founder of the *European Cervical Spine Society*, Mario Boni (1922–1986) [161], honored by Pierre Kehr at the first combined meeting in Strasbourg in 1985. In 1963, inspired by Fernstrom's ball, Hjalmar Reitz (?–1996) and Mauritius Joubert (1918–2002) adapted the technique to the cervical spine, without much success [162]. It would take more than 20 years for Brian Cummins (1933–2003) to propose a new metal–metal pair [163], followed by new generations based on Vincent Bryan's invention of a polyurethane core between two porous titanium plates [164, 165], and finally the "ball and socket" models [166]. Vincent Pointillart, renowned advocate of cervical mobility restoration and member of the original Bryan prosthesis team, is to be credited with one of the extremely rare papers on a prototype implant failure in 2001 [167].

3.7 Deformity Surgery

3.7.1 Instrumented Correction

The first attempts at deformity surgery date back to the nineteenth century, with Jules Guérin (1801–1886), also known as public health pioneer [168], who proposed multiple myotomies, which were rapidly criticized by Joseph-François Malgaigne (1806–1865) [169]. In 1895, François Calot proposed stabilization using interspinous ties combined with plaster cast correction. The famous German surgeon Richard von Volkmann (1830–1889) is credited with the first rib resection in connection with scoliotic surgical treatment [170]. In 1958, Paul Harrington (1911–1980), faced with a large population of poliomyelitis patients and the inadequate results of orthopedic treatment and the first vertebral fusions, was the first to develop a system suitable for scoliosis instrumentation [171]. Composed of stainless steel hooks and rods mounted in distraction, its assembly enables spinal curvature to be corrected in the frontal plane. These results are improved by the addition of bone grafting combined with immobilization in a postoperative plaster cast corset for 6–8 months. However, despite satisfactory correction of the frontal curvature, this correction is unfortunately frequently lost, and the technique results in postoperative flatbacks. This technological revolution was accompanied by the creation of the venerable *Scoliosis Research Society* (SRS), whose first symposium was held on June 10, 1966 in Minneapolis under the impetus of David Levine and John Moe (1906–1988). In 1972, Eduardo Luque (1931–2002) introduced segmental spinal instrumentation [172], faced with several concerns in the management of scoliosis: the cost of rods and postoperative immobilization that was difficult to tolerate in Mexico's tropical climate. His implant (sublaminar steel wires connected to two L-shaped rods) was an undeniable success, as for the first time it allowed patients to avoid the need for a postoperative corrective corset. In 1975, Yves Cotrel (1925–2019) suffered cardiac arrest, bringing his career as a surgeon to an abrupt end. An eminently imaginative mind, he returned to his files and looked into the correction of scoliosis and the need for prolonged postoperative immobilization. He went on to develop a series of innovations, including a roughened rod with a worked surface, and open clasps enabling a multisegmental grip on the spine, resulting in three-dimensional correction in the horizontal plane. In 1983, at the Hôpital Saint-Vincent-de-Paul in Paris, he and Jean Dubousset, whom he had met through Pierre Queneau, operated on the first patient to be lifted on the third day without a cast or corset. The CD (COTREL-DUBOUSSET) was born [173]. To this day, it revolutionizes the surgical management of spinal deformities.

3.7.2 The Birth of Spino-pelvic Alignment

The etymology of the spinal universe revolves around the notion of rotating geometric shapes. While the first notions of concavity and convexity of curvatures certainly date back to Hippocratic times, the term vertebra from the Latin *vertere* (to turn) is found in the early writings of Celsus (34 BC–14 AD), and the terms scoliosis from the Greek curvature, kyphosis or hunchback, and lordosis or anterior curvature, are attributed to Galen of Pergamon. The father of orthopedics himself, Nicolas Andry (1658–1742), who coined the word by combining the roots *orthos* or straight and *paedion* or child, was already suggesting the treatment of scoliosis, illustrated by his symbol of the constrained tree [22]. In 1780, the horizontal plane was first described by engineer Magny, who skillfully emphasized vertebral rotation as the *primum movens* of scoliotic disease, the source of three-dimensional deformity [169]. It was William Adams (1820–1900) in 1882 who, using a series of cadaveric images based on Gideon Mantell's (1790–1852) anatomical study of scoliosis, precisely measured the angles and established the link between rotation and gibbosity [174]. At the beginning of the twentieth century, the development of radiography enabled the analysis of deformity in living subjects and saw the birth of vertebral radio-geometry in 1948 at the *Hospital for Special Surgery,* introduced by John Cobb (1903–1967) [175]. Alain Delmas (1910–1990), dean of Paris Medical Faculty and prolific anatomist, continuing the work of Henri Rouviere (1876–1952), suggests in 1953 a first classification of sagittal posture from his personal collection, describing L3 as the apex of the lumbar lordosis [176]. Pierre Stagnara (1917–1995) is credited with the birth of sagittal balance and his classification of different radiographic spinal profiles. In 1982, he demonstrated the reciprocal changes between curves, establishing the first sagittal plane reference table [177]. The sacrosanct pelvimetry was first invented by During J. in a forgotten publication submitted in *Spine* in 1980 and published in 1985, probably because of the complexity of his geometric proposal [178]. Ginette Duval-Beaupere (1928–2023) and Jean Legaye, at the beginning of the 1990s, proposed to include the pelvis in the analysis of spinal curvatures and popularized the pelvic trigonometry, composed of three major angles: pelvic incidence, sacral slope, and pelvic tilt [179, 180]. The importance of the pelvis, described as the pelvic vertebra by Jean Dubousset, as well as other concepts such as the inverted pendulum and the cone of economy, contributed greatly to a paradigm shift in the perception of static and dynamic skeletal equilibrium [181]. Radiological global alignment of the spine was introduced in 1991 by Itoi, analyzing posture in osteoporotic patients [182]. In 1997, Paolo Mangione and Jacques Sénégas (1938–2025) published two landmark articles, introducing the concept of the pelvi-femoral angle, the dynamic junction between pelvis and lower limbs, and the course of pelvic incidence during developmental growth [183, 184]. In the 2000s, Pierre Roussouly continued the work of the Lyon school with his classification of different types of back and introduced a forward-looking notion of degenerative lesion development [185]. He is also associated with the concept of balance compensation underlined by Cédric Barrey and Jean-Charles Le-Huec [186–188]. In the United States, Lawrence Lenke is a leading authority with his famous and complex coronal classification of adolescent scoliosis [189]. Between 2005 and 2007, the inestimable Virginie Lafage, accompanied by Jean-Pierre Farcy, Frank Schwab, and Abdelkrim Benchick el Fegoun (1975–2021) published their work on the radio-clinical correlations [190, 191] initiated by Roger Jackson in 1989 [192]. This naturally led to the SRS-SCHWAB classification, widely used in the surgical community. In 2009, Jean-Marc Vital alongside Olivier Gille and Nicolas Aurouer proposed the first work on computerized preoperative planning, which transforms the surgical plan by simulating postoperative radiographic alignment [193]. In 2019, the *European Spine Study Group*, including Ferran Pellise and Ibrahim Obeid, together with the *International Spine Study Group*, including Shay Bess and Chritopher Ames, proposed a deployable model predicting outcomes in the setting of deformity surgery in 2022, paving the way for artificial intelligence [194].

3.7.3 Thoracolumbar Osteotomy Techniques

One of the leading articles on scoliosis is that of Alex Mc Lennan (1872–1953), who in 1922 outlined the various etiologies of the disease and proposed a technique for excavating the apical vertebra in the convexity, recognized as the first vertebral resection [195]. In 1945, Marius Smith-Petersen (1886–1953) described the first posterior technique in rheumatoid arthritis [196], supplemented in 1946 by an anterior approach with grafting by E. La Chapelle [197]. A series of 120 patients published in 1949 by A. Law reported the postoperative death of ten patients, prompting John Adams (1913–2011) in 1951 to propose a lateral decubitus technique on a dedicated table, together with recommendations for risk management [198]. At the time, there was no instrumented fusion, and patients were generally immobilized for a year. The first description of a three-column osteotomy is attributed to Vincent Scudese in 1963 [199]. From 1984 to

1987, the pioneering Alberto Ponte (1926–2023), who had spent a year with John Cobb (1903–1967) and founded the first dedicated spinal surgery department in Italy, perfected a "pedicle-to-pedicle" posterior osteotomy technique indicated for Scheuermann's disease but extended to other indications [200]. In 1984, Charles Heinig (1929–2019) invented the "eggshell" osteotomy technique [201]. In 1985, Eivind Thomasen, a Danish surgeon, developed a transpedicular osteotomy offering improved correction and fusion rates, particularly when combined with instrumentation [202]. The postoperative flat-back syndrome, epidemic since the popularization of the Harrington technique, is described in 1988 by Michael LaGrone [203], leads to an exponential worldwide increase in lordotic reconstruction osteotomy techniques. In 2015, Frank Schwab described a comprehensive classification of spinal osteotomies [204].

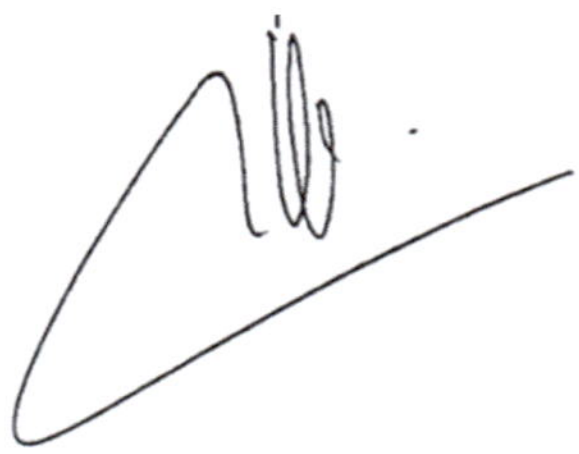

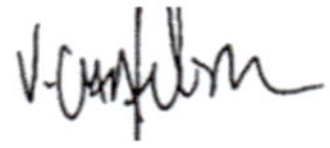

References

1. Van Middendorp JJ, Sanchez GM, Burridge AL. The Edwin Smith papyrus: a clinical reappraisal of the oldest known document on spinal injuries. Eur Spine J. 2010;19:1815–23.
2. Knoeller SM, Seifried C. Historical Perspective History of Spinal Surgery. Spine. 25:2838.
3. Gruber P, Boeni T. History of spinal disorders. Spinal Disorders: Fundamentals of Diagnosis and Treatment. 2008;1–37.
4. Kumar K. Spinal Deformity and Axial Traction. Spine (Phila Pa 1976) [Internet]. 1996;21(5):653–5. Available from: http://journals.lww.com/00007632-199603010-00024
5. Marketos SG, Skiadas P. Hippocrates. Spine (Phila Pa 1976) [Internet]. 1999;24(13):1381. Available from: http://journals.lww.com/00007632-199907010-00018
6. Marketos SG, Skiadas PK. The modern hippocratic tradition. Spine (Phila Pa 1976) [Internet]. 1999;24(11):1159–63. Available from: http://journals.lww.com/00007632-199906010-00019
7. Acar F, Naderi S, Guvencer M, Türe U, Arda MN. Herophilus of Chalcedon: a pioneer in neuroscience. Neurosurgery. 2005;56(4):861.
8. Marketos SG, Skiadas PK. Galen: a pioneer of spine research. Spine (Phila Pa 1976). 24(22):2358–62.
9. Markatos K, Korres D, Kaseta MK, Karamanou M, Androutsos G. Paul of Aegina (625–690): his work and his contribution to neurologic surgery: trephinations and laminectomies in the dark ages. In: World neurosurgery, vol. 109. Elsevier Inc; 2018. p. 338–41.
10. Er U, Naderi S. Paulus Aegineta. Spine (Phila Pa 1976) [Internet]. 2013;38(8):692–5. Available from: http://journals.lww.com/00007632-201304150-00010
11. Markatos K. Paul of Aegina (ca 625–690 AD), his work and his contribution to the treatment of spine disorders: the first routine laminectomy in the recorded history [Internet]. 2017. Available from: https://www.researchgate.net/publication/314050790
12. Gurunluoglu R, Gurunluoglu A. Paul of Aegina: Landmark in surgical progress. World J Surg. 2003;27:18–25.
13. René Briau. d'Egine P. Chirurgie de Paul d'Egine: texte grec restitué et collationné sur tous les manuscrits de la Bibliothèque impériale, accompagné des variantes de ces manuscrits et de celles des deux éditions de Venise et de Bale, ainsi que de notes philologiques et médicales. V. Masson. 1855.
14. Ai-Rodhan NRF, Fox JL, Nrf AR, Ai-Zahrawi FJ, Neurosurgery A. Al-Zahrawi and Arabian Neurosurgery, 936–1013 AD. Surg Neurol. 1986;26:92.
15. Amr SS, Tbakhi A. Abu Al Qasim Al Zahrawi (Albucasis): Pioneer of Modern Surgery. Ann Saudi Med [Internet]. 2007;27(3):220–1. Available from: http://www.annsaudimed.net/doi/10.5144/0256-4947.2007.220
16. Naderi S, Acar F, Mertol T, Arda MN. Functional anatomy of the spine by Avicenna in his eleventh century treatise Al-Qanun fi al-Tibb (The Canons of Medicine). Neurosurgery. 2003;52(6):1449.
17. Amundsen DW. Medieval canon law on medical and surgical practice by the clergy. Bull Hist Med [Internet]. 1978;52(1):22–44. Available from: http://www.ncbi.nlm.nih.gov/pubmed/352450
18. BULLOUGH VL. Training of the nonuniversity-educated medical practitioners in the later middle ages. J Hist Med Allied Sci [Internet]. 1959;XIV(10):446–58. Available from: https://academic.oup.com/jhmas/article-lookup/doi/10.1093/jhmas/XIV.10.446
19. Cumston CG. Henry De Mondeville, the man and his writings: with translation of several chapters of his works. Buffalo Medical J [Internet].

1903;42(7):486–504. Available from: http://www.ncbi.nlm.nih.gov/pubmed/36885983
20. Ghosh SK. Henri de Mondeville (1260–1320): Medieval French Anatomist and Surgeon EPONYM. Eur J Anat. 2015;19
21. Macdougall SC. The surgeon and the saints: Henri de Mondeville on divine healing. J Mediev Hist [Internet]. 2000;26(3):253–67. Available from: https://www.tandfonline.com/doi/full/10.1016/S0304-4181%2800%2900007-5
22. Gruber P, Boeni T. History of spinal disorders. In: Spinal Disorders [Internet]. Berlin/Heidelberg: Springer; 2008. p. 1–37. Available from: http://link.springer.com/10.1007/978-3-540-69091-7_1.
23. Splavski B, Rotim K, Boop FA, Gienapp AJ, Arnautović KI. Ambroise Paré: his contribution to the future advancement of neurosurgery and the hardships of his times affecting his life and brilliant career. In: World neurosurgery, vol. 134. Elsevier Inc; 2020. p. 233–9.
24. Banerjee AD, Nanda A. Ambroise Paré and 16th century neurosurgery. Br J Neurosurg. 2011;25(2):193–6.
25. Ruisinger MM. Misreading pictures: Fabricius Hildanus (1560–1634) and the cure of spinal dislocation. J Hist Neurosci. 2005;14:334–40.
26. Geraud O. Sur un coup de feu à l'épine. In: Mémoires de l'Académie royale de chirurgie. Paris: Delaguette; 1753. p. 515–7.
27. Hanigan WC, Sloffer C. Nelson's wound: treatment of spinal cord injury in 19th and early 20th century military conflicts. Neurosurg Focus [Internet]. 2004;16(1):1–13. Available from: https://thejns.org/view/journals/neurosurg-focus/16/1/foc.2004.16.1.5.xml
28. Louis A. Remarques et observations sur la fracture et la luxation des vertèbres; Mémoire lu à la séance publique de l'Académie royale de chirurgie, le 18 avril 1774, par Louis, secrétaire-perpétuel de cette Societé. In: Archives Générales de Médecine. Paris; 1836. p. 397–429.
29. Armour D. Lettsomian Lecture on the surgery of the spinal cord and its membranes. Lancet [Internet]. 1927;209(5400):423–30. Available from: https://linkinghub.elsevier.com/retrieve/pii/S0140673600729527
30. Silver J. History of cervical spine surgery: From nihilism to advanced reconstructive surgery. In: Spinal Cord., vol. 52. Nature Publishing Group; 2014. p. 339.
31. Lister J. On the Antiseptic Principle in the Practice of Surgery. BMJ [Internet]. 1867;2(351):246–8. Available from: https://www.bmj.com/lookup/doi/10.1136/bmj.2.351.246
32. Hayward G. An account of a case of fracture and dislocation of the spine. New England J Medicine Sur Collateral Branches Sci [Internet]. 1815;4(1):1–3. Available from: http://www.nejm.org/doi/abs/10.1056/NEJM181501010040101
33. Bell C. Injury of the Spine Marrow from the hurt on the Spine. In: Barrington E, Haswell G, editors. Institutes of surgery: arranged in the order of the lectures delivered. Philadelphia: University of Edinburgh; 1843. p. 94–7.
34. Burch D. Astley Paston Cooper (1768–1841): anatomist, radical and surgeon. J R Soc Med. 2010;103(12):505–8.
35. Weiner MF, Silver JR. The contribution to our understanding of spinal disorders by the great Windmill Street School of Anatomy, vol. 49. Spinal Cord; 2011. p. 323–32.
36. Markham JW. The history of laminectomy prior to 1866. Bull Hist Med [Internet]. 1952;26(4):375–84. [cited 2024 Apr 12] Available from: http://www.ncbi.nlm.nih.gov/pubmed/14954289
37. Smith AG. ARTICLE IX.–Account of a Case in which Portions of Three Dorsal Vertebrae were removed for the relief of Paralysis from Fracture, with partial success. North Amer Med Sur J (1826–1831). 1829;8(15):94.
38. Knopf SA, William T, Morton G. The discoverer and revealer of surgical anesthesia: a plea for his place in the hall of fame. Boston Med Surg J [Internet]. 1920;183(11):317–21. Available from: http://www.nejm.org/doi/abs/10.1056/NEJM192009091831101
39. Ruch TC. Charles Edouard Brown-Séquard (1817–1894). Yale J Biol Med [Internet]. 1946;18(4):227–38. Available from: http://www.ncbi.nlm.nih.gov/pubmed/21434249
40. Hutchison J. Case of exception of portions of the eighth, ninth and tenth dorsal vertebrae; with a tabular summary of twenty cases in which the operation has been made. American Medical Times: Weekly Series New York J Med. 1861;3(2):19–22.
41. Macewen W. An address on the surgery of the brain and spinal cord. Br Med J [Internet]. 1888;2(1441):302–9. Available from: http://www.ncbi.nlm.nih.gov/pubmed/20752403
42. Keller T. Victor horsley's surgery for cervical caries and fracture. Spine (Phila Pa 1976) [Internet]. 1996;21(3):398–401. Available from: http://journals.lww.com/00007632-199602010-00030
43. Gowers WR, Horsley V. A case of tumour of the spinal cord. Removal Recovery Med Chir Trans [Internet]. 1888;71:377–430.11. Available from: http://www.ncbi.nlm.nih.gov/pubmed/20896735
44. Tan TC, Black PML. Sir Victor Horsley (1857–1916): pioneer of neurological surgery. Neurosurgery [Internet]. 2002;50(3):607–12. Available from: http://journals.lww.com/00006123-200203000-00032
45. Erichsen JE. Injuries of the spine. In: The science and art of surgery: being a treatise on surgical injuries, diseases, and operations. 5th ed. Lea, HC; 1869. p. 374–5.
46. Brand RA. Sir William Arbuthnot Lane, 1856–1943. Clin Orthop Relat Res [Internet]. 2009;467(8):1939–43. Available from: https://journals.lww.com/00003086-200908000-00002

47. Arbuthnot LW. Case of Spondylolisthesis Associated with Progressive Paraplegia; Laminectomy. Lancet [Internet]. 1893;141(3635):991–2. Available from: https://linkinghub.elsevier.com/retrieve/pii/S0140673602039697
48. Ray BS. The development of neurosurgery in New York City. Bull N Y Acad Med [Internet]. 1979;55(10):916–38. Available from: http://www.ncbi.nlm.nih.gov/pubmed/295681
49. Taylor AS. Unilateral laminectomy. Ann Surg [Internet]. 1910;51(4):529–33. Available from: http://journals.lww.com/00000658-191004000-00010
50. Stookey B. Compression of the spinal cord due to ventr extradural cervical chondromas. Arch Neurol Psychiatry [Internet]. 1928;20(2):275. Available from: http://archneurpsyc.jamanetwork.com/article.aspx?doi=10.1001/archneurpsyc.1928.02210140043003
51. Scarff JE. Byron Stookey 1887–1966. Trans Am Neurol Assoc [Internet]. 1967;92:304–5. Available from: http://www.ncbi.nlm.nih.gov/pubmed/4939098
52. Hirabayashi K, Watanabe K, Wakano K, Suzuki N, Satomi K, Ishii Y. Expansive open-door laminoplasty for cervical spinal stenotic myelopathy. Spine (Phila Pa 1976) [Internet]. 1983;8(7):693–9. Available from: http://www.ncbi.nlm.nih.gov/pubmed/6420895
53. Hirabayashi K, Watanabe K. A review of my invention of expansive laminoplasty. Neurospine. 2019;16(3):379–82.
54. Hirabayashi K, Satomi K. Operative procedure and results of expansive open-door laminoplasty. Spine (Phila Pa 1976) [Internet]. 1988;13(7):870–6. Available from: http://www.ncbi.nlm.nih.gov/pubmed/3143157
55. Senegas J, Etchevers JP, Vital JM, Baulny D, Grenier F. Recalibration of the lumbar canal, an alternative to laminectomy in the treatment of lumbar canal stenosis. Rev Chir Orthop Reparatrice Appar Mot [Internet]. 1988;74(1):15–22. Available from: http://www.ncbi.nlm.nih.gov/pubmed/2967989
56. Cannon AH. Wilhelm Conrad Roentgen. Q Bull Northwest Univ Med Sch [Internet]. 1959;33(2):146–51. Available from: http://www.ncbi.nlm.nih.gov/pubmed/13668030
57. Röntgen WC. On a new kind of rays. Science (1979) [Internet]. 1896;3(59):227–31. Available from: https://www.science.org/doi/10.1126/science.3.59.227
58. Sicard JA, Forestier J. Diagnostic et thérapeutique par le lipiodol: clinique et radiologie. Paris: Masson; 1928.
59. Bonnemain B. History of contrast media: celebrating the centenary of the use of Lipiodol in radiology. Erciyes Med J. 2021;
60. Bonnemain B, Guerbet M. The history of Lipiodol (1901–1994) or How a medication may evolve with the times. Rev Hist Pharm (Paris). 1995;42(305):159–70.
61. Hounsfield GN. Computed medical imaging. Science (1979) [Internet]. 1980;210(4465):22–8. Available from: https://www.science.org/doi/10.1126/science.6997993
62. Hounsfield GN. Computerized transverse axial scanning (tomography): Part I. Description of system. British J Radiol. 1973;46
63. Oldendorf WH, Crandall PH. Bilateral Cerebral Circulation Curves Obtained by Intravenous Injection of Radioisotopes. J Neurosurg [Internet]. 1961;18(2):195–200. Available from: https://thejns.org/view/journals/j-neurosurg/18/2/article-p195.xml
64. Bloch F. Nuclear Induction. Physical Review [Internet]. 1946;70(7–8):460–74. Available from: https://link.aps.org/doi/10.1103/PhysRev.70.460
65. Charpak G, Bouclier R, Bressani T, Favier J, Zupančič Č. The use of multiwire proportional counters to select and localize charged particles. Nucl Instrum Methods [Internet]. 1968;62(3):262–8. Available from: https://linkinghub.elsevier.com/retrieve/pii/0029554X68903716
66. Dubousset J, Charpak G, Dorion I, Skalli W, Lavaste F, Deguise J, et al. Une nouvelle imagerie Ostéo-Articulaire basse dose en position debout: le système EOS A new 2D and 3D imaging approach to musculo-skeletal physiology and pathology with low-dose radiation and the standing position: the EOS system. Bull Acad Natle Méd. 2004;189:287, 287–97.
67. Cotugno D. De ischiade nervosa commentarius. Napoli: Fratres Simonios; 1764.
68. Lasègue C. Consideration sur la sciatique. In: Archives générales de médecine. Paris; 1864. p. 558–80.
69. Forst JJ. Contribution à l'étude clinique de la sciatique [Internet]. Paris; 1881. [cited 2024 Apr 13]. Available from: https://archive.org/details/BIUSante_TPAR1881x033/mode/2up?view=theater
70. Lazarevic LK. Ischias postica cotunnii. In: Archivum Serbicum pro universa scientia et arte medica recipienda; 1880. p. 23–5.
71. De Beurmann L. Note sur un signe peu connu de la sciatique: recherches expérimentales. Archives de physiologie normale et pathologique. 1884;16:375–80.
72. Chaudhary K. The History behind the Discovery of Root Tension Signs and the Invention of the Lumbar Discectomy Surgery. J Orthop Case Rep. 2021;11(1):121–6.
73. Drača S. Foreign scientists on the contribution of Serbian physician and scientist Dr. Lazar K. Lazarević to medical science. Srp Arh Celok Lek. 2016;144(1–2):111–5.
74. Virchow R. Untersuchungen über die Entwickelung des Schädelgrundes im gesunden und krankhaften zustand: und über den einfluss derselben auf

Schädelform, Gesichtsbildung und Gehirnbau. Berlin: G. Reimer; 1857.
75. Kocher T. Die Läsionen des Rückenmarks bei Verletzungen der Wirbelsäule. Min Grenzgeb Med u Chir. 1896;1:482–660.
76. Goldthwait JE. The Lumbo-sacral articulation; an explanation of many cases of "Lumbago," "Sciatica" and Paraplegia. Boston Med Surg J [Internet] 1911 ;164(11):365–372. Available from: http://www.nejm.org/doi/abs/10.1056/NEJM191103161641101.
77. Oppenheim H, Krause F. Ueber Einklemmung bzw. Strangulation der Cauda equina. DMW - Deutsche Medizinische Wochenschrift [Internet]. 1909;35(16):697–700. Available from: http://www.thieme-connect.de/DOI/DOI?10.1055/s-0029-1201407
78. Adson AW. Results of the removal of tumors of the spinal cord. Arch Neurol Psychiatry [Internet]. 1922;8(5):520. Available from: http://archneurpsyc.jamanetwork.com/article.aspx?doi=10.1001/archneurpsyc.1922.02190170067004
79. Dandy WE. Loose cartilage from intervertebral disk simulating tumor of the spinal cord. Archives of Surgery [Internet]. 1929;19(4):660. Available from: http://archsurg.jamanetwork.com/article.aspx?doi=10.1001/archsurg.1929.01150040096003
80. Stienen MN, Surbeck W, Tröhler U, Hildebrandt G. Little-known Swiss contributions to the description, diagnosis, and surgery of lumbar disc disease before the Mixter and Barr era: Historical vignette. J Neurosurg Spine. 2013;19:767–73.
81. Blamoutier A. Nerve root compression by lumbar disc herniation: a French discovery? In: Orthopaedics and traumatology: surgery and research, vol. 105. Elsevier Masson SAS; 2019. p. 335–8.
82. Mixter WJ, Barr JS. Rupture of the Intervertebral Disc with Involvement of the Spinal Canal. New England J Med [Internet]. 1934;211(5):210–5. Available from: http://www.nejm.org/doi/abs/10.1056/NEJM193408022110506
83. Parisien RC, Ball PA. Historical Perspective William Jason Mixter (1880–1958). Spine (Phila Pa 1976) [Internet]. 1998;23(21):2363–6. Available from: http://journals.lww.com/00007632-199811010-00024
84. Love JG. Protruded Intervertebral Disc (Fibrocartilage). Proc R Soc Med [Internet]. 1939;32(12):1697–721. Available from: http://journals.sagepub.com/doi/10.1177/003591573903201244
85. Love JG. Protruded intervertebral disks. J Am Med Assoc [Internet]. 1939;113(23) Available from: http://jama.jamanetwork.com/article.aspx?doi=10.1001/jama.1939.02800480015005
86. Yasargil MG. Microsurgical operation of herniated Lumbar disc; 1977. p. 81. Available from: http://link.springer.com/10.1007/978-3-642-66578-3_16
87. Caspar W, Campbell B, Barbier DD, Kretschmmer R, Gotfried Y. The Caspar microsurgical discectomy and comparison with a conventional standard lumbar disc procedure. Neurosurgery [Internet]. 1991:78. Available from: http://journals.lww.com/00006123-199101000-00013
88. Caspar W. A new surgical procedure for lumbar disc herniation causing less tissue damage through a microsurgical approach; 1977. p. 74–80. Available from: http://link.springer.com/10.1007/978-3-642-66578-3_15
89. Pitzen T, Barbier D, Papavero L. Wolfhard Caspar (1938-2019): A Pioneer of Spinal Microsurgery. Spine (Phila Pa 1976). 2020;45(9):563–4.
90. Mayer HM. A History of endoscopic lumbar spine surgery: what have we learnt? vol. 2019. BioMed Research International. Hindawi Limited; 2019.
91. Sachs B, Fraenkel J. Progressive ankylotic rigidity of the spine (Spondylose rhizomélique). J Nerv Ment Dis [Internet]. 1900;27(1):1–15. Available from: http://journals.lww.com/00005053-190001000-00001
92. Bailey P, Casamajor L. Osteo-arthritis of the spine as a cause of compression of the spinal cord and its roots: With reports of five cases. J Nerv Ment Dis [Internet]. 1911;38(10):588–609. [cited 2024 Apr 14] Available from: https://journals.lww.com/jonmd/citation/1911/10000/OSTEO_ARTHRITIS_OF_THE_SPINE_AS_A_CAUSE_OF.2.aspx
93. Charles AE, Albert Elsberg MD. (1871–1948): Father of Spinal Cord Surgery. Neurosurgery [Internet]. 1987;20(5):811–4. Available from: http://journals.lww.com/00006123-198705000-00027
94. Ohry A. Charles Albert Elsberg (1871–1948) and his forgotten contributions to the treatment of Spinal Cord Injured patients. Spinal Cord Ser Cases. 2021;7(1)
95. Dyck P, Doyle JB. "Bicycle test" of van Gelderen in diagnosis of intermittent cauda equina compression syndrome. J Neurosurg [Internet]. 1977;46(5):667–70. Available from: https://thejns.org/view/journals/j-neurosurg/46/5/article-p667.xml
96. Verbiest H. A radicular syndrome from developmental narrowing of the lumbar vertebral canal. J Bone Joint Surg Br [Internet]. 1954;36-B(2):230–7. Available from: https://online.boneandjoint.org.uk/doi/10.1302/0301-620X.36B2.230
97. Hadra BE. The classic: wiring of the vertebrae as a means of immobilization in fracture and potts' disease. Clin Orthop Relat Res [Internet]. 2007;460:11–3. Available from: https://journals.lww.com/00003086-200707000-00004
98. Calot F. Note sur la correction opératoire des scolioses graves [Internet]. Paris: Masson; 1897. [cited 2024 Apr 14]. Available from: https://gallica.bnf.fr/ark:/12148/bpt6k56206803.texteImage
99. Lange F, Peltier LF. The classic. Support for the spondylitic spine by means of buried steel bars, attached to the vertebrae. By Fritz Lange 1910. Clin Orthop Relat Res [Internet]. 1986;203:3–6. Available from: http://www.ncbi.nlm.nih.gov/pubmed/3514031

100. Miller DJ, Vitale MG, Russell A. Hibbs: Pioneer of Spinal Fusion, vol. 40. Spine. Lippincott Williams and Wilkins; 2015. p. 1311–3.
101. Albee FH. Transplantation of a portion of the tibia into the spine for pott's disease. J Am Med Assoc [Internet]. 1911;LVII(11):885. Available from: http://jama.jamanetwork.com/article.aspx?doi=10.1001/jama.1911.04260090107012
102. Dossani RH, Shaughnessy J, Kalakoti P, Nanda A. William Edward Gallie (1882-1959): Father of the Gallie wiring technique for atlantoaxial arthrodesis. J Neurosurg. 2018;128(3):938–41.
103. Gallie WE. Fifty years of orthopedic surgery. Med Clin North Am. 1957;41(4):1101–9.
104. Cleveland M, Bosworth DM, Thompson FR. Pseudarthrosis in the lumbosacral spine. J Bone Joint Surg Am [Internet]. 1948;30A(2):302–12. Available from: http://www.ncbi.nlm.nih.gov/pubmed/18912293
105. Peek RD, Wiltse LL. History of Spinal Fusion. In: Spinal Fusion [Internet]. New York, NY: Springer; 1990. p. 3–8. Available from: http://link.springer.com/10.1007/978-1-4612-3272-8_1.
106. King D. Internal fixation for lumbosacral fusion. The American Journal of Surgery [Internet]. 1944;66(3):357–61. Available from: https://linkinghub.elsevier.com/retrieve/pii/S0002961044902011
107. Thompson WAL, Ralston EL. Pseudarthrosis following spine fusion. J Bone Joint Surg Am [Internet]. 1949;31A(2):400–5. Available from: http://www.ncbi.nlm.nih.gov/pubmed/18116573
108. Boucher HH. A method of spinal fusion. J Bone Joint Surg Br [Internet]. 1959;41-B(2):248–59. Available from: https://online.boneandjoint.org.uk/doi/10.1302/0301-620X.41B2.248
109. Levine DB. The Hospital for Special Surgery affiliates with Cornell University Medical College and New York Hospital, 1951; Philip D. Wilson retires as Surgeon-in-Chief, 1955. HSS J. 2009;5(2):83–91.
110. Thakur JD, Wild E, Menger R, Hefner M, Adeeb N, Kalakoti P, et al. George chance and Frank Holdsworth: understanding spinal instability and the evolution of modern spine injury classification systems. In: Neurosurgery, vol. 86. Oxford University Press; 2020. p. E509–16.
111. Denis F. Spinal instability as defined by the three-column spine concept in acute spinal trauma. Clin Orthop Relat Res [Internet]. 1984;189:65–76. Available from: http://www.ncbi.nlm.nih.gov/pubmed/6478705
112. Louis R. Spinal stability as defined by the three-column spine concept. Anat Clin [Internet]. 1985;7(1):33–42. Available from: http://www.ncbi.nlm.nih.gov/pubmed/3994851
113. Magerl F, Aebi M, Gertzbein SD, Harms J, Nazarian S. A comprehensive classification of thoracic and lumbar injuries. Eur Spine J [Internet]. 1994;3(4):184–201. Available from: http://www.ncbi.nlm.nih.gov/pubmed/7866834
114. Mazel C. The contribution of Raymond Roy-Camille to spine surgery. ArgoSpine News & Journal [Internet]. 2008;19(1):97–102. Available from: http://link.springer.com/10.1007/BF03041187
115. Roy-Camille R, Saillant G, Mazel C. Plating of thoracic, thoracolumbar, and lumbar injuries with pedicle screw plates. Orthop Clin North Am [Internet]. 1986;17(1):147–59. Available from: http://www.ncbi.nlm.nih.gov/pubmed/3945476
116. Janssen ME. Remembering Fritz Magerl. Global Spine J SAGE Publications Ltd. 2021;11:275–6.
117. Makarevich SV. Historical aspects of transpedicular fixation of the spine: literature review. Hirurgiâ pozvonočnika [Internet]. 2018;15(4):95–106. Available from: https://www.spinesurgery.ru/jour/article/view/1520
118. Abbott Byrd III, J. 94 The synergy spinal system. In: Kim DH, Vaccaro AR, Fessler RG, editors. Spinal instrumentation: surgical techniques [Internet]. Stuttgart: Georg Thieme Verlag; 2005. Available from: http://www.thieme-connect.de/DOI/DOI?10.1055/b-0034-75918.
119. Sénégas J, Vital JM, Pointillart V, Mangione P. Long-term actuarial survivorship analysis of an interspinous stabilization system. Eur Spine J [Internet]. 2007;16(8):1279–87. Available from: http://www.ncbi.nlm.nih.gov/pubmed/17426988
120. Grevitt MP, Gardner ADH, Spilsbury J, Shackleford IM, Baskerville R, Pursell LM, et al. The Graf stabilisation system: early results in 50 patients. European Spine J [Internet]. 1995;4(3):169–75. Available from: http://link.springer.com/10.1007/BF00298241
121. Briggs Y, Milligan PR. Chip fusion of the low back following exploration of the spinal canal. J Bone Joint Surg. 1944;26(1):125–30.
122. Cloward RB. The Treatment of Ruptured Lumbar Intervertebral Discs by Vertebral Body Fusion. J Neurosurg [Internet]. 1953;10(2):154–68. Available from: https://thejns.org/view/journals/j--neurosurg/10/2/article-p154.xml
123. Lin PM. A Technical Modification of Cloward's Posterior Lumbar Interbody Fusion. Neurosurgery [Internet]. 1977;1(2):118–24. Available from: http://journals.lww.com/00006123-197709000-00006
124. Steffee AD, Sitkowski DJ. Posterior lumbar interbody fusion and plates. Clin Orthop Relat Res [Internet]. 1988;227:99–102. Available from: http://www.ncbi.nlm.nih.gov/pubmed/3338227
125. Brantigan JW, Steffee AD. A carbon fiber implant to aid interbody lumbar fusion. Two-year clinical results in the first 26 patients. Spine (Phila Pa 1976). [Internet]. 1993;18(14):2106–7. Available from: http://www.ncbi.nlm.nih.gov/pubmed/8272967
126. Harms J, Stoltze D. The indications and principles of correction of post-traumatic deformities. Eur Spine J [Internet]. 1992;1(3):142–51. Available from: http://www.ncbi.nlm.nih.gov/pubmed/20054929
127. Pott P. Farther remarks on the useless state of the lower limbs, in consequence of a curvature of the

spine: being a supplement to a former treatise on that subject. 1782. Clin Orthop Relat Res. 2007;460:4–9.
128. Müller W. Transperitoneale Freilegung der Wirbelsäule bei tuberkulöser Spondylitis. Deutsche Zeitschrift für Chirurgie [Internet]. 1906;85(1):128–35. Available from: http://link.springer.com/10.1007/BF02894985
129. Ito H, Asami G. Lumbosacral sympathetic ganglionectomy its value as a therapeutic measure for thromboangiitis obliteranS. Am J Surg. 1932;15(1):26–38.
130. Capener N. Spondylolisthesis. British J Sur [Internet]. 1932;19(75):374–86. Available from: https://academic.oup.com/bjs/article/19/75/374/6220775
131. Burns BH. An operation for spondylolisthesis. The Lancet [Internet]. 1933;221(5728):1233. Available from: https://linkinghub.elsevier.com/retrieve/pii/S0140673600857244
132. Mercer W. Spondylolisthesis: With a Description of a New Method of Operative Treatment and Notes of Ten Cases. Edinb Med J [Internet]. 1936;43(9):545–72. Available from: http://www.ncbi.nlm.nih.gov/pubmed/29648170
133. Lane JD, Moore ES. Transperitoneal approach to the intervertebral disc in the lumbar area. Ann Surg [Internet]. 1948;127(3):537–51. Available from: http://journals.lww.com/00000658-194803000-00013
134. Merle D'Aubigne R, Cauchoix J, Faulong. Anterior transperitoneal arthrodesis in the therapy of spondylolisthesis. Rev Orthop Chir Appar Mot [Internet]. 1950;36(6):490–4. Available from: http://www.ncbi.nlm.nih.gov/pubmed/14816925
135. Southwick WO, Robinson RA. Surgical approaches to the vertebral bodies in the cervical and lumbar regions. J Bone Joint Surg Am [Internet]. 1957;39-A(3):631–44. Available from: http://www.ncbi.nlm.nih.gov/pubmed/13428808
136. Harmon P. Anterior Extraperitoneal Lumbar Disk Excision and Vertebral Body Fusion. Clin Orthop. 1960;18:169–98.
137. Hodgson AR, Wong SK. A description of a technic and evaluation of results in anterior spinal fusion for deranged intervertebral disk and spondylolisthesis. Clin Orthop Relat Res [Internet]. 1968;56:133–62. Available from: http://www.ncbi.nlm.nih.gov/pubmed/5652772
138. Dwyer AF, Newton NC, Sherwood AA. An anterior approach to scoliosis. A preliminary report. Clin Orthop Relat Res [Internet]. 1969;62:192–202. Available from: http://www.ncbi.nlm.nih.gov/pubmed/5774835
139. Kuslich SD, Ulstrom CL, Griffith SL, Ahern JW, Dowdle JD. The Bagby and Kuslich method of lumbar interbody fusion. History, techniques, and 2-year follow-up results of a United States prospective, multicenter trial. Spine (Phila Pa 1976) [Internet]. 1998;23(11):1267–78. discussion 1279. Available from: http://www.ncbi.nlm.nih.gov/pubmed/9636981
140. Wagner PC, Grant BD, Bagby GW, Gallina AM, Sande RD, Ratzlaff M. Evaluation of Cervical Spinal Fusion as a Treatment in the Equine "Wobbler" Syndrome. Veterinary Surgery [Internet]. 1979;8(3):84–8. Available from: https://onlinelibrary.wiley.com/doi/10.1111/j.1532-950X.1979.tb00614.x
141. Oxland TR, Grant B. Obituary - Dr George W Bagby. Int Orthop. 2017;41(4):857–8.
142. Ray CD. Threaded titanium cages for lumbar interbody fusions. Spine (Phila Pa 1976) [Internet]. 1997;22(6):667–79; discussion 679–80. Available from: http://www.ncbi.nlm.nih.gov/pubmed/9089940
143. O'Brien JP, Dawson MH, Heard CW, Momberger G, Speck G, Weatherly CR. Simultaneous combined anterior and posterior fusion. A surgical solution for failed spinal surgery with a brief review of the first 150 patients. Clin Orthop Relat Res [Internet]. 1986;203:191–5. Available from: http://www.ncbi.nlm.nih.gov/pubmed/2937594
144. Choy WJ, Abi-Hanna D, Cassar LP, Hardcastle P, Phan K, Mobbs RJ. History of integral fixation for anterior lumbar interbody fusion (ALIF): the hartshill horseshoe. In: World Neurosurgery, vol. 129. Elsevier Inc.; 2019. p. 394–400.
145. Madan SS, Boeree NR. Comparison of instrumented anterior interbody fusion with instrumented circumferential lumbar fusion. Eur Spine J. 2003;12(6):567–75.
146. Kim DY, Kwon OH, Park JY. Comparison Between 3-DimensionalPrinted Titanium and Polyetheretherketone Cages: 1-Year Outcome After Minimally Invasive Transforaminal Interbody Fusion. Neurospine. 2022;19(3):524–32.
147. Deng Z, Zou Q, Wang L, Wang L, Xiu P, Feng G, et al. Comparison between three-dimensional printed titanium and PEEK cages for cervical and lumbar interbody fusion: a prospective controlled trial. Orthop Surg. 2023;15(11):2889–900.
148. Kurtz SM, Devine JN. PEEK biomaterials in trauma, orthopedic, and spinal implants. Biomaterials [Internet]. 2007;28(32):4845–69. Available from: https://linkinghub.elsevier.com/retrieve/pii/S0142961207005467
149. Williams DF, McNamara A, Turner RM. Potential of polyetheretherketone (PEEK) and carbon-fibre-reinforced PEEK in medical applications. J Mater Sci Lett [Internet]. 1987;6(2):188–90. Available from: http://link.springer.com/10.1007/BF01728981
150. Fisahn C, Burgess B, Iwanaga J, Chapman JR, Oskouian RJ, Tubbs RS. Ulf Fernström (1915–1985) and his contributions to the development of artificial disc replacements. In: World neurosurgery, vol. 98. Elsevier Inc.; 2017. p. 278–80.
151. Rydevik B, Hansson T, Szpalski M, Aebi M, Gunzburg R. Alf Nachemson, MD, PhD, 1931-2006: An exceptional pioneer in spine care. Vol. 16, European Spine J. Springer; 2007. pp. 303–305.

152. Enker P, Steffee A, Mcmillin C, Keppler L, Biscup R, Miller S. Artificial disc replacement. Preliminary report with a 3-year minimum follow-up. Spine (Phila Pa 1976) [Internet]. 1993;18(8):1061–70. Available from: http://www.ncbi.nlm.nih.gov/pubmed/8367774
153. Büttner-Janz K, Schellnack K, Zippel H. Biomechanics of the SB Charité lumbar intervertebral disc endoprosthesis. Int Orthop [Internet]. 1989;13(3):173–6. Available from: http://link.springer.com/10.1007/BF00268042
154. Szpalski M, Gunzburg R, Mayer M. Spine arthroplasty: A historical review. In: European Spine J, vol. 11. Springer; 2002.
155. Errico TJ. Lumbar disc arthroplasty. In: Clinical Orthopaedics and Related Research. Lippincott Williams and Wilkins; 2005. p. 106–17.
156. Dereymaker A, Mulier J. Nouvelle cure chirurgicale des discopathies cervicales: la méniscectomie par voie ventrale, suivie d'arthrodèse par greffe intercorporéale. Neurochirurgie. 1956;2:233–4.
157. Bartels RHMA, Goffin J. Albert Dereymaeker and Joseph Cyriel Mulier's description of anterior cervical discectomy with fusion in 1955. J Neurosurg Spine [Internet]. 2018;28(4):395–400. Available from: https://thejns.org/view/journals/j-neurosurg-spine/28/4/article-p395.xml
158. Cloward RB. The anterior approach for removal of ruptured cervical disks. J Neurosurg [Internet]. 1958;15(6):602–17. Available from: https://thejns.org/view/journals/j-neurosurg/15/6/article-p602.xml
159. Smith GW, Robinson RA. The treatment of certain cervical-spine disorders by anterior removal of the intervertebral disc and interbody fusion. J Bone Joint Surg Am [Internet]. 1958;40-A(3):607–24. Available from: http://www.ncbi.nlm.nih.gov/pubmed/13539086
160. Caspar W, Barbier DD, Klara PM. Anterior cervical fusion and Caspar plate stabilization for cervical trauma. Neurosurgery [Internet]. 1989;25(4):491–502. Available from: http://www.ncbi.nlm.nih.gov/pubmed/2797387
161. Boni M, Cherubino P, Denaro V, Benazzo F. Multiple subtotal somatectomy. Technique and evaluation of a series of 39 cases. Spine (Phila Pa 1976) [Internet]. 1984;9(4):358–62. Available from: http://www.ncbi.nlm.nih.gov/pubmed/6474249
162. Reitz H, Joubert MJ. Intractable headache and cervico-brachialgia treated by complete replacement of cervical intervertebral discs with a metal prosthesis. S Afr Med J [Internet]. 1964;7(38):881–4. Available from: http://www.ncbi.nlm.nih.gov/pubmed/14227712
163. Cummins BH, Robertson JT, Gill SS. Surgical experience with an implanted artificial cervical joint. J Neurosurg [Internet]. 1998;88(6):943–8. Available from: https://thejns.org/view/journals/j--neurosurg/88/6/article-p943.xml
164. Bryan VE. Cervical motion segment replacement. Eur Spine J. 2002;11(SUPPL. 2):S92.
165. Heller JG, Sasso RC, Papadopoulos SM, Anderson PA, Fessler RG, Hacker RJ, et al. Comparison of BRYAN cervical disc arthroplasty with anterior cervical decompression and fusion: clinical and radiographic results of a randomized, controlled, clinical trial. Spine (Phila Pa 1976) [Internet]. 2009;34(2):101–7. Available from: http://www.ncbi.nlm.nih.gov/pubmed/19112337
166. Derman PB, Zigler JE. Cervical disc arthroplasty: rationale and history. Int J Spine Surg. 2020;14(s2):S5–13.
167. Pointillart V. Cervical disc prosthesis in humans: first failure. Spine (Phila Pa 1976) [Internet]. 2001;26(5):E90–2. Available from: http://www.ncbi.nlm.nih.gov/pubmed/11242398
168. Masic I. The most influential scientists in the development of public health (1): Jules Rene Guerin (1801–1886). In: Materia Socio-Medica, vol. 31. Academy of Medical Sciences in Bosnia and Herzegovina; 2019. p. 150.
169. Rey JC. Histoire du traitement de la scoliose. In: Histoire des sciences médicales organe officiel de la société française d'histoire de la médecine; 2008. p. 21–8.
170. Willy C, Schneider P, Engelhardt M, Hargens AR, Mubarak SJ. Richard von Volkmann: surgeon and Renaissance man. Clin Orthop Relat Res. 2008;466(2):500–6.
171. Harrington PR. Treatment of scoliosis. Correction and internal fixation by spine instrumentation. J Bone Joint Surg Am [Internet]. 1962;44-A:591–610. Available from: http://www.ncbi.nlm.nih.gov/pubmed/14036052
172. Luque ER. Segmental spinal instrumentation for correction of scoliosis. Clin Orthop Relat Res [Internet]. 1982;163:192–8. Available from: http://www.ncbi.nlm.nih.gov/pubmed/7067252
173. Cotrel Y, Dubousset J. A new technic for segmental spinal osteosynthesis using the posterior approach. Rev Chir Orthop Reparatrice Appar Mot [Internet]. 1984;70(6):489–94. Available from: http://www.ncbi.nlm.nih.gov/pubmed/6239334
174. Adams W. Lectures on the pathology and treatment of lateral and other forms of curvature of the spine. J. & A. Churchill; 1882.
175. Botterbush KS, Zhang JK, Chimakurty PS, Mercier P, Mattei TA. The life and legacy of John Robert Cobb: the man behind the angle. J Neurosurg Spine [Internet]. 2023;1:1–8. Available from: https://thejns.org/view/journals/j-neurosurg-spine/aop/article-10.3171-2023.7.SPINE23146/article-10.3171-2023.7.SPINE23146.xml
176. Delmas A, Depreux R. Spinal curves and intervertebral foramina. Rev Rhum Mal Osteoartic. 1953;20(1):25–9.
177. Stagnara P, Claude De Mauroy J, Dran G, Gonon GP, Costanzo G, Dimnet J, et al. Reciprocal Angulation of Vertebral Bodies in a Sagittal Plane: Approach to References for the Evaluation of Kyphosis and Lordosis. Spine (Phila Pa 1976) [Internet].

1982;7(4):335–42. Available from: http://journals.lww.com/00007632-198207000-00003
178. During J, Goudfrooij H, Keessen W, Beeker TW, Crowe A. Toward standards for posture. Postural characteristics of the lower back system in normal and pathologic conditions. Spine (Phila Pa 1976) [Internet]. 1985;10(1):83–7. Available from: http://www.ncbi.nlm.nih.gov/pubmed/3157224
179. Legaye J, Duval-Beaupère G, Hecquet J, Marty C, Duval-Beaupère G, Hecquet J, et al. Pelvic incidence: a fundamental pelvic parameter for three-dimensional regulation of spinal sagittal curves. Eur Spine J. 1998;7:99.
180. Duval-Beaupère G, Schmidt C, Cosson P. A barycentremetric study of the sagittal shape of spine and pelvis: The conditions required for an economic standing position. Ann Biomed Eng [Internet]. 1992;20(4):451–62. Available from: http://link.springer.com/10.1007/BF02368136
181. Dubousset J. The Pelvic Vertebra, the Cephalic Vertebra and the Concept of the Chain of Balance. In: Spinal Anatomy. Cham: Springer; 2020. p. 171–87.
182. Itoi E. Roentgenographic Analysis of Posture in Spinal Osteoporotics. Spine (Phila Pa 1976) [Internet]. 1991;16(7):750–6. Available from: http://journals.lww.com/00007632-199107000-00011
183. Mangione P, Gomez D, Senegas J, Mangione P, Gomez D, Senegas J. Study of the course of the incidence angle during growth. Eur Spine J. 1997;6:163.
184. Mangione P, Sénégas J. Sagittal balance of the spine. Rev Chir Orthop Reparatrice Appar Mot. 1997;83(1):22–32.
185. Roussouly P, Gollogly S, Berthonnaud E, Dimnet J. Classification of the normal variation in the sagittal alignment of the human lumbar spine and pelvis in the standing position. Spine (Phila Pa 1976). 2005;30(3):346–53.
186. Le Huec JC, Thompson W, Mohsinaly Y, Barrey C, Faundez A. Sagittal balance of the spine. Eur Spine J. 2019;28(9):1889–905.
187. Barrey C, Roussouly P, Perrin G, Le Huec JC. Sagittal balance disorders in severe degenerative spine. Can we identify the compensatory mechanisms? Eur Spine J. 2011;20(S5):626–33.
188. Barrey C, Roussouly P, Le Huec JC, D'Acunzi G, Perrin G. Compensatory mechanisms contributing to keep the sagittal balance of the spine. Eur Spine J. 2013;22(S6):834–41.
189. Lenke LG, Betz RR, Harms J, Bridwell KH, Clements DH, Lowe TG, et al. Adolescent idiopathic scoliosis: a new classification to determine extent of spinal arthrodesis. J Bone Joint Surg Am. 2001;83(8):1169–81.
190. Schwab F, Benchick el-Fegoun A, Gamez L, Goodman H, Farcy JP. A Lumbar classification of scoliosis in the adult patient: preliminary approach. Spine (Phila Pa 1976). 2005;30(14):1670–3.
191. Schwab F, Lafage V, Farcy JP, Bridwell K, Glassman S, Ondra S, et al. Surgical Rates and Operative Outcome Analysis in Thoracolumbar and Lumbar Major Adult Scoliosis. Spine (Phila Pa 1976). 2007;32(24):2723–30.
192. Jackson RP, Simons EH, Stripinis D. Coronal and Sagittal Plane Spinal Deformities Correlating with Back Pain and Pulmonary Function in Adult Idiopathic Scoliosis. Spine (Phila Pa 1976). 1989;14(12):1391–7.
193. Aurouer N, Obeid I, Gille O, Pointillart V, Vital JM. Computerized preoperative planning for correction of sagittal deformity of the spine. Surg Radiol Anat. 2009;31(10):781–92.
194. Ames CP, Smith JS, Pellisé F, Kelly MP, Gum JL, Alanay A, et al. Development of deployable predictive models for minimal clinically important difference achievement across the commonly used health-related quality of life instruments in adult spinal deformity surgery. Spine (Phila Pa 1976). 2019;44(16):1144–53.
195. Scoliosis MLA. The. Br Med J. 1922;2(3227):864–6.
196. Smith-Petersen MN, Larson CB, Aufranc OE. Osteotomy of the spine for correction of flexion deformity in rheumatoid arthritis. Clin Orthop Relat Res. 1969;66:6–9.
197. La Chapelle EH. Osteotomy of the lumbar spine for correction of kyphosis in a case of ankylosing spondylarthritis. J Bone Joint Surg Am. 1946;28(4):851–8.
198. Adams JC. Technique, dangers and safeguards in osteotomy of the spine. J Bone Joint Surg Br. 1952;34-B(2):226–32.
199. Scudese VA. Vertebral wedge osteotomy. JAMA. 1963;186(7):627.
200. Ponte A, Orlando G, Siccardi GL. The true ponte osteotomy: by the one who developed it. Spine Deform. 2018;6(1):2–11.
201. Murrey DB, Brigham CD, Kiebzak GM, Finger F, Chewning SJ. Transpedicular decompression and pedicle subtraction osteotomy (Eggshell procedure). Spine (Phila Pa 1976). 2002;27(21):2338–45.
202. Thomasen E. Vertebral osteotomy for correction of kyphosis in ankylosing spondylitis. Clin Orthop Relat Res. 1985;194:142–52.
203. La GMO. Loss of lumbar lordosis: a complication of spinal fusion for scoliosis. Orthop Clin N Am. 1988;19(2):383–93.
204. Schwab F, Blondel B, Chay E, Demakakos J, Lenke L, Tropiano P, et al. The comprehensive anatomical spinal osteotomy classification. Neurosurgery. 2015;76(Supplement 1):S33–41.

Epidemiology of Spinal Diseases, Spine Surgeons, and Spinal Procedures

Paul Roblot, Arthur Durouchoux, Cèdre Adine-Leboucher, Louis Chaix, and Jean-Rodolphe Vignes

1 Introduction

Spine surgery is shared between different surgeons as orthopedic, neurological, pediatric, eventually trauma surgeons, and involves several medical specialties as anesthesiologists and rehabilitation specialists. Indeed, this part of surgery concerns degenerative, traumatic, deformative, oncological, and functional subspecialties. Most of the surgeons are specialized in one or two subspecialties, especially trauma surgeons.

As other specialties, spine surgery is highly dependent on localization around the world. The geography and the local demography may influence surgical spinal cares, such as the instrumentation and the rate of procedures [72]. The number of surgeries seem to have increased during the last decade [13, 15, 43]. Considering the aging of the population, it is likely that the health demand in spine surgery will increase, especially in the elderly [32, 52]. Then, the health-care system will have to adapt. Nowadays, spine surgery is managed mostly by orthopedic surgeons in most of the countries detailed [54, 55]. The surgical demography is changing, but some countries remain having no neurosurgeon, as well as no specialized orthopedic spinal surgeon. This disparity is a huge challenge for the global spinal surgery societies and for some local general surgeons.

The surgical procedures are also changing, depending on the local resources and the surgeons' demography. Indeed, Western Europe, North America, and Asia usually perform mostly endoscopic, minimal invasive, and instrumented surgeries, while Africa, and especially sub-Sharian Africa, prefers noninstrumented surgery [41, 57]. Such procedures depend on the surgeons and resources, but must adapt to the patients, who are not the same in different continents. These differences may be explained by several factors such as the available resources, but likely by the complains and the anatomy of the patients. This part aims to detail the current demography of spinal diseases, spinal procedures, and spinal surgeons.

P. Roblot
Neurosurgery Department A, University Hospital of Bordeaux, Bordeaux, France

Neurosurgery Departement, Centre Hospitalier Territorial Gaston-Bourret, Nouméa, Nouvelle-Calédonie, France
e-mail: paul.roblot@cht.nc

A. Durouchoux · C. Adine-Leboucher · L. Chaix
J.-R. Vignes (✉)
Neurosurgery Departement, Centre Hospitalier Territorial Gaston-Bourret, Nouméa, Nouvelle-Calédonie, France

University of Bordeaux, Bordeaux, France
e-mail: arthur.dourouchoux@chu-bordeaux.fr; cedre.adine-leboucher@etu.u-bordeaux.fr; louis.chaix@etu.u-bordeaux.fr; jean-rodolphe.vignes@chu-bordeaux.fr

C. Y. Barrey (ed.), *Spine Surgery*, SFCR Experts Series 1,
https://doi.org/10.1007/978-3-031-85446-0_2

2 Spinal Diseases

2.1 Degenerative Spinal Diseases

Between 1990 and 2020, musculoskeletal disorders more than doubled, and expectations are another doubling between 2020 and 2050. Among these disorders, low back pain and neck pain are the most frequent. For example, low back pain, which is the main cause of disability after cardiovascular diseases, as well as pulmonary restrictions, will concern more than 800 million people in 2050 [22]. Then, it is likely that spinal surgeons will be more and more sollicited [24]. Degenerative spinal diseases, encompassing spondylolisthesis, disc degeneration, and lumbar stenosis are highly dependent on geographical considerations. The prevalence rates are decreasing in Central Europe, Eastern Europe and Central Asia, stable in Western Europe and America or Australasia. Overall, among spinal surgeries, degenerative spinal diseases are around 80% of the spinal surgeries performed in France (mostly lumbar) [23]. The number of cases will then likely follow the global population, with major increase in Asia and Africa. Considering the global ageing of the population, these specific patients will require major health demands and should be anticipated [22].

Lumbar Degenerative Spinal Diseases

The most frequent incidence of newly diagnosed lumbar degenerative spinal disease is in Europe (5.7%), followed by North America (4.5%) and the lowest incidence in Africa (2.4%). These rates are the highest for spondylolisthesis (0.83%), disc degeneration (8.6%), and spinal stenosis (2.2%) in Europe, with substantial differences with Africa, the whole Asia, and North and South America. Indeed, degenerative spinal diseases are mostly diagnosed in high-income countries. These data suffered from a huge bias of publication, since the large majority of studies of provided by high-income countries [63]. Moreover, it is likely that the access for diagnosis and treatment of nonlethal disability, especially in low-income countries, is limited for a huge part of the patients. This disparity, between low and middle versus high-income countries, even if the first ones will have to manage four times as much total patients for degenerative spinal disease as high-income countries, is a huge challenge for the spinal surgeon's workforce.

Cervical Degenerative Spinal Diseases

The global repartition of neck pain is completely different than the repartition of lumbar degenerative diseases. The highest prevalence rates are observed in North Africa and the Middle East, and the lowest in Australasia, mostly forecasted cases in females. Populations changes, such as growth, seem to increase the absolute number of cases, without changing the prevalence rates, whereas the population ageing in South America increases the prevalence rate [90].

The cervical disc degeneration is less studies, with few data provided. These pathologies are more frequently diagnosed in patients in the fifth decade, and mostly induced by spondylosis or road traffic accidents [26, 44]. The current precise incidence of cervical degenerative myelopathy or radiculopathy is unknown. It is likely that the cases diagnosed concerned only a few part of the patients of suffering such conditions worldwide. An estimation for cervical degenerative myelopathy is around 4 case per 100,000 persons each year [61].

A specific kind of cervical degenerative myelopathy is usually diagnosed in the Japanese patients by ossification of ligamentum flavum. This disease mostly affects the thoracic spine, but often the cervical spine too [91].

Global disparities are likely to follows the disparities for lumbar degenerative diseases, with even less data. Considering the ageing of the global population, it is likely that the incidence will increase for cervical myelopathy, more than cervical radiculopathy due to disc herniation.

2.2 Spinal Cord Injuries

Considering the spinal cord injuries, a slight decrease has been observed in that prevalence rate between 1990 and 2019, but with an increase in global absolute number of patients. Moreover, considering the ageing and the growth of the global population, spinal cord injuries concern older patients nowadays than before, likely inducing more health issues [70]. The overall global incidence is around 10 cases per 100,000 persons each year, with almost 800,000 new cases annually worldwide, with higher incidence in Africa (13.6) and the lowest in Europe (3.4). These injuries are still mostly encountered in low- and middle-income countries, where the road safety is poor [46].

However, spinal injuries affect two main patterns of patients. Young patients with low sociodemographic index are mostly injured by road traffic accidents, while older patients, mostly women, suffer from spinal fractures induced by falls. These last patients are becoming more frequent, and the surgical techniques are following this progression [6, 30].

2.3 Spinal Infections

Tuberculosis—Pott's Disease

Tuberculosis affects a large part of the global population. Spinal tuberculosis concerns about 1% of the patients [83]. In low- and middle-income countries, Pott's disease is a very frequent cause of admission, especially when HIV prevalence is important. When health services have not a systematic way to report tuberculosis, its incidence is difficult to estimate accurately [25]. Considering the WHO data, major incidences of tuberculosis are observed in Africa and South-East Asia [95]. For example, India seems to present one-third of all the patients presenting Pott's disease. Moreover, countries with high prevalence of HIV infection are likely to suffer from a high incidence of Pott's disease. In high-income countries, some populations are at higher risk such as migrants from endemic areas and intravenous substance users. However, incidence rates are ten times lower in Europe than in Africa [25, 84]. Among patients with active tuberculosis involving the spine, there is a high incidence of kyphosis and neurological complications in the following months and years, leading to a significant rate of surgical interventions [19, 53, 81].

Nowadays, Pott's disease affects mostly young patients in low- and middle-income countries. This diagnosis leads the search for an occurrence of HIV infection.

Pyogenic Spondylodiscitis

Pyogenic infections of the spine are mostly due to *Staphylococcus aureus* or Gram-negative bacteria. Spondylodiscitis affects patients usually older than 50, and mainly in the lumbar spine. The incidence of this spinal infection is increasing in the Western Europe, whereas spinal tuberculosis is decreasing [28, 32, 79]. This infection affects mostly the elderly and will likely be impacted by the ageing of the population. For example, the observed incidence of spondylodiscitis was 31.9 cases per 1000 persons each year for people in the 90+ age group against 9.5 cases for the whole population in Germany. This incidence increased by 106% between 2005 and 2021, more than the population grew dramatically surpassing the predictions based on the population growth. This increase is most likely explained by the ageing population, the rise of diabetes, and the rise of immunosuppressed patients [21].

2.4 Spinal Deformations

Scoliosis is usually diagnosed in the first decades, and it depends on social, economic, and racial features. The incidence of idiopathic scoliosis is described usually by school-screening. The current overall incidence is around 1–3%, with the highest incidence between 10 and 14%, especially in females [39, 45, 76]. Children growing in an urban environment present higher rates of scoliosis than rural population [77]. The data about incidence of scoliosis in low-income countries are rare. However, it seems that the incidence is similar to other continents, with contradictory data about the influence of race in incidence, allowing no conclusion [3, 39, 80, 94]. No real difference in the incidence of idiopathic scoliosis between the regions in the world has been observed due to the absence of difference or the lack of data in some continents. Infantile and neuromuscular scoliosis are less frequent, needing specific medical considerations. The idiopathic scoliosis is twice as frequent as neuromuscular scoliosis, and far more frequent than congenital scoliosis (4.5/100,000 individuals vs. 0.7/100,000). It is likely that there is a lack of data about neurogenic scoliosis, since low- and middle-income countries are only beginning to adopt legislation for folic acid administration during pregnancy, with higher rates of dysraphism [8].

2.5 Spinal Tumors

Spinal Metastasis

The spine is the most common site for solid cancer bony metastases [17]. The WHO planned a 60% increase in newly diagnosed cancers in the world, with nearly 30 million new cancers diagnosed in 2040 [74]. Then, recent estimations evaluate the incidence rate from 10 to 30/100,000 individuals each year, including 8/100,000 with spinal cord compression. As other diseases, the elderly is the most concerned, with a major increase in the 85+ [73, 93]. Prostatic cancer will be the most solid cancer responsible for bony metastasis, which is likely related to the improvement of systemic treatments [85].

Spinal Primitive Tumors

This type of tumors includes bony tumors and tumor of central nervous system. The last ones are very rare, with epidemiological data provided solely by high-income countries. For example, between 2003 and 2007, the WHO registered only 18 cases of operated intradural intramedullary tumors in Africa, and 2359 cases in Europe. Intraspinal tumors, including intramedullary and extramedullary, are more frequent in females than males with respective incidence rates of 0.3/100,000 per year, and 0.5/100,000 for females. Among them, meningiomas are the most encountered tumor, being intradural extramedullary. Among the intramedullary tumors, the most frequent are astrocytomas and ependymomas. The incidence rates for all intradural intramedullary tumors are much lower than other spinal tumors (0.18/100,000 in Europe, 0.21/100,000 in North America) [1, 11, 34].

Primary bone tumors are rare diseases, even more involving the spine. The two most tumors are osteosarcoma and Ewing sarcoma. All primary bone tumors represents only 0.2% of all neoplasms and are majorly diagnosed in Caucasian males [71, 92].

2.6 Spinal Inflammation

Rheumatoid arthritis may affect the spine in two principal ways: an atlantoaxial subluxation and lumbar scoliosis. Thirty percent of the patients diagnosed for a rheumatoid arthritis are presenting a lumbar scoliosis. The lack of remission of the disease may lead to a scoliosis progression and is a predictive factor for atlantoaxial subluxation [12, 36, 37]. Even in the absence of prospective epidemiological study, it is likely that the frequence of such patients will decrease, following the improvement of treatments, and such spinal deformations will be diagnosed in the elderly with longer disease duration.

3 Spinal Surgeons

3.1 Specialties and Geographical Trends

One surgeon can take care of 147,000 people. The global population reached 8 billion in 2022. Then, the worldwide workforce of spine surgeons should be around 54,000 spine surgeons [51, 56]. The global demography of spinal surgeons is very irregular. This specific surgery is shared by both orthopedic and neurological surgeons. Among them, two main scientific societies are pooling those surgeons: the World Federation of Neurosurgical Societies and the AO Spine (Arbeitgemeinschaft für Osteosynthesefragen). Then, among these we may describe the global presence of spine surgeons. The AO Spine estimates the number of worldwide spine surgeons around 12,000 and the global neurosurgical workforce is estimated around 73,000 [29].

However, these numbers are only estimations since there is no specific register of spine surgeons.

In Europe, spine surgeons are associated in the Eurospine. This society brings together orthopedists and neurosurgeons involved in the spine surgery. Its members are mostly orthopedists (352/549—64.1%) rather than neurosurgeons [96]. In the United States, this distribution seems similar with 55% of orthopedic surgeons in the new generation of spine surgeons [60].

Japan and South Korea have seen the number of spine surgeons increasing during the last decades. However, in Japan, spine surgeries increased more than the number of spine surgeons (2.4 times between 2003 and 2017 against 1.5 times) [43, 48]. In the same way, the US needs for spine surgeons is increasing, and the current need for spine surgeons is evaluated 20% more than the current surgeons' number [51].

In low- and middle-income countries, these numbers are poorly described. Even the number of spine surgeons seem unidentified. However, the low rate of spinal pathologies diagnosed and treated seem to reveal a likely severe lack of access to spinal surgical care, as well as spinal surgeons. For example, Central African Republic has neurosurgeon of nearly five million [97]. The World Spine Care charity illustrates these needs since it has been solicited to install spine care programs in several African countries, Brazil, Peru, Argentina, India, and Vietnam [31].

Then, the major changes in spinal surgery with technical devices and advanced expertise in high-income countries are likely increasing the global disparities with low- and middle-income countries.

3.2 Gender Trends

Even if the gender disparities remain in this subspecialty, women are becoming more frequent in spine surgery in the recent years. Before the 60 s, no woman was graduated in neurosurgery. Nowadays, this subspecialty is highly masculine. Only 8–25% of spine surgeons in America are women [2, 9, 64, 65]. Orthopedic surgery is one of the last specialties to correct the lack of gender diversity, needing governmental programs to correct such disparity [47]. These differences have been likely influenced by the common gender discriminations [20, 58]. However, female spine surgeons are becoming more and more present in the specialty, and such inequality will decrease, even if the predictions are really too slow [69, 70]. This evolution may lead to a diversification of surgeons, and likely improve surgical treatment since female surgeons have lower rates of severe postoperative complications, including death [87].

4 Spinal Surgeries

The number of spinal surgeries globally significantly increased for at least a decade [42, 43]. However, the geographical disparities in surgical techniques are major and is probably not totally due to the variations in patients' anatomy.

The first spinal surgeries to correct a deformation were performed in the nineteenth century. Considering the results and a following lawsuit, this surgery has been erased from the practice until the end of the century [78]. The current surgery for spinal diseases began in the middle of the twentieth century with Harrington, with the first instrumented correction's surgeries, then the discectomy by Caspar and Yazargil (1977), followed by Harms and Roy-Camille plates (1982–1983), and since the last two decades the CT-guided instrumentation, minimally invasive surgery, and robotic spinal surgery [86].

The first evolutions in surgical approaches to the spine were developed mostly for lumbar surgery. In the 1980s, the first endoscopic approach were developed for lumbar decompression [38]. Then, these techniques' popularity increased and became usual. Nowadays, these techniques are used in most of the high-income countries [4].

Given the improvement of optics and techniques in the operative room, the endoscopic surgery has been developed, after lumbar surgery, for the cervical spine and for both anterior and posterior approaches [5, 14, 68]. Even if the minimally invasive and endoscopic techniques are promising and reducing the skin incisions, the length of stay, the rehabilitation duration, Europe and North America seem to use less of these contemporary techniques than Asia, especially Japan and South Korea, and South America [41]. Indeed, North America and even more Europe have lately developing such techniques, and most of the surgeons do not use these techniques in their regular practice [50].

The minimally invasive techniques are increasing with developing programs of international training courses, but the open surgery remains the standard for people who have access to spinal surgery in low- and middle-income countries, since the endoscopic or microscopic surgical approaches require expensive surgical devices [35, 49]. The two most frequent approaches to operate the cervical spine are anterior, called Smith–Robinson approach, and posterior. These two well-known approaches are the most used in Europe and North and South America [27]. The anterior approach, which involves removing a problematic disc, may lead to the placement of a cage (fusion) or a prothesis (arthroplasty) [27]. The last decade has been describing inconsistent results about the difference between these techniques [27, 67, 82, 88]. The posterior approach can be performed by both open and minimally invasive techniques. The last one remains rare since the anterior approach has been replacing posterior fusions.

Nowadays, percutaneous and minimal invasive surgeries have been replacing classical open approaches minimize surgical morbidity. Cervical approaches are both minimally invasive, with anterior and the reduced skin incision, and posterior, with percutaneous surgeries, since the intraoperative navigation devices exist [18].

Thoracic and lumbar fractures and stenosis are now usually managed using percutaneous and minimal invasive techniques [7, 33]. Adult thoracolumbar deformations are also treated with minimal invasive techniques, with less significant differences than fractures or decompressions [16].

Scoliosis is and has been managed with the Cotrel-Dubousset technique, using multiple screws and corrections in an open approach, and is now starting to be managed by vertebral body tethering, a new technique using videothoracoscopy to insert lateral screws in the main part of the scoliosis. The results are still debated due to the high rate of complications [10, 59, 62, 66].

Considering the discectomy and fusion techniques, the current techniques are now using minimal invasive techniques for both thoracic and lumbar approaches. Thoracic discectomies and fusions are performed by a working portal tubular retractor with a transmuscular approach or videothoracoscopy using an intrathoracic approach [40, 75]. Lumbar approaches may differ depending on the level. Different techniques are described as the anterior retroperitoneal approach: lateral, oblique, and posterior lumbar interbody fusions. All these techniques are now available with tubular retractors and then minimal invasive approaches. The current trend appears to be the use of navigation and robotic devices, though further studies and technical improvements are needed to better determine their cost-effectiveness and improve clinical outcome [89].

5 Conclusion

Spinal diseases will become increasingly challenging to manage with the current workforce of spinal surgeons. Degenerative spinal diseases are expected to double between 2025 and 2050. Consequently, spine surgery societies and spine surgeons will need to adapt their demographics and practices to ensure care for as many patients as possible. This evolution will require more surgeons, and the inclusion of women spine surgeons is not only encouraged but necessary to expand the workforce.

The disparities in surgical techniques, surgeons' demographic features, and access to spinal surgical care should be more precisely assessed before imagining solutions to ensure spinal care for all patients around the world.

Declarations This study has not been published before; it is not under consideration for publication anywhere else; its publication has been approved by all coauthors, and at the institute where the work has been carried out.

Conflict of Interest Disclosures *All authors declare: no support from any organization for this study; no financial relationships with any organizations that might have an interest in the submitted work.*

Funding/Support None.

Role of the Funder/Sponsor N/A.

Additional Contributions None.

Ethics approval N/A.

Consent to Participate N/A.

Consent for Publication N/A.

Availability of Data and Material Dr. Roblot had full access to all the data in the study and takes responsibility for the integrity of the data and the accuracy of the data analysis. Data are available on request to the corresponding author.

Code Availability N/A.

References

1. Abd-El-Barr MM, Huang KT, Moses ZB, et al. Recent advances in intradural spinal tumors. Neuro-Oncology. 2018;20:729–42. https://doi.org/10.1093/neuonc/nox230.
2. Abosch A, Rutka JT. Women in neurosurgery: inequality redux. J Neurosurg. 2018;129:277–81. https://doi.org/10.3171/2018.4.JNS172878.
3. Adegoke B, Akinpelu A, Taylor B Adolescent idiopathic scoliosis in Ibadan, Nigeria.
4. Ahn Y. A historical review of endoscopic spinal discectomy. World Neurosurg. 2021;145:591–6. https://doi.org/10.1016/j.wneu.2020.08.008.
5. Ahn Y, Lee S-H, Shin S-W. Percutaneous endoscopic cervical discectomy: clinical outcome and radiographic changes. Photomed Laser Surg. 2005;23:362–8. https://doi.org/10.1089/pho.2005.23.362.
6. Algahtany M, McFaull S, Chen L, et al. The changing etiology and epidemiology of traumatic spinal injury: a population-based study. World Neurosurg. 2021;149:e116–27. https://doi.org/10.1016/j.wneu.2021.02.066.
7. An B, Li X-C, Zhou C-P, et al. Percutaneous full endoscopic posterior decompression of thoracic myelopathy caused by ossification of the ligamentum flavum. Eur Spine J. 2019;28:492–501. https://doi.org/10.1007/s00586-018-05866-2.
8. Atta CAM, Fiest KM, Frolkis AD, et al. Global birth prevalence of Spina Bifida by folic acid fortification status: a systematic review and meta-analysis. Am J Public Health. 2016;106:e24–34. https://doi.org/10.2105/AJPH.2015.302902.
9. Balasubramanian SC, Palanisamy D, Bakhti S, et al. Women in neurosurgery (WIN): barriers to progress, world win directory and the way forward. Asian J Neurosurg. 2020;15:828–32. https://doi.org/10.4103/ajns.AJNS_108_20.
10. Barone G, Giudici F, Manzini F, et al. Adolescent idiopathic scoliosis surgery: postoperative functional outcomes at 32 years mean follow-up. Children (Basel). 2023;11:52. https://doi.org/10.3390/children11010052.
11. Bell JS, Koffie RM, Rattani A, et al. Global incidence of brain and spinal tumors by geographic region and income level based on cancer registry data. J Clin Neurosci. 2019;66:121–7. https://doi.org/10.1016/j.jocn.2019.05.003.
12. Bettaieb H, Ferjani HL, Ben Nessib D, et al. Predictors factors of atlanto-axial subluxation in Tunisian patients with rheumatoid arthritis. Musculoskeletal Care. 2023;21:968–75. https://doi.org/10.1002/msc.1759.
13. Bhargava S, Sharma M, Dietz N, et al. Demographics and outcomes of spine surgery in octogenarians and nonagenarians: a comparison of the national inpatient sample, Marketscan and national surgical quality improvement program databases. Cureus. 11:e6195. https://doi.org/10.7759/cureus.6195.
14. Carr DA, Abecassis IJ, Hofstetter CP. Full endoscopic unilateral laminotomy for bilateral decompression of the cervical spine: surgical technique and early experience. J Spine Surg. 2020;6:447–56. https://doi.org/10.21037/jss.2020.01.03.
15. Chapon R, Meyblum J, Simon L, et al. Global French spine surgery activity: executive report of demographics data and trend; 2022. https://doi.org/10.21203/rs.3.rs-1260367/v1.
16. Chou D, Lafage V, Chan AY, et al. Patient outcomes after circumferential minimally invasive surgery compared with those of open correction for adult spinal deformity: initial analysis of prospectively collected data. J Neurosurg Spine. 2022;36:203–14. https://doi.org/10.3171/2021.3.SPINE201825.
17. Coleman RE. Clinical features of metastatic bone disease and risk of skeletal morbidity. Clin Cancer Res. 2006;12:6243s–9s. https://doi.org/10.1158/1078-0432.CCR-06-0931.
18. Coric D, Rossi V. Percutaneous Posterior Cervical Pedicle Instrumentation (C1 to C7) With Navigation Guidance: Early Series of 27 Cases. Global Spine J. 2022;12:27S–33S. https://doi.org/10.1177/21925682211029215.
19. Diomandé M, Coulibaly Y, Goua JJ, et al. Pott's disease in Abidjan: experience of the department of rheumatology of university teaching hospital of Cocody: about 420 cases. Tunis Med. 2023;101:19–25.
20. Falavigna A, Ramos MB, de Farias FAC, et al. Perception of gender discrimination among spine surgeons across Latin America: a web-based survey.

Spine J. 2022;22:49–57. https://doi.org/10.1016/j.spinee.2021.04.009.

21. Fantoni M, Trecarichi EM, Rossi B, et al. Epidemiological and clinical features of pyogenic spondylodiscitis. Eur Rev Med Pharmacol Sci. 2012;16(Suppl 2):2–7.
22. Ferreira ML, de Luca K, Haile LM, et al. Global, regional, and national burden of low back pain, 1990–2020, its attributable risk factors, and projections to 2050: a systematic analysis of the Global Burden of Disease Study 2021. The Lancet Rheumatol. 2023;5:e316–29. https://doi.org/10.1016/S2665-9913(23)00098-X.
23. Garcia R, Bezin J, Grobost P, Vignes J-R. Complications neurologiques, à un an de la chirurgie du rachis pour pathologie dégénérative, en 2018, en France. J Epidemiol Population Health. 2024;72:202230. https://doi.org/10.1016/j.jeph.2024.202230.
24. Gill TK, Mittinty MM, March LM, et al. Global, regional, and national burden of other musculoskeletal disorders, 1990–2020, and projections to 2050: a systematic analysis of the Global Burden of Disease Study 2021. Lancet Rheumatol. 2023;5:e670–82. https://doi.org/10.1016/S2665-9913(23)00232-1.
25. Glaziou P, Floyd K, Raviglione MC. Global Epidemiology of Tuberculosis. Semin Respir Crit Care Med. 2018;39:271–85. https://doi.org/10.1055/s-0038-1651492.
26. Goacher E, Phillips R, Mowforth OD, et al. Hospitalisation for degenerative cervical myelopathy in England: insights from the National Health Service Hospital Episode Statistics 2012 to 2019. Acta Neurochir. 2022;164:1535–41. https://doi.org/10.1007/s00701-022-05219-5.
27. Goedmakers CMW, de Vries F, Bosscher L, et al. Long-term results of the NECK trial-implanting a disc prosthesis after cervical anterior discectomy cannot prevent adjacent segment disease: five-year clinical follow-up of a double-blinded randomised controlled trial. Spine J. 2023;23:350–60. https://doi.org/10.1016/j.spinee.2022.11.006.
28. Grammatico L, Baron S, Rusch E, et al. Epidemiology of vertebral osteomyelitis (VO) in France: analysis of hospital-discharge data 2002–2003. Epidemiol Infect. 2008;136:653–60. https://doi.org/10.1017/S0950268807008850.
29. Gupta S, Gal ZT, Athni TS, et al. Mapping the global neurosurgery workforce. Part 1: Consultant neurosurgeon density. J Neurosurg. 2024;141:1–9. https://doi.org/10.3171/2023.9.JNS231615.
30. Haizel-Cobbina J, Thakkar R, Still M, et al. Global epidemiology of pediatric traumatic spine injury: a systematic review and meta-analysis. World Neurosurg. 2023;178:172–180.e3. https://doi.org/10.1016/j.wneu.2023.07.051.
31. Haldeman S, Nordin M, Outerbridge G, et al. Creating a sustainable model of spine care in underserved communities: the World Spine Care (WSC) charity. Spine J. 2015;15:2303–11. https://doi.org/10.1016/j.spinee.2015.06.046.
32. Heck VJ, Klug K, Prasse T, et al. Projections From Surgical Use Models in Germany Suggest a Rising Number of Spinal Fusions in Patients 75 Years and Older Will Challenge Healthcare Systems Worldwide. Clin Orthop Relat Res. 2023;481:1610–9. https://doi.org/10.1097/CORR.0000000000002576.
33. Heintel TM, Berglehner A, Meffert R. Accuracy of percutaneous pedicle screws for thoracic and lumbar spine fractures: a prospective trial. Eur Spine J. 2013;22:495–502. https://doi.org/10.1007/s00586-012-2476-8.
34. Helseth A, Mørk SJ. Primary intraspinal neoplasms in Norway, 1955 to 1986. A population-based survey of 467 patients. J Neurosurg. 1989;71:842–5. https://doi.org/10.3171/jns.1989.71.6.0842.
35. Henderson L, McDonald S, Eames N. The ever increasing demand for metastatic spinal surgery. Ulster Med J. 2012;81:156–7.
36. Honda S, Murata K, Fujibayashi S, et al. Effect of high disease activity on spinal sagittal malalignment in patients with rheumatoid arthritis. J Neurosurg Spine. 2024:1–9. https://doi.org/10.3171/2024.1.SPINE231199.
37. Honda S, Murata K, Otsuki B, et al. Active rheumatoid arthritis and scoliosis: a mid-term cohort study. Spine (Phila Pa 1976). 2024; https://doi.org/10.1097/BRS.0000000000005035.
38. Kambin P, Schaffer JL. Percutaneous lumbar discectomy: review of 100 patients and current practice. Clin Orthop Relat Res. 1989;238:24.
39. Kebaish KM, Neubauer PR, Voros GD, et al. Scoliosis in adults aged forty years and older: prevalence and relationship to age, race, and gender. Spine (Phila Pa 1976). 2011;36:731–6. https://doi.org/10.1097/BRS.0b013e3181e9f120.
40. Khoo LT, Smith ZA, Asgarzadie F, et al. Minimally invasive extracavitary approach for thoracic discectomy and interbody fusion: 1-year clinical and radiographic outcomes in 13 patients compared with a cohort of traditional anterior transthoracic approaches. J Neurosurg Spine. 2011;14:250–60. https://doi.org/10.3171/2010.10.SPINE09456.
41. Kim J-S, Yeung A, Lokanath YK, Lewandrowski K-U. Is Asia truly a hotspot of contemporary minimally invasive and endoscopic spinal surgery? J Spine Surg. 2020;6:S224–36. https://doi.org/10.21037/jss.2019.12.13.
42. Kobayashi K, Ando K, Nishida Y, et al. Epidemiological trends in spine surgery over 10 years in a multicenter database. Eur Spine J. 2018;27:1698–703. https://doi.org/10.1007/s00586-018-5513-4.
43. Kobayashi K, Sato K, Kato F, et al. Trends in the numbers of spine surgeries and spine surgeons over the past 15 years. Nagoya J Med Sci. 2022;84:155–62. https://doi.org/10.18999/nagjms.84.1.155.
44. Kolenkiewicz M, Włodarczyk A, Wojtkiewicz J. Diagnosis and Incidence of Spondylosis and Cervical Disc Disorders in the University Clinical Hospital in Olsztyn, in Years 2011–2015.

Biomed Res Int. 2018;2018:5643839. https://doi.org/10.1155/2018/5643839.
45. Konieczny MR, Senyurt H, Krauspe R. Epidemiology of adolescent idiopathic scoliosis. J Child Orthop. 2013;7:3–9. https://doi.org/10.1007/s11832-012-0457-4.
46. Kumar R, Lim J, Mekary RA, et al. Traumatic Spinal Injury: Global Epidemiology and Worldwide Volume. World Neurosurg. 2018;113:e345–63. https://doi.org/10.1016/j.wneu.2018.02.033.
47. Lattanza LL, Meszaros-Dearolf L, O'Connor MI, et al. The Perry Initiative's Medical Student Outreach Program Recruits Women into Orthopaedic Residency. Clin Orthop Relat Res. 2016;474:1962–6. https://doi.org/10.1007/s11999-016-4908-y.
48. Lee SE, Jahng T-A, Kim K-J, et al. Research articles published by Korean spine surgeons: Scientific progress and the increase in spine surgery. J Clin Neurosci. 2017;36:6–11. https://doi.org/10.1016/j.jocn.2016.10.025.
49. Leidinger A, Extremera P, Kim EE, et al. The challenges and opportunities of global neurosurgery in East Africa: the neurosurgery education and development model. Neurosurg Focus. 2018;45:E8. https://doi.org/10.3171/2018.7.FOCUS18287.
50. Lewandrowski K-U, Soriano-Sánchez J-A, Zhang X, et al. Regional variations in acceptance, and utilization of minimally invasive spinal surgery techniques among spine surgeons: results of a global survey. J Spine Surg. 2020;6:S260–74. https://doi.org/10.21037/jss.2019.09.31.
51. Lifton J. The demand for spine surgeons. Spine J. 2008;8:1042–4. https://doi.org/10.1016/j.spinee.2008.01.002.
52. Mani K, Kleinbart E, Goldman SN, et al. Projections of single-level and multilevel spinal instrumentation procedure volume and associated costs for Medicare patients to 2050. J Am Acad Orthop Surg Glob Res Rev. 2024;8:e24.00053. https://doi.org/10.5435/JAAOSGlobal-D-24-00053.
53. Mansoer J, Scheele S, Floyd K, et al. New methods for estimating the tuberculosis case detection rate in high-HIV prevalence countries: the example of Kenya. Bull World Health Organ. 2009;87(186–192):192A–B. https://doi.org/10.2471/blt.08.051474.
54. Minhas SV, Chow I, Patel AA, Kim JYS. Surgeon specialty differences in single-level anterior cervical discectomy and fusion. Spine (Phila Pa 1976). 2014;39:1648–55. https://doi.org/10.1097/BRS.0000000000000499.
55. Moore ML, Singh R, McQueen K, et al. Workforce trends in spinal surgery: geographic distribution and primary specialty characteristics from 2012 to 2017. World Neurosurg. 2021;156:e392–7. https://doi.org/10.1016/j.wneu.2021.09.073.
56. Nations U Day of 8 Billion. https://www.un.org/en/dayof8billion. Zugegriffen: 08. Juni 2024.
57. Park BE. Surgical treatment of degenerative lumbar spine disease in rural Sub-Saharan Africa: a retrospective study of 450 cases and its future implications. World Neurosurg. 2016;87:417–21. https://doi.org/10.1016/j.wneu.2015.11.077.
58. Pechlivanidou E, Antonopoulos I, Margariti RE. Gender equality challenges in orthopaedic surgery: a systematic review. Int Orthop. 2023;47:2143–71. https://doi.org/10.1007/s00264-023-05876-w.
59. Piazzolla A, Solarino G, De Giorgi S, et al. Cotrel-Dubousset instrumentation in neuromuscular scoliosis. Eur Spine J. 2011;20(Suppl 1):S75–84. https://doi.org/10.1007/s00586-011-1758-x.
60. Post AF, Dai JB, Li AY, et al. Workforce analysis of spine surgeons involved with neurological and orthopedic surgery residency training. World Neurosurg. 2019;122:e147–55. https://doi.org/10.1016/j.wneu.2018.09.152.
61. Radcliff KE, Curry EP, Trimba R, et al. High incidence of undiagnosed cervical myelopathy in patients with hip fracture compared with controls. J Orthop Trauma. 2016;30:189–93. https://doi.org/10.1097/BOT.0000000000000485.
62. Raitio A, Syvänen J, Helenius I. Vertebral body tethering: indications, surgical technique, and a systematic review of published results. J Clin Med. 2022;11:2576. https://doi.org/10.3390/jcm11092576.
63. Ravindra VM, Senglaub SS, Rattani A, et al. Degenerative lumbar spine disease: estimating global incidence and worldwide volume. Global Spine J. 2018;8:784–94. https://doi.org/10.1177/2192568218770769.
64. Renfrow JJ, Rodriguez A, Liu A, et al. Positive trends in neurosurgery enrollment and attrition: analysis of the 2000–2009 female neurosurgery resident cohort. J Neurosurg. 2016;124:834–9. https://doi.org/10.3171/2015.3.JNS142313.
65. Rohde RS, Wolf JM, Adams JE. Where are the women in orthopaedic surgery? Clin Orthop Relat Res. 2016;474:1950–6. https://doi.org/10.1007/s11999-016-4827-y.
66. Roser MJ, Askin GN, Labrom RD, et al. Vertebral body tethering for idiopathic scoliosis: a systematic review and meta-analysis. Spine Deform. 2023;11:1297–307. https://doi.org/10.1007/s43390-023-00723-9.
67. Rožanković M, Marasanov SM, Vukić M. Cervical disk replacement with discover versus fusion in a single-level cervical disk disease: a prospective single-center randomized trial with a minimum 2-year follow-up. Clin Spine Surg. 2017;30:E515–22. https://doi.org/10.1097/BSD.0000000000000170.
68. Ruetten S, Komp M, Merk H, Godolias G. A new full-endoscopic technique for cervical posterior foraminotomy in the treatment of lateral disc herniations using 6.9-mm endoscopes: prospective 2-year results of 87 patients. Minim Invasive Neurosurg. 2007;50:219–26. https://doi.org/10.1055/s-2007-985860.
69. Saadé S, Delafontaine A, Cattan J, et al. Attractiveness and gender dynamics in surgical specialties: a comparative analysis of French medical graduates

(2017–2022). BMC Med Educ. 2024;24:197. https://doi.org/10.1186/s12909-024-05174-y.
70. Safdarian M, Trinka E, Rahimi-Movaghar V, et al. Global, regional, and national burden of spinal cord injury, 1990–2019: a systematic analysis for the Global Burden of Disease Study 2019. Lancet Neurol. 2023;22:1026–47. https://doi.org/10.1016/S1474-4422(23)00287-9.
71. Sakhrekar R, Iorio C, Yoon S, et al. Philosophies and surgical techniques for Ewing's sarcoma of spine with review of literature. J Orthop Case Rep. 2024;14:168–75. https://doi.org/10.13107/jocr.2024.v14.i03.4330.
72. Schallmo MS, Cook RW, Weiner JA, et al. Do demographic factors of spine surgeons affect the rate at which spinal fusion is performed on patients? Spine (Phila Pa 1976). 2017;42:1261–6. https://doi.org/10.1097/BRS.0000000000002060.
73. Shakil H, Malhotra AK, Badhiwala JH, et al. Contemporary trends in the incidence and timing of spinal metastases: a population-based study. Neuro-Oncol Adv. 2024;6:vdae051. https://doi.org/10.1093/noajnl/vdae051.
74. Siegel RL, Miller KD, Wagle NS, Jemal A. Cancer statistics, 2023. CA Cancer J Clin. 2023;73:17–48. https://doi.org/10.3322/caac.21763.
75. Singh R, Gonzales-Portillo GS, Nguyen B, et al. Anterior thoracic Diskectomy and fusion: surgical technique and anatomic considerations. World Neurosurg. 2022;166:89. https://doi.org/10.1016/j.wneu.2022.07.052.
76. de Souza FI, Di Ferreira RB, Labres D, et al. Epidemiology of adolescent idiopathic scoliosis in students of the public schools in Goiânia-GO. Acta Ortop Bras. 2013;21:223–5. https://doi.org/10.1590/S1413-78522013000400008.
77. Sung S, Chae H-W, Lee HS, et al. Incidence and surgery rate of idiopathic scoliosis: a nationwide database study. Int J Environ Res Public Health. 2021;18:8152. https://doi.org/10.3390/ijerph18158152.
78. Tarpada SP, Morris MT, Burton DA. Spinal fusion surgery: a historical perspective. J Orthop. 2017;14:134–6. https://doi.org/10.1016/j.jor.2016.10.029.
79. Thavarajasingam SG, Subbiah Ponniah H, Philipps R, et al. Increasing incidence of spondylodiscitis in England: An analysis of the national health service (NHS) hospital episode statistics from 2012 to 2021. Brain Spine. 2023;3:101733. https://doi.org/10.1016/j.bas.2023.101733.
80. du Toit A, Tawa N, Leibbrandt DC, et al. Current knowledge of idiopathic scoliosis among practising physiotherapists in South Africa. S Afr J Physiother. 2020;76:1500. https://doi.org/10.4102/sajp.v76i1.1500.
81. Toloba Y, Diallo S, Maiga Y, et al. Spinal tuberculosis (Pott's disease): epidemiological, clinical, radiological and evolutionary aspects at the University Hospital of Point G. Mali Med. 2011;26:8–11.
82. Tu T-H, Wang C-Y, Chen Y-C, Wu J-C. Multilevel cervical disc arthroplasty: a review of optimal surgical management and future directions. J Neurosurg Spine. 2023;38:372–81. https://doi.org/10.3171/2022.11.SPINE22880.
83. Tuli SM. Historical aspects of Pott's disease (spinal tuberculosis) management. Eur Spine J. 2013;22:529–38. https://doi.org/10.1007/s00586-012-2388-7.
84. Varatharajah S, Charles Y-P, Buy X, et al. Update on the surgical management of Pott's disease. Orthop Traumatol Surg Res. 2014;100:229–35. https://doi.org/10.1016/j.otsr.2013.09.013.
85. Vogelzang NJ, Beer TM, Gerritsen W, et al. Efficacy and safety of autologous dendritic cell-based immunotherapy, docetaxel, and prednisone vs placebo in patients with metastatic castration-resistant prostate cancer: the VIABLE phase 3 randomized clinical trial. JAMA Oncol. 2022;8:546–52. https://doi.org/10.1001/jamaoncol.2021.7298.
86. Walker CT, Kakarla UK, Chang SW, Sonntag VKH. History and advances in spinal neurosurgery. J Neurosurg Spine. 2019;31:775–85. https://doi.org/10.3171/2019.9.SPINE181362.
87. Wallis CJD, Jerath A, Aminoltejari K, et al. Surgeon sex and long-term postoperative outcomes among patients undergoing common surgeries. JAMA Surg. 2023;158:1185–94. https://doi.org/10.1001/jamasurg.2023.3744.
88. Wang Q-L, Tu Z-M, Hu P, et al. Long-term results comparing cervical disc arthroplasty to anterior cervical discectomy and fusion: a systematic review and meta-analysis of randomized controlled trials. Orthop Surg. 2020;12:16–30. https://doi.org/10.1111/os.12585.
89. Wang TY, Park C, Dalton T, et al. Robotic navigation in spine surgery: where are we now and where are we going? J Clin Neurosci. 2021;94:298–304. https://doi.org/10.1016/j.jocn.2021.10.034.
90. Wu A-M, Cross M, Elliott JM, et al. Global, regional, and national burden of neck pain, 1990–2020, and projections to 2050: a systematic analysis of the Global Burden of Disease Study 2021. Lancet Rheumatol. 2024;6:e142–55. https://doi.org/10.1016/S2665-9913(23)00321-1.
91. Xu P, Wang C, He H, et al. Spinal balance failure: a potential cause of spinal ligament ossification. Med Hypotheses. 2011;76:908–10. https://doi.org/10.1016/j.mehy.2011.03.006.
92. Yang J, Lou S, Yao T. Trends in primary malignant bone cancer incidence and mortality in the United

States, 2000–2017: a population-based study. J Bone Oncol. 2024;46:100607. https://doi.org/10.1016/j.jbo.2024.100607.
93. Zaikova O, Giercksky K-E, Fosså SD, et al. A population-based study of spinal metastatic disease in South-East Norway. Clin Oncol (R Coll Radiol). 2009;21:753–9. https://doi.org/10.1016/j.clon.2009.09.023.
94. Zavatsky JM, Peters AJ, Nahvi FA, et al. Disease severity and treatment in adolescent idiopathic scoliosis: the impact of race and economic status. Spine J. 2015;15:939–43. https://doi.org/10.1016/j.spinee.2013.06.043.
95. 1.1 TB incidence. https://www.who.int/teams/global-tuberculosis-programme/tb-reports/global-tuberculosis-report-2023/tb-disease-burden/1-1-tb-incidence. Zugegriffen: 02. Juni 2024.
96. EUROSPINE member directory. https://www.eurospine.org/about-us/membership/members-directory/. Zugegriffen: 05. Juni 2024.
97. Global Neurosurgical Workforce Map - About WFNS | WFNS. https://wfns.org/menu/61/global-neurosurgical-workforce-map. Zugegriffen: 08. Juni 2024.

Living Anatomy of the Spine

Olivier Hamel and Jean-Marc Vital

The knowledge of the normal anatomy of the spine, as well as its spatial and temporal variations, is essential for understanding all steps of spinal pathology diagnosis and treatment.

The anatomy usually described, and with which the reader is familiar, is that of the young adult, a state that is in reality only very transient.

We will therefore study the morphogenesis and growth that lead to this state in adulthood, then its degeneration into its physiological form in a continuum that we consider to be a "living anatomy" of the spine.

1 Morphogenesis

The first key event in spinal morphogenesis is gastrulation, which takes place at the beginning of the third week and leads to the establishment of the three laminae (entoblast, mesoblast, and ectoblast), but also induces what will become the median line and define the craniocaudal axis (Fig. 1).

Mesoblast formation on the primitive midline gives rise to the notochordal process, which at the end of the third week, after a transitional opening toward the entoblast, becomes the notochordal plate and then the notochord at the beginning of the fourth week (Figs. 2 and 3).

In a cranial–caudal direction, axial mesoblast induces the formation of the neural plate, within the ectoblast, which gives rise to the neural tube (Figs. 4 and 5), future central nervous system, and neural crests themselves at the origin of numerous structures (sensory and vegetative ganglia, adrenals, melanocytes, etc.).

On either side of the notochord, at the same time and also in a craniocaudal way, para-axial mesoblast condense to form the axial skeleton. This mesoblast segments himself into rounded formations called somitomeres (Fig. 6), most of which become somites (the first seven somitomeres disappear). In humans, by the fifth week, 42–44 pairs of somites are paired on either side of the median notochord. After regression of the first somitomeres, only 37 remain:

- 4 pairs of occipital somites,
- 8 pairs of cervical somites,
- 12 pairs of thoracic somites,
- 5 pairs of lumbar somites,
- 5 pairs of sacral somites,
- 3 pairs of coccygeal somites.

Each somite has three divisions: sclerotomes, myotomes, and dermatomes. Sclerotomes arise from the ventromedial portion of the somite, and these cells condense (Figs. 7 and 8), depending

O. Hamel (✉)
Clinique des Cèdres, Toulouse, France

J.-M. Vital
Centre DOSCEA, Bayonne, France

C. Y. Barrey (ed.), *Spine Surgery*, SFCR Experts Series 1,
https://doi.org/10.1007/978-3-031-85446-0_3

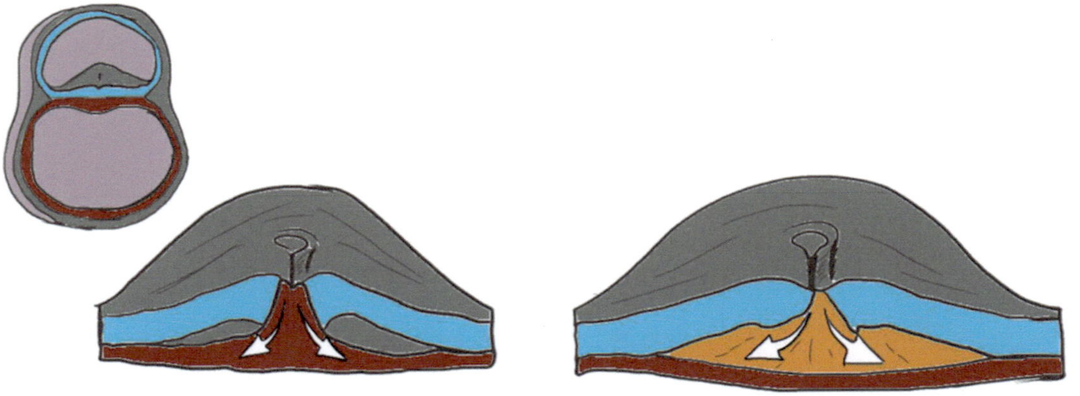

Fig. 1 Gastrulation event (third week) on a section of embryo passing from two to three laminae

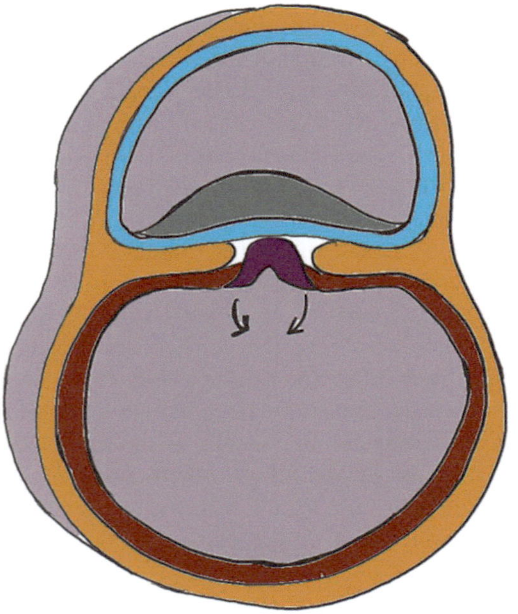

Fig. 2 Formation of the notochordal process on a section of embryo

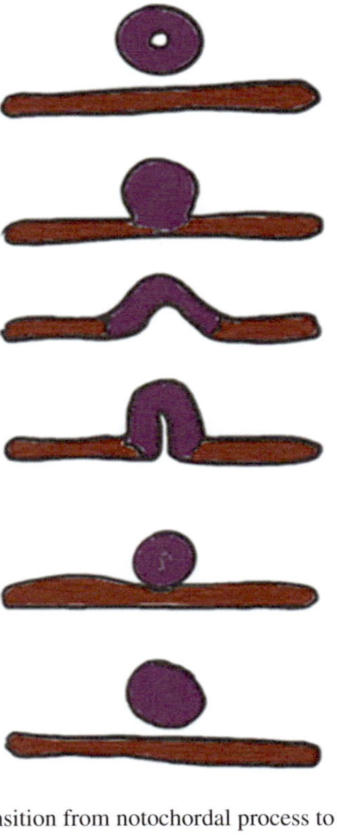

Fig. 3 Transition from notochordal process to notochord

on the molecular signal and its origin, around the notochord in the ventral portion (future disco-corporeal system) and around the neural tube in the dorsal portion (future dorsal vertebral arch). The spinous processes respond to a different molecular signal. The neural tube, derived from ectoblast, is therefore formed before the vertebrae, from mesoblast, which will protect it within a central spinal canal.

The other decisive event in spinal morphology and its relationship with the nervous system is resegmentation, transition from the somitic to the vertebral stage. In an area of less active cell proliferation, the somites divide into a cranial half and a caudal half. Cells from adjacent somite

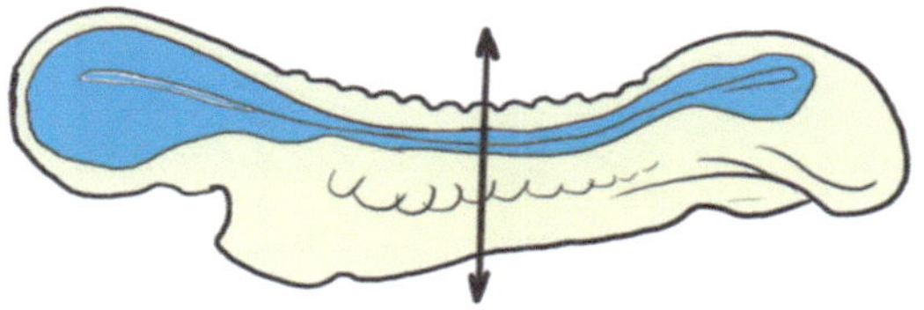

Fig. 4 Dorsal view of an embryo (third week) showing the neural plate

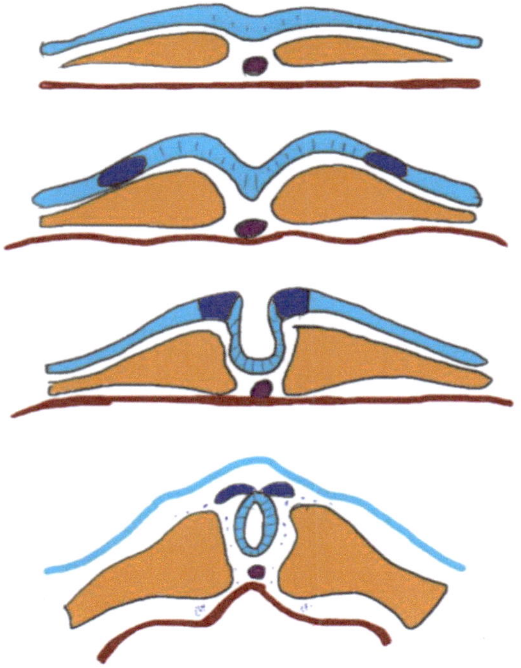

Fig. 5 Transition from neural plate to neural tube, formation of neural crests

halves recombine to give rise to a single vertebral draft (Fig. 9). This new segmentation allows the spinal roots to pass between each vertebra within the intervertebral foramina. The seven cervical vertebrae are formed from eight somites. The fourth occipital somite leads to the proatlas, which is involved in the formation of the first cervical vertebra (Fig. 10). This explains the particular conformation of the first two cervical vertebrae, but also the existence of eight cervical spinal roots: the first between the occiput and the first cervical vertebra; the eighth between the seventh cervical vertebra and the first thoracic vertebra.

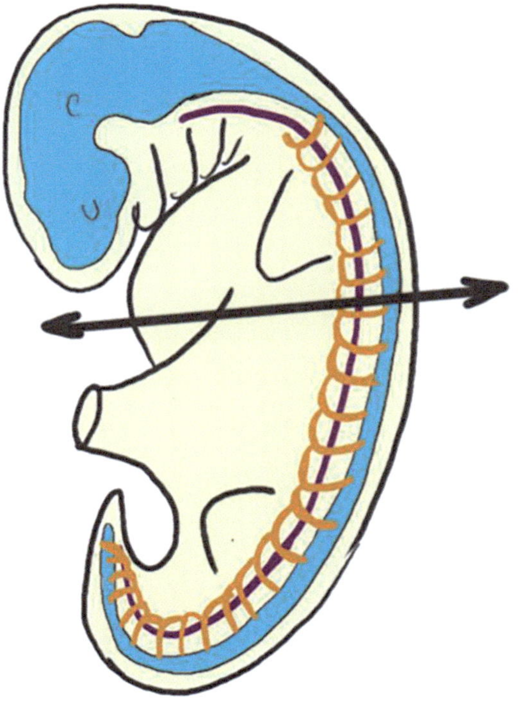

Fig. 6 Lateral view of an embryo (fourth week) showing the neural tube, notochord, and somites

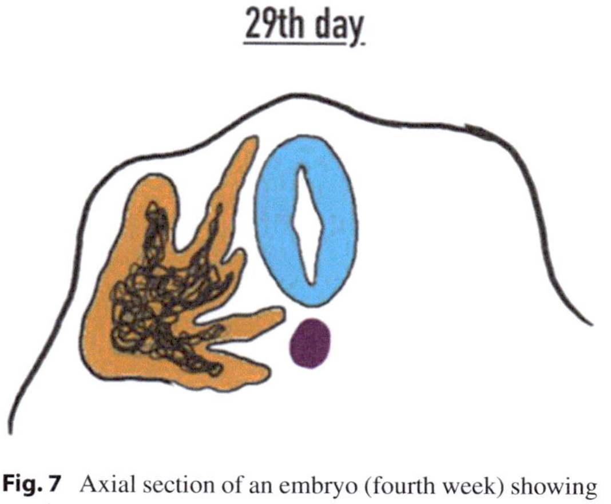

Fig. 7 Axial section of an embryo (fourth week) showing condensation of a sclerotome around the notochord and the neural tube

The notochord disappears within vertebrae consisting of these two hemisomites. A stigma remains from the fusion of the two hemisomites in the center of the vertebral body: Hahn's cleft, which will be occupied by the basivertebral vessels.

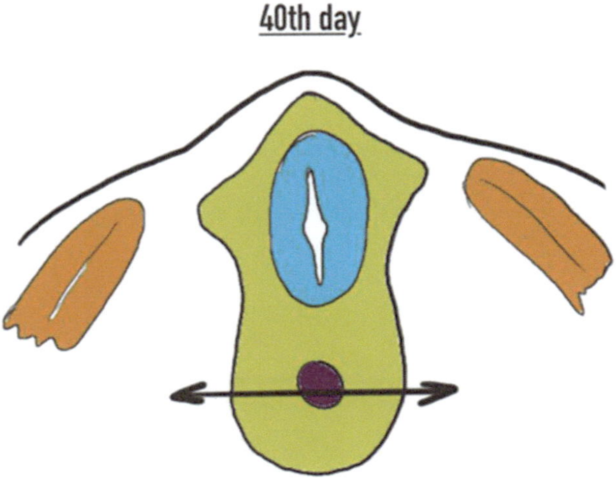

Fig. 8 Axial section (40th day) showing formation of a vertebrae

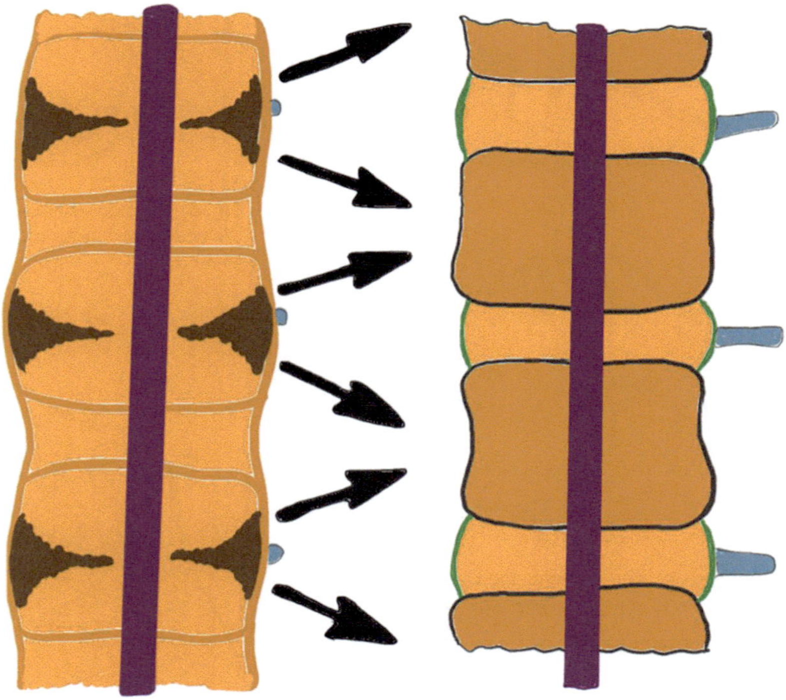

Fig. 9 Coronal section of the spine showing the phenomena of resegmentation

A few notochord cells remain in the nucleus pulposus of the intervertebral disc (IVD). The fibrous annulus of the disc is made up of cells left behind during somite division, receiving tissue contributions from both hemisomites, but it seems that the main contribution comes from its caudal half (i.e., the future cranial part of the vertebra). It is soon possible to distinguish a concentric peripheral organization surrounding an area of notochordal cartilage (Fig. 11). The annulus fibrosus is the first organized element of the IVD, before any mechanical stress. The position of the chordal remnants is initially central, then becomes more dorsal, either as a result of greater development of the ventral perinotochordal components or as a result of embryonic kyphosis.

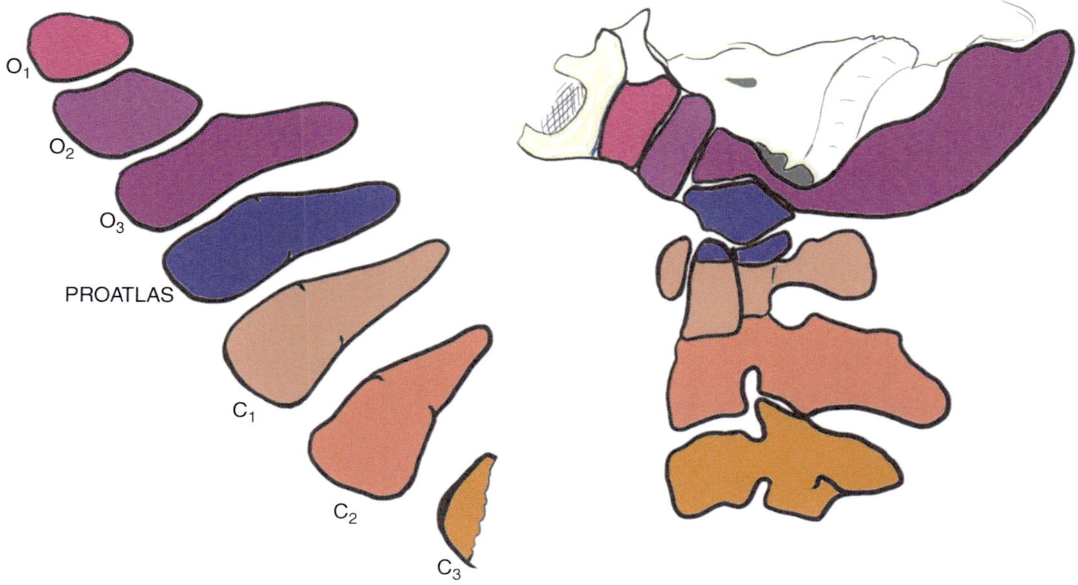

Fig. 10 Specificity of craniocervical junction embryology from occipital somites

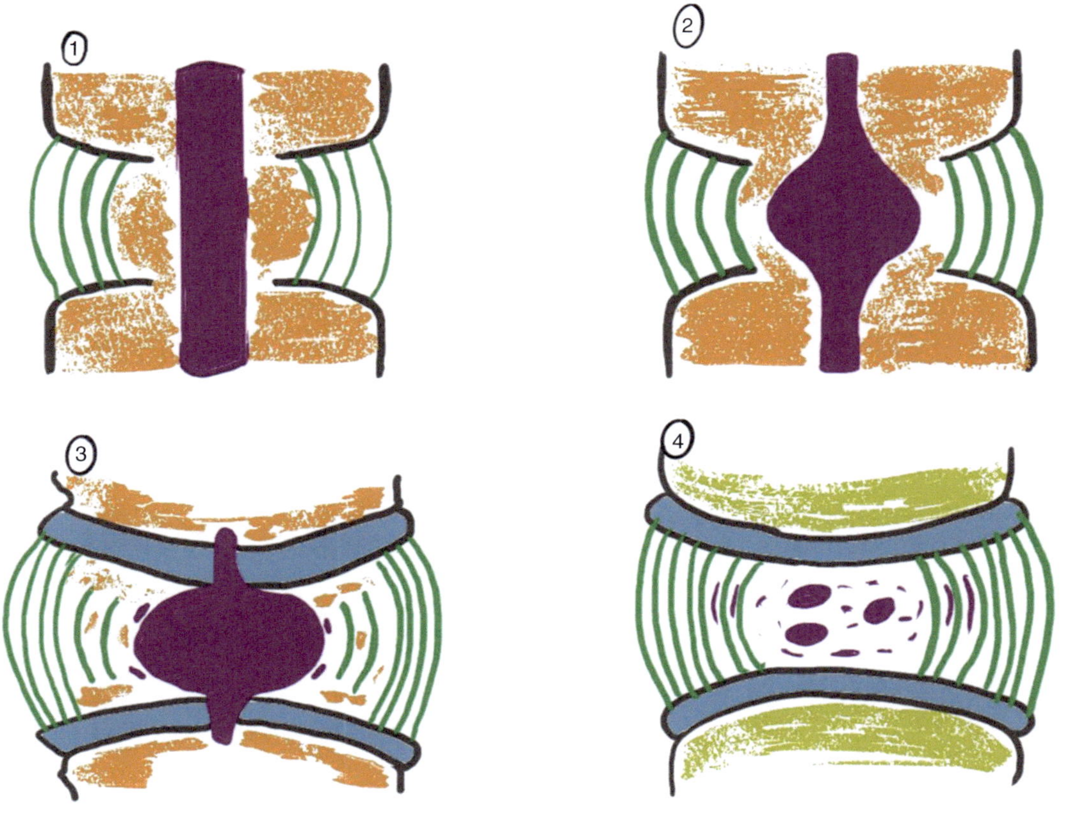

Fig. 11 Formation of the intervertebral disc

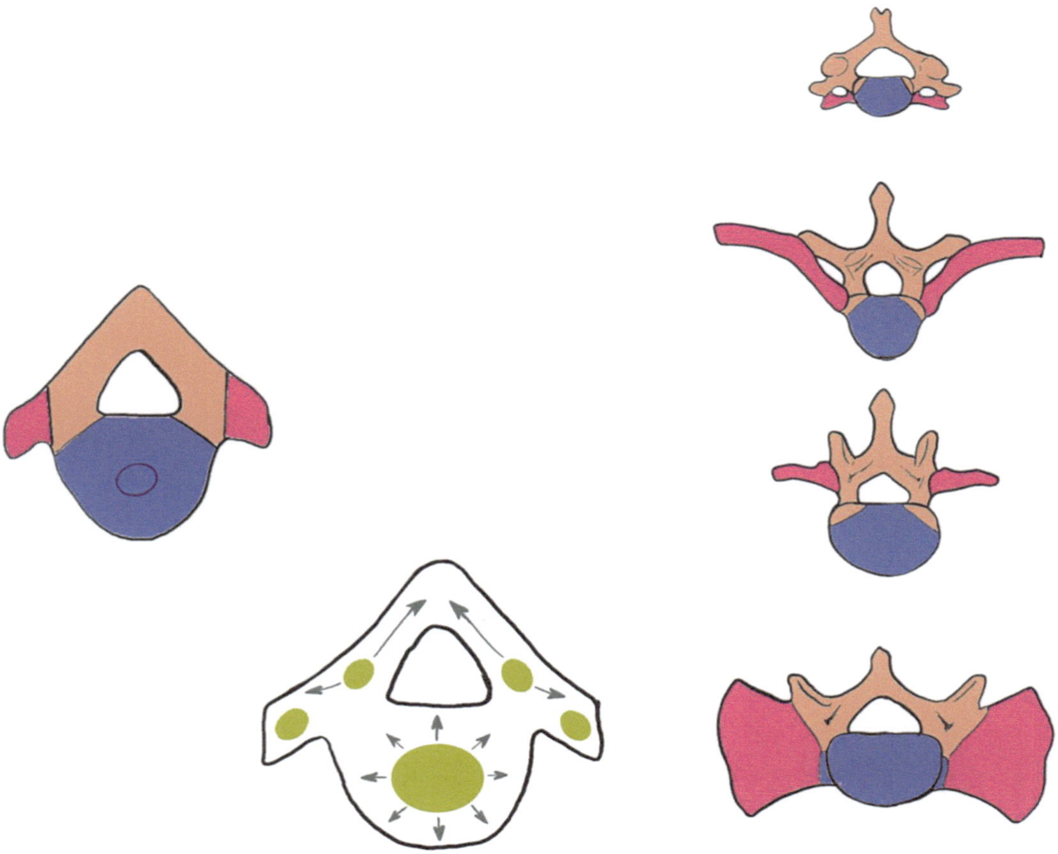

Fig. 12 Evolution of lateral condensations considering the different vertebral segments

The vertebral drafts are marked by small lateral condensations at the level of the dorsal arch. These will develop in different ways depending on the segment under consideration (Fig. 12):

- In the cervical region, they form the ventral part of the transverse processes,
- In the thoracic region, they lengthen to form the ribs,
- In the lumbar region, it forms the costiform processes,
- At the level of the first two or three sacral pieces, it gives lateral masses forming the sacral alae.

These mesenchymal cells from the sclerotomes also give rise to ligamentous and meningeal structures.

All these stages may be marked by a disturbance in segmentation, which will lead to variations in the number of mobile vertebrae or their bony expansions (occipitalization of the atlas, sacralization of L5 or, more rarely, lumbar sacralization of S1, mega-transverse processes of C7 or even cervical ribs, lumbar ribs, etc.).

From the third month, five primary ossification centers appear, a process that begins at the end of the embryonic period: the first, ventral, within the vertebral body, two dorsal on either side of the median line, one on the future pedicle, and the other on the future lamina. The corporeal nucleus is separated from the others by the neurocentral synchondroses (Fig. 12). Thus, within the vertebra, mesenchymal tissue is replaced by cartilage tissue and finally by bone tissue, which corresponds to an enchondral ossification.

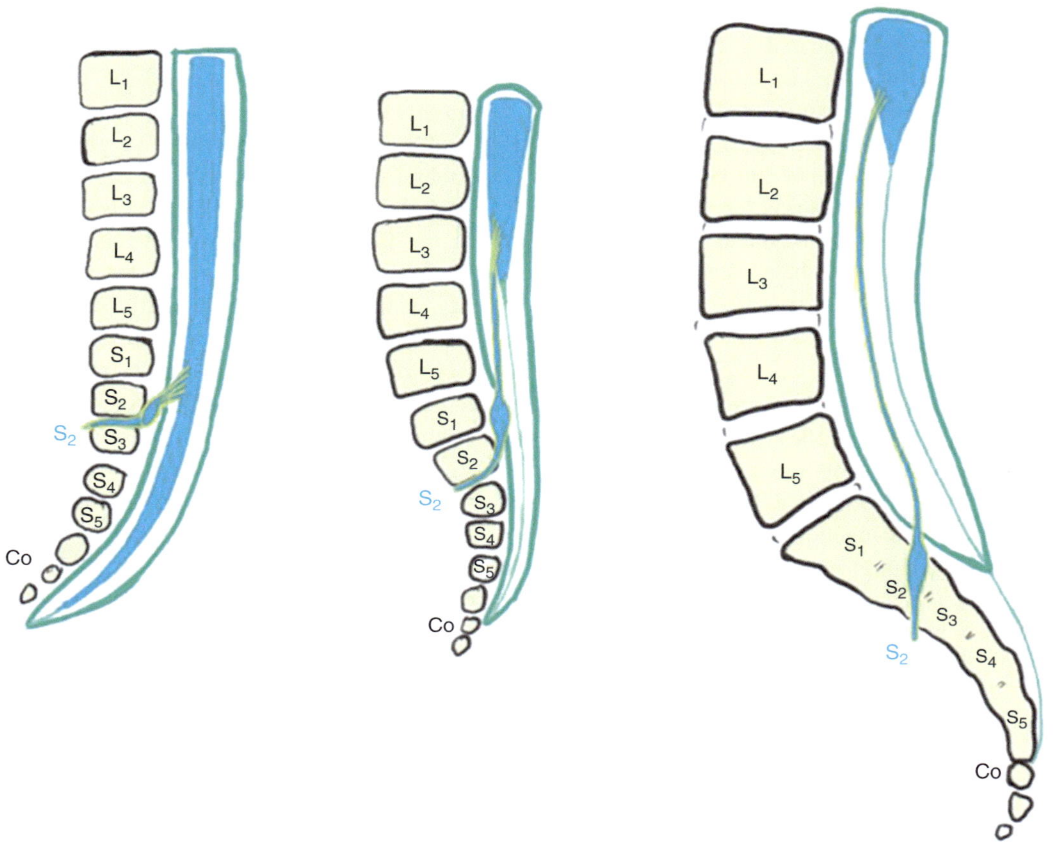

Fig. 13 Sagittal view of the spine showing the differential growth between spine and neural tube

Morphology of the spine is thus obtained and growth begins, which will be even greater after birth. While the spinal column continues to grow, the neural tube slows considerably. This differential growth explains the position of the conus medullaris at L3 level at birth. It also explains the arrangement of the spinal roots, which become vertical in a craniocaudal direction until the formation of the cauda equina, which brings together the lumbosacral roots downstream of the conus medullaris. The position of the spinal roots within the intervertebral foramen, still in this craniocaudal direction, becomes increasingly cranial for the same reason (Fig. 13).

2 Growth

The postnatal period is marked by ossification and two predominant growth phases: the first 5 years and puberty. At 1 year of age, the sagittal curves are established in the erect position, although it is sometimes mentioned that the lumbar lordosis already exist in the fetus.

By the age of 5, the spinal column has grown as much as it will grow throughout the rest of its growth, including the further acceleration during puberty. The vertebral body will double in size from 10 to 17 years old.

At birth, each vertebra is constituted by three bony parts (body, right and left dorsal arches) joined by cartilage. The last sacral vertebrae and the coccygeal vertebrae are completely cartilaginous, and only begin to ossify during childhood. The primary bony core of the body (centrum), shaped like a coffee bean, is the same height as the intervertebral space. At the age of 4, the vertebra is rectangular with beveled anterior angles.

Two types of cartilages play a particular role in this growth:

- neurocentral cartilage, located at the junction of the centrum and the neural arch, which is gradually becoming more dorsal (Fig. 14). This cartilage is known as bipolar because it is located at the junction between the two primary ossification nuclei. It is most active in the first 5–6 years of life, but the age at which it closes is debated, ranging from 6 to 16 years depending on the author. Closure occurs first in the cervical region, then in the lumbar region, and finally in the thoracic region. However, it is important to differentiate between the end of activity and closure. The neurocentral cartilage is involved both in the anteroposterior dimension of the spinal canal, which is therefore fixed at an early stage, and in the growth in height of the posterior third of the vertebral body.
- the annular ring (marginal listel), which is a secondary ossification nucleus and not a growth plate, has a later action. This annular ring is located between the centrum and the discs (Fig. 15). It appears at 2 years of age, ossifies from back to front and fuses with the vertebral body at around 17–18 years of age. It partially ensures the growth in height of the vertebral body. It is strongly adherent to the peripheral part of the IVD (Sharpey fibers) and to the longitudinal ligaments, but is weakly adherent to the core of the vertebral body, which explains the possibility of separation between the annular ring and the centrum, a separation described as "epiphyseal." The final stage in the ossification of the vertebral body is the fusion of the centrum and annular ring. This fusion begins at the age of 14 but is completed only by the age of 25, and leads to the limbus vertebra.

The first two cervical vertebrae are an exception from the embryonic period, when an occipital sclerotome is involved in their formation. Their growth also escapes the rules described above. C1 (atlas) is marked by three ossification nuclei: two lateral nuclei that become the lateral masses and a ventral nucleus that participates in the formation of the entire ring. Ossification of C2 (axis) begins at 5 months in utero with the neural arch and body nuclei, similar to those of the other vertebrae, but the odontoid process is initially formed by two nuclei, which fuse secondarily on the median line, and a nucleus corresponding to the tip of the odontoid, which ossifies at 6 years and fuses at around 12 years (Fig. 16).

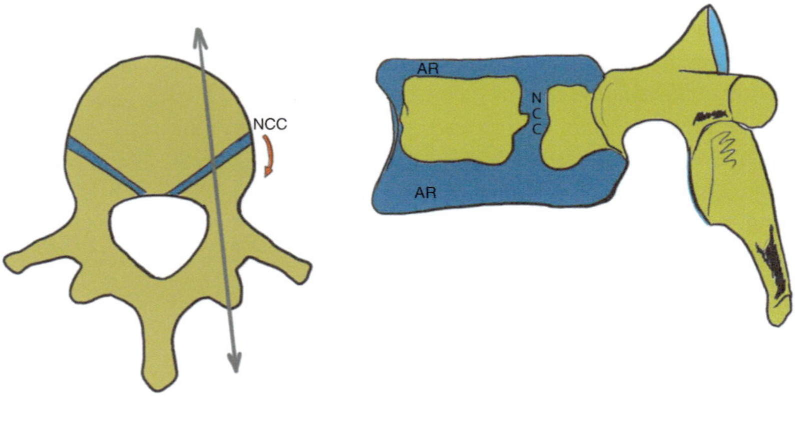

Fig. 14 Neurocentral cartilage on axial and sagittal paramedian views

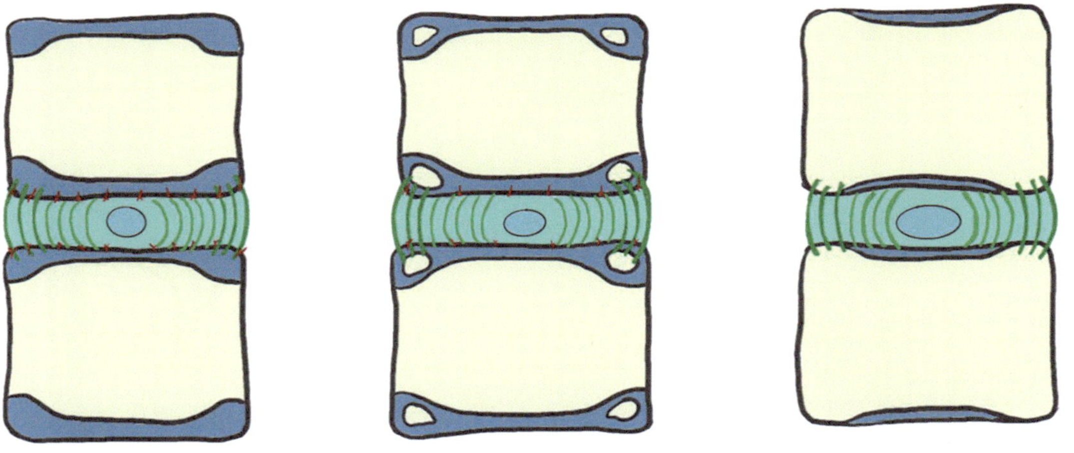

Fig. 15 Annular ring (marginal listel) and intervertebral disc maturation on coronal views

Fig. 16 Ossification nuclei and growth cartilages of atlas and axis

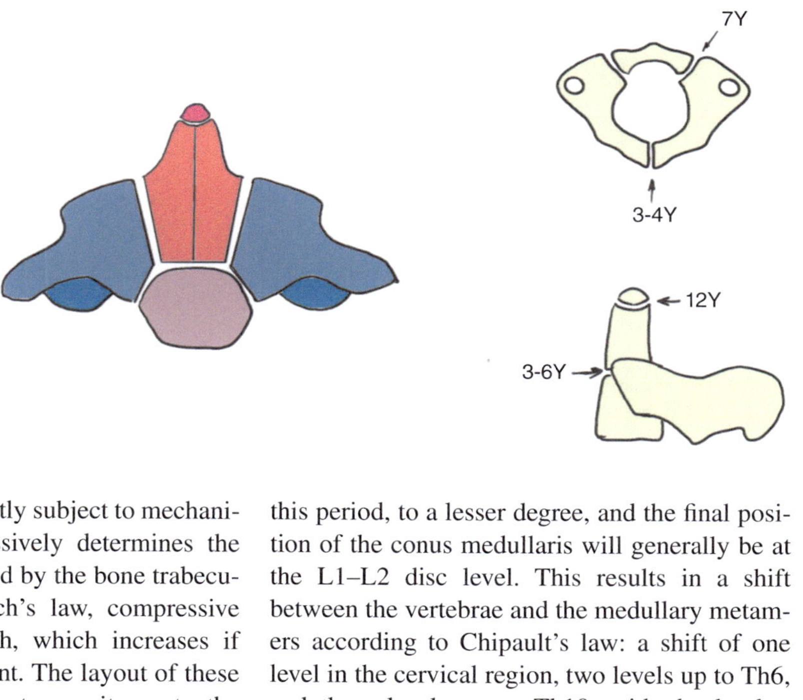

Bone growth is constantly subject to mechanical stress, which progressively determines the "lines of force" represented by the bone trabeculae. According to Delpech's law, compressive stress slows down growth, which increases if compressive stress is absent. The layout of these trabeculae is linked either to gravity or to the traction exerted by the muscles on the bone processes during movement (Fig. 17). This arrangement tells us what will become the zone of weakness (ventral part of the vertebral body) and the most resistant zone (pedicle) of the vertebrae (Fig. 18).

The differential growth between the vertebral column and the spinal cord also occurs during this period, to a lesser degree, and the final position of the conus medullaris will generally be at the L1–L2 disc level. This results in a shift between the vertebrae and the medullary metamers according to Chipault's law: a shift of one level in the cervical region, two levels up to Th6, and three levels up to Th10, with the lumbar metamers facing Th11 and Th12 and the sacral metamers facing L1 (Fig. 19).

Maturation process also concerns IVD. From birth to the end of growth, this process is marked by two phenomena: the first is peripheral, with the disappearance of the vessels from the annular ring (between 3 and 10 years), replaced by a diffusion system that allows exchanges between the

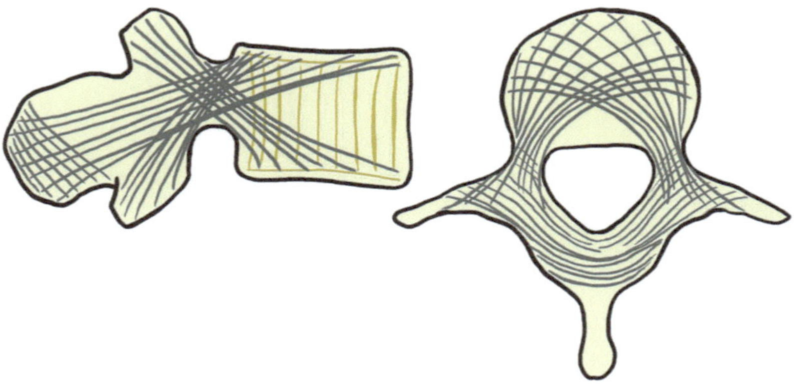

Fig. 17 Bony trabeculae on axial and sagittal paramedian views

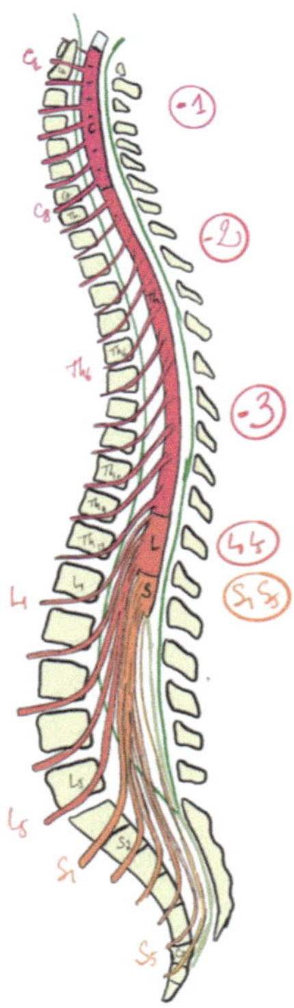

Fig. 18 Chipault's law

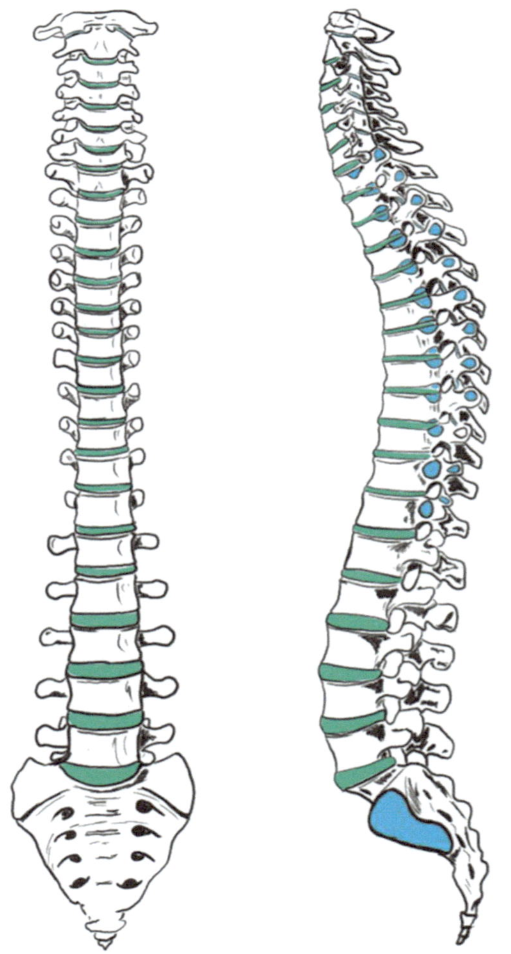

Fig. 19 Normal result of spinal construction (AP and lateral views)

IVD and the vertebral body (Fig. 15); the second is central, with the gradual disappearance of the notochordal cells, replaced by cells with a chondrocytic phenotype. It is also during this period (between 4 and 8 years of age) that the nucleus pulposus of the IVD changes from a round to an elliptical shape.

3 Adulthood: A Temporary Anatomy

The anatomy of the spine, considered as normal, is defined as that of the young adult (Fig. 19). The spinal column is usually made up of a stack of 32 vertebrae, all different but divided into five segments: 7 cervical vertebrae, which together usually form a lordosis, 12 thoracic vertebrae arranged in a kyphosis, 5 lumbar vertebrae arranged in a lordosis, 5 sacral vertebrae fused together in a kyphosis, and a 3-pieces coccygeal appendage, the remains of a tail found in most mammals. Junction's zones between these different segments, and above all between the skull and the spine, have specific anatomical features that give rise to specific pathological conditions.

The vertebrae are linked together (with the exception of the sacral vertebrae) by a disco-ligament system known as the functional spinal unit (FSU). These curvatures, which provide an energy-efficient sagittal balance for upright posture, will have an influence on possible degenerative changes. For example, low lumbar lordosis leads to more IVD degeneration, while high lordosis will generate more stress on the dorsal arches and their joints.

As soon as the formation of the spine is completed, an ineluctable degeneration begins. In fact, the IVD, the centerpiece of the FSU, undergoes its first constitutional alteration, through loss of hydration, as early as adolescence, even before the annular ring has completely fused to the body. The IVD is the first tissue in the human body to degenerate.

This leads to progressive, synchronized remodeling of the IVD and adjacent vertebral endplates (Fig. 20). Signs of disc degeneration on MRI are present in over 80% of asymptomatic subjects, and in almost a third of subjects under the age of 30. The notion of "disc degeneration" is particularly complex to define insofar it can be considered as a physiological phenomenon, like all

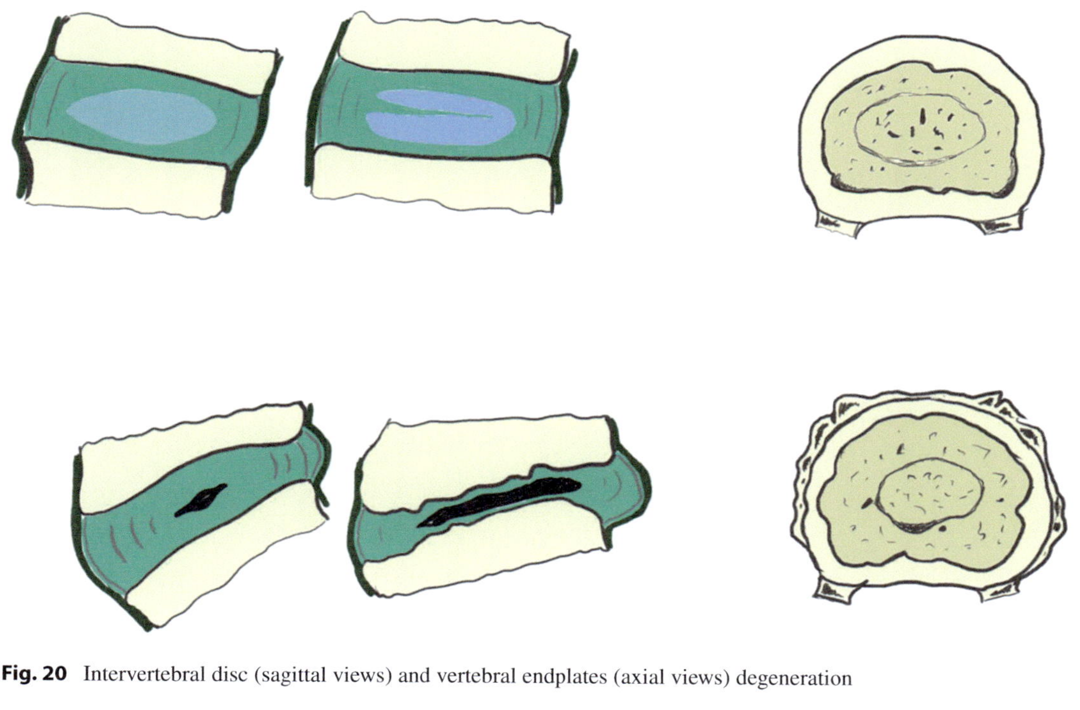

Fig. 20 Intervertebral disc (sagittal views) and vertebral endplates (axial views) degeneration

ageing. It can therefore be difficult to differentiate pathological degeneration from physiological senescence, which are both identical processes.

Mechanical stress that cause disc damages is also responsible for changes to the vertebral endplates. A particular form of this is uncarthrosis, which affects only the lower cervical vertebrae. The impact of mechanical stress can be very particular if it occurs before ossification of the annular ring.

Evolution of the vertebral endplates also compromises the disco-corporeal exchanges that are essential for the survival of the IVD. The result is a loss of differentiation between the annulus fibrosus and the nucleus pulposus, which coincides with a loss of IVD biomechanical properties. In addition, there is a progressive thickening of the ligamentous structures, particularly the yellow ligament, whose elasticity is reduced. This is followed by a reduction in disc height which, particularly in the lumbar region, leads to a loss of lordosis, since the discs at this level are normally higher at the anterior part than at the posterior part. The concomitant hypertrophy of the zygapophyseal joints and spinous processes increases the kyphosis-inducing process of ageing (Fig. 21).

Finally, the natural evolution, particularly of the most mobile segments, is the reduction in the caliber of the canals (central spinal canal and intervertebral foramen), consequence of the loss of disc height, and ligament thickening. This narrowing is just as physiological as disc degeneration; nevertheless, the nervous system remains protected for a long time by the initial size of these spaces and by the safety and sliding elements constituted by intradural cerebrospinal fluid and extradural (epidural) fat (Fig. 21).

A segmental anatomy therefore emerges from the embryonic period to adolescence, with many possible variations in the number of these segments, their dimensions, their arrangement in the frontal or sagittal plane, and so on, some of which potentially promote pathological evolutions. The subsequent evolution of this anatomy, which is subjected to numerous intrinsic and extrinsic factors, should most often be considered as normal. It is for these reasons that, over and above an analysis of what can be visualized at time *T*, the practitioner must understand how a symptomatic spine was formed, grew, and degenerated.

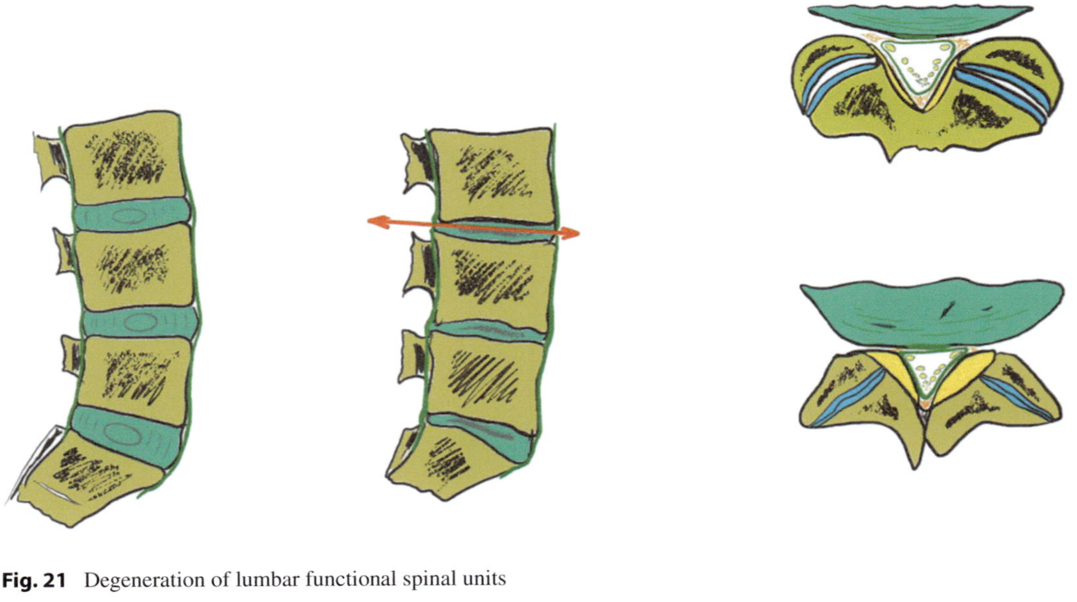

Fig. 21 Degeneration of lumbar functional spinal units

Bibliography

1. Bogduk N. Anatomie clinique du rachis lombal et sacré. Paris: Elsevier; 2005. p. 340.
2. Colombier P, Clouet J, Hamel O, Lescaudron L, Guicheux J. The lumbar intervertebral disc: from embryonic development to degeneration. Joint Bone Spine. 2014;81(2):125–9.
3. Diméglio A, Canavese F. The growing spine: how spinal deformities influence normal spine and thoracic spine growth. Eur Spine J. 2012;21:64–70.
4. Kim SJ, Lee TH, Lim SM. Prevalence of disc degeneration in asymptomatic Korean subjects. Part 1: Lumbar Spine. J Korean Neurosurg Soc. 2013;53(1):31–8.
5. Larsen WJ. Embryologie humaine. Bruxelles: De Boeck Université; 1996. p. 479.
6. Lee TH, Kim SJ, Lim SM. Prevalence of disc degeneration in asymptomatic Korean subjects. Part 2: Cervical spine. J Korean Neurosurg Soc. 2013;53(2):89–95.
7. Paturet G. Anatomie Humaine Tome II: Ostéologie, arthrologie, myologie (à l'exclusion de celles des membres). Paris: Masson; 1951. p. 994.
8. Peacock A. Observations on the prenatal development of the intervertebral disc in man. J Anat. 1951;85(3):260–74.
9. Peacock A. Post-natal structure of intervertebral disc in man. J Anat. 1952;86(2):162–79.
10. Roughley PJ. Biology of intervertebral disc aging and degeneration. Involvement of the extracellular matrix. Spine. 2004;29(23):2691–9.
11. Vital JM, Beguiristain JL, Algara C, Villas C, Lavignolle B, Grenier N, Sénégas J. The neurocental cartilage: anatomy, physiology and physiopathology. Surg Radiol Anat. 1989;11:324–8.
12. Vital JM. Anatomie de la colonne vertébrale – Nouveaux concepts. Montpellier: Sauramps Médical; 2016. p. 675.

Biomechanical Insights and Innovations in Spinal Pathology and Surgical Interventions

Tanguy Vendeuvre and Arnaud Germaneau

1 Introduction

The spine is a fundamental structure of the human body, playing a central role in supporting and protecting the central nervous system while allowing significant mobility. From a biomechanical perspective, the spine can be compared to a ship's mast due to its load-bearing and stabilizing functions (Fig. 1). It is designed to maintain balance and withstand the forces exerted during daily movements and physical loads. This analogy highlights how forces are distributed along the spine, and how surrounding structures, such as muscles, ligaments, and intervertebral discs, contribute to maintaining the integrity of this complex system [1–3].

In clinical settings, understanding spinal biomechanics is crucial for diagnosing and treating a variety of pathologies, including spinal deformities, vertebral fractures, and degenerative conditions [4–6]. These ailments affect a large portion of the population and can significantly impact patients' quality of life. Recent imaging techniques and numerical modeling have provided new insights into the complex interactions of forces acting on the spine, improving both diagnostic and therapeutic approaches.

The spine is subjected to various mechanical forces and moments that determine its behavior under stress:

- **Compression forces**: Compression forces act along the vertical axis of the spine, especially when standing or lifting loads. These forces are primarily supported by the vertebral bodies and intervertebral discs, which act as shock absorbers, absorbing and redistributing loads along the spine. Recent studies have shown that intervertebral discs play a critical role in redistributing these loads, but their capacity to do so can decline with age, leading to increased stress on the vertebrae [7, 8].
- **Tensile forces**: During movements such as stretching or suspension, the spine undergoes tensile forces that tend to separate the vertebrae. These forces are primarily resisted by ligaments and muscles, which limit excessive movement and stabilize the spine [3, 9].
- **Shear forces**: Shear forces occur when opposing parallel forces act on the spine, such as during translational or twisting movements. These forces are particularly critical at the intervertebral discs, where they can lead to significant displacements or deformations [10].

T. Vendeuvre (✉)
CHU de Poitiers, Department of Orthopaedic surgery and Traumatology, Poitiers, France

Institut Pprime UPR 3346, CNRS – Université de Poitiers – ISAE-ENSMA, Poitiers, France
e-mail: tanguy.vendeuvre@chu-poitiers.fr

A. Germaneau
Institut Pprime UPR 3346, CNRS – Université de Poitiers – ISAE-ENSMA, Poitiers, France
e-mail: arnaud.germaneau@univ-poitiers.fr

C. Y. Barrey (ed.), *Spine Surgery*, SFCR Experts Series 1,
https://doi.org/10.1007/978-3-031-85446-0_4

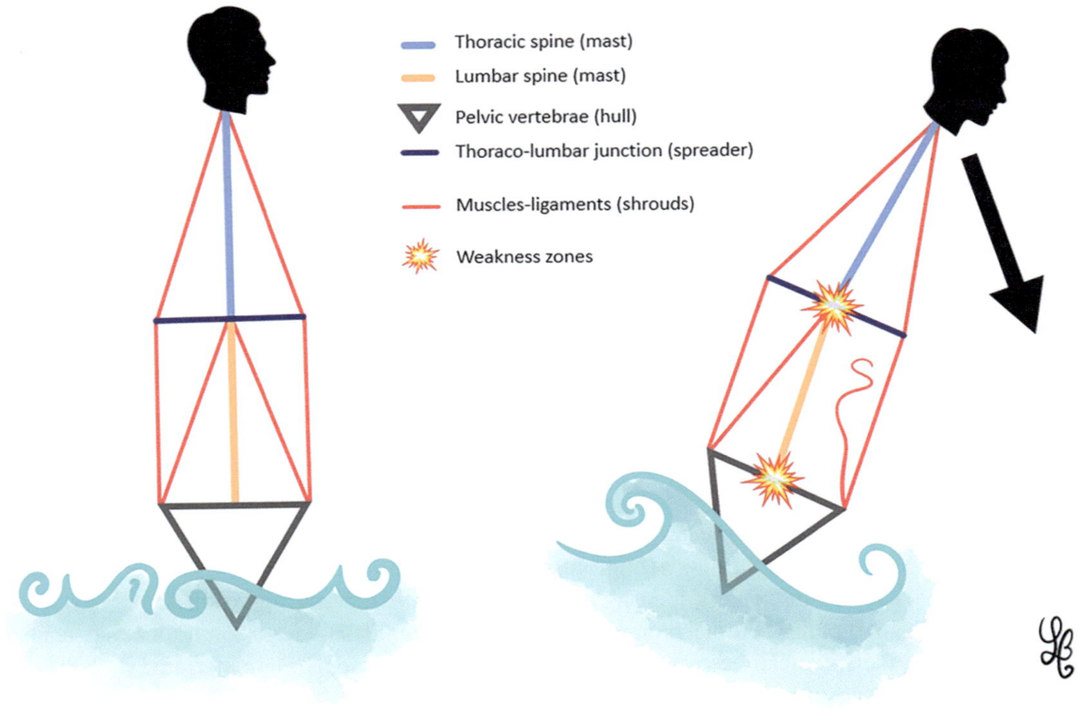

Fig. 1 Illustration of spinal balance through the analogy of a sailboat's equilibrium

The **moments of force**, which represent the rotational or twisting effect induced by these applied forces, are particularly relevant in the analysis of flexion, extension, and rotational movements of the spine:

- **Flexion moment**: This occurs when a force acts on the spine in the sagittal plane, generating a moment that bends the spine forward (flexion) or backward (extension). These moments are mostly supported by the posterior structures of the spine, such as the facet joints and interspinous ligaments, which bear most of the strain during these movements [8].
- **Torsion moment**: Rotational movements around the vertical axis of the spine, such as during trunk rotations, generate torsion moments. These moments place significant strain on the intervertebral discs and ligaments and can lead to injuries when forces exceed the tissue's capacity to adapt [11, 12].

Understanding these forces and moments is essential for grasping how the spine maintains its balance and stability, and how disruptions in these forces can lead to pathologies or injuries. The spine's ability to resist these forces depends on the quality of bone tissue, intervertebral discs, and the coordination of stabilizing muscles [3, 12].

An analogy can be made to a ship (Fig. 1): the triangular hull could represent the pelvic vertebra (as described by Dubousset), while the shrouds represent the musculoskeletal chains. The relationship with the lower limbs (in this case, the sea and waves) influences the hull's position and the distribution of stresses on the mast. Sailing enthusiasts can easily recognize the mast's breaking points based on the height of the waves and the strength of the wind.

The weak points in the spine include the lumbar spine junctions (L4–L5, L5–S1) and the sacroiliac joints, as well as the thoracolumbar junction, analogous in this metaphor to a spreader. A weakness or rupture in the stabilizing elements (the shrouds) leads to excessive stress on the mast, and the mast's resistance depends on the spine's geometry and bone quality.

Surgical interventions on the spine present major challenges due to the complexity of the vertebral column and the need to preserve its function while correcting abnormalities. Postoperative complications can include residual spinal deformity, persistent pain, and degeneration of adjacent spinal segments. These issues raise important questions about the effectiveness of current surgical techniques and underscore the need for better biomechanical evaluation before surgical intervention [13, 14].

Moreover, recent advances in imaging and numerical modeling technologies, such as finite element models (FEM), offer new possibilities for more accurate predictions of postoperative outcomes and allow for personalized treatments based on the specific anatomical and biomechanical characteristics of each patient. These tools not only improve surgical planning but also help reduce the risk of complications by adjusting interventions according to individual biomechanical constraints [15–17].

The central issue in spinal biomechanics lies in the delicate balance between correcting structural abnormalities and maintaining spinal function. How can a deformity be effectively corrected without introducing new harmful mechanical stresses? How can the spine's reactions to surgical interventions be predicted? And, most importantly, how can therapeutic strategies be developed that are both effective and sustainable in the long term?

These questions are particularly relevant as patients' expectations for postoperative quality of life continue to rise. It is becoming increasingly important to understand the complex interactions between the forces applied to the spine, the mechanical properties of tissues, and the body's biomechanical responses. This chapter will explore these issues by delving into the various methods of biomechanical characterization, both in vivo and in vitro, as well as recent advances in numerical modeling and artificial intelligence.

2 Characterization of Spinal Geometry Access to Spinal Geometry: Volumetric Image Segmentation

Accurate characterization of spinal geometry is crucial for understanding how mechanical stresses are distributed throughout the structure under different loading conditions. It relies on advanced imaging techniques and volumetric image segmentation methods, which allow for detailed extraction of geometric information from spinal structures. This data is essential for biomechanical studies and for planning surgical interventions. With recent advances in imaging, new methods have improved the accuracy and detail of these geometric reconstructions. Techniques such as computed tomography (CT) and magnetic resonance imaging (MRI) have become indispensable tools for obtaining precise images of the spine's anatomy, and their integration with sophisticated segmentation algorithms allows for the generation of three-dimensional (3D) models of the spine.

2.1 CT Scan and Bone Structure Segmentation

Computed tomography (CT) scans are widely used to capture fine cross-sectional images of the spine, providing high-resolution views of bone structures. CT segmentation involves isolating and reconstructing bones, such as vertebrae, into 3D models using semiautomatic or automatic algorithms (Fig. 2). Techniques such as active contours and statistical shape models help to reliably define bone contours, making it easier to conduct biomechanical analyses or prepare for surgical procedures [18, 19]. The precision offered by CT scans makes them an interesting tool for assessing bone density and structural integrity.

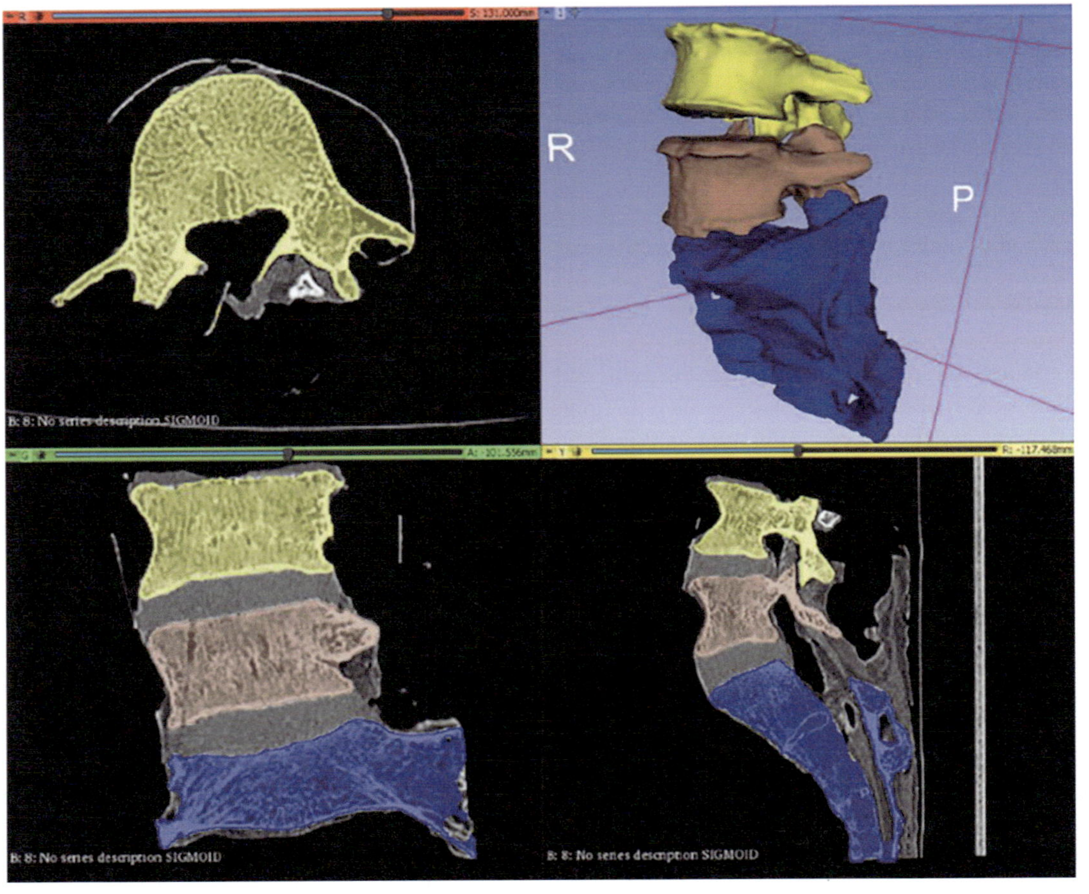

Fig. 2 Example of segmentation process performed on a lumbar spine specimen

2.2 MRI and Soft Tissue Segmentation

Magnetic resonance imaging (MRI) is essential for visualizing soft tissues of the spine, including intervertebral discs, ligaments, and the spinal cord. Volumetric segmentation techniques applied to MRI allow precise delineation of these structures, facilitating deeper understanding of the interactions between intervertebral discs and vertebrae, as well as the surrounding ligaments [20]. With the help of machine learning algorithms and intensity-based segmentation methods [21], MRI segmentation has become more accurate, enabling clinicians to construct 3D models of the spine that include soft tissue components. This is especially useful in assessing the biomechanical properties of intervertebral discs and their degeneration, which is a common issue in older patients or those suffering from spinal disorders. Advances in MRI technology, combined with elastography, have also enabled the measurement of tissue stiffness, which is vital for understanding the mechanical behavior of spinal discs and other soft tissues [22]. This provides clinicians with a noninvasive way to detect early signs of degeneration, offering a more proactive approach to managing spinal health.

2.3 Ultrasound and Real-Time Dynamic Segmentation

Although less commonly used for static spinal reconstructions, ultrasound plays a significant role in the dynamic evaluation of spinal structures. Unlike MRI or CT, which are typically used for static imaging, ultrasound can capture real-time images, making it valuable for studying the dynamic behavior of the spine, such as during motion. Recent developments in ultrasound technology have introduced volumetric segmentation methods that can be applied in real time, allowing for continuous tracking of vertebral and muscular movements. These capabilities are particularly beneficial for evaluating conditions such as dynamic instability or for monitoring the efficacy of treatments in real time [23]. Algorithms designed to segment ultrasound images focus on identifying interfaces between bones and muscles, allowing clinicians to monitor changes in spinal alignment during physical activities [24]. Real-time segmentation can provide insights into how certain postures or movements affect the spine, and can be used to guide rehabilitation exercises for patients recovering from spinal injuries.

3 Material Properties of the Spine Methods for Characterizing Mechanical Properties

Understanding the material properties of the spine, including bones, intervertebral discs, and soft tissues, is essential for assessing mechanical behavior under various stress conditions. These properties are critical for developing accurate biomechanical models and improving therapeutic interventions, including surgical techniques and implant design. Recent advancements in imaging and testing methods have enabled more precise characterization of these properties, leading to better predictive models and clinical outcomes.

3.1 CT Scan and Bone Density

Computed tomography (CT) remains a cornerstone in evaluating the mechanical properties of spinal bones. CT-derived bone mineral density (BMD) is crucial for predicting bone strength and fracture risk, particularly in individuals with osteoporosis. By measuring Hounsfield units, CT scans can provide an estimate of bone mineral density (BMD), which correlates directly with bone strength [25–27]. This capability is particularly important for predicting the mechanical behavior of bones, assessing fracture risk, and identifying weaknesses in patients with osteoporosis. More recent studies have emphasized the use of CT imaging in conjunction with finite element models (FEM) to simulate the biomechanical response of spinal vertebrae under different loading conditions. Incorporating BMD data into FEM models helps to better predict how vertebrae will react to forces such as compression, torsion, and bending, thereby enabling more personalized treatment plans. Incorporating BMD from CT into FEM allows clinicians to better anticipate mechanical failures, such as vertebral fractures, especially in patients with degenerative conditions such as osteoporosis [28]. Integration of data from imaging and modeling has improved the accuracy of spinal surgery planning. CT imaging can also detect age-related changes in bone structure, which are critical for understanding fracture risk and planning preventive interventions.

3.2 Elastography with MRI and Ultrasound

The mechanical properties of soft tissues in the spine, such as intervertebral discs and ligaments, are equally important in maintaining spinal stability. Elastography, performed using MRI or ultrasound, is an emerging technique for noninvasively measuring the stiffness of these tissues [29]. It has proven especially useful for detecting early signs of disc degeneration, which can lead to structural instability. By measuring tissue stiffness through shear wave propagation, elastography enables clinicians to assess the mechanical properties of intervertebral discs and other spinal tissues without invasive procedures [30]. This makes it a valuable tool for early diagnosis and prevention of degenerative disc disease. MRI-based elastography is increasingly being used to assess tissue integrity, predict the progression of disc degeneration, and aid in surgical decision-making [22].

3.3 Development of Transfer Laws Between Imaging and Mechanical Properties

One of the ongoing challenges in spinal biomechanics is the translation of imaging data into mechanical properties that can be directly used in predictive models. Transfer laws bridge this gap by correlating metrics obtained from imaging—such as bone density or tissue stiffness—with mechanical parameters such as elasticity, strength, and failure thresholds [31]. Transfer laws enable the creation of patient-specific finite element models that accurately reflect individual spinal properties. This approach is particularly useful in preoperative planning, allowing for a more customized surgical approach based on the unique biomechanics of each patient [32].

4 Boundary Conditions

Understanding the boundary conditions and in vivo measurements of the spine is essential for accurately predicting spinal behavior under physiological loads. These conditions represent the forces and constraints acting on the spine during normal activities and provide the basis for developing realistic biomechanical models. With recent technological advances, a variety of tools and techniques have been developed to more precisely capture in vivo spinal dynamics, facilitating better diagnosis and treatment of spinal disorders.

4.1 In Vivo Measurements

In vivo measurements are crucial for understanding the mechanical forces and movements applied to the spine under real-life conditions. These measurements allow researchers to observe how the spine responds to various loads and postures, and help clinicians to assess spinal stability and function [33]. The data collected is particularly valuable for diagnosing spinal pathologies such as scoliosis, kyphosis, or degenerative disc disease. Recent advancements have led to the development of more sophisticated in vivo measurement systems, such as time-of-flight (TOF) cameras, motion capture systems, and EOS imaging, which provide more accurate and less invasive ways to measure spinal dynamics [34]. These techniques have allowed for real-time, noninvasive assessments of spinal motion, particularly during dynamic activities such as walking or lifting. These data are essential for developing customized rehabilitation and surgical interventions based on an individual's specific biomechanical profile.

4.2 Scoliometer and Inclinometer: Angular Measurements

Traditional tools such as the scoliometer and inclinometer (Fig. 3) remain useful for measuring the angular deformations of the spine, particularly in screening for conditions such as scoliosis. The scoliometer is a simple, noninvasive tool that measures the lateral curvature of the spine, helping to detect early scoliosis in young patients. The inclinometer, on the other hand, is commonly used to measure the range of motion of the spine in different planes, including flexion, extension, and lateral bending. Although these tools are straightforward, they have been integrated with more advanced technologies to enhance their accuracy and reliability. Digital inclinometers and scoliometers, for instance, now incorporate electronic sensors to provide real-time data, which can be stored and analyzed using computer software [35]. Recent innovations include 3D reconstruction techniques combined with inclinometry to offer more accurate measurements of spinal deformities in patients with scoliosis and other spinal conditions [36].

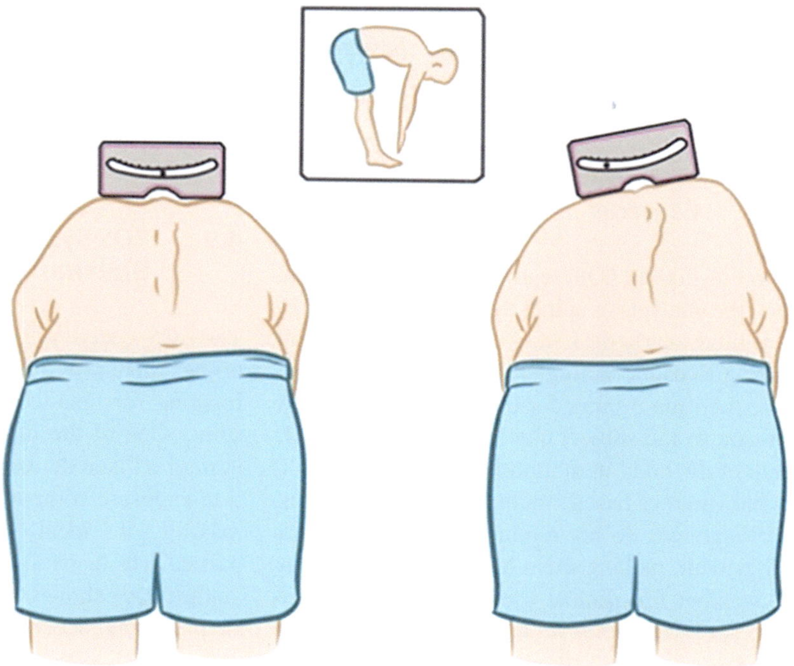

Fig. 3 Angular measurements with an inclinometer

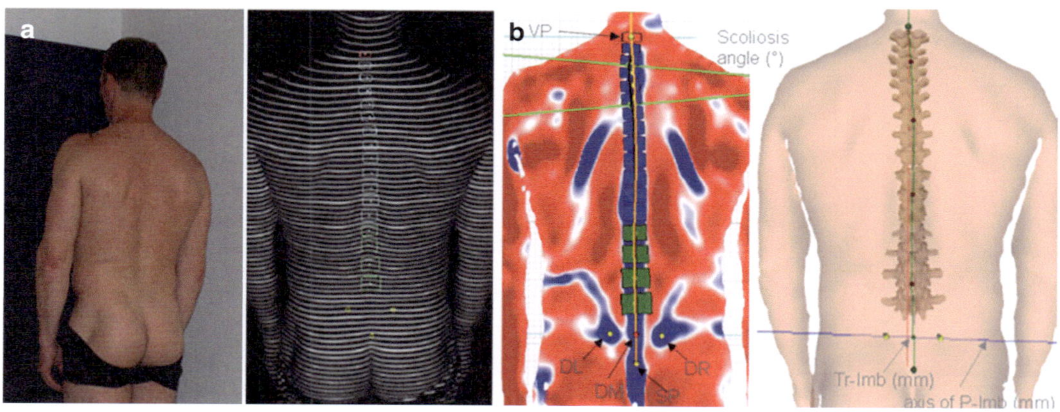

Fig. 4 Raster method (**a**) and 3D reconstruction of the back (**b**) [37]

4.3 Moiré and Raster: Surface Techniques

Moiré optical techniques and raster methods are commonly used for noninvasive surface analysis of the back (Fig. 4) [37]. These techniques help to visualize the topography of the spine and to detect deformities such as scoliosis or kyphosis. The moiré method involves projecting a grid of lines onto the patient's back, and the resulting distortions reveal three-dimensional deformations of the spine [38]. Recent improvements in moiré technology have focused on increasing accuracy and reducing the influence of external factors such as lighting or patient posture. Raster methods, similar to moiré, are now frequently combined with computer algorithms to create high-resolution 3D reconstructions of spinal curvature [39, 40]. Moiré and raster techniques are increasingly used in conjunction with EOS imaging and motion capture systems to provide comprehensive assessments of spinal posture and movement [41].

4.4 Motion Analysis Using TOF Cameras

Time-of-flight (TOF) cameras have revolutionized the analysis of spinal movement by allowing real-time, markerless tracking of body segments during dynamic activities. These cameras measure the time it takes for light to travel from the camera to the subject and back, providing a 3D map of the body in motion (Fig. 5). Unlike traditional marker-based motion capture systems, TOF cameras do not require direct contact with the patient, making them less invasive and more convenient for clinical use [42]. These systems are especially useful for analyzing spinal motion in real time during functional activities such as walking or sitting. Data from TOF cameras is often integrated with finite element models to better understand the forces acting on the spine during different movements.

4.5 EOS System: Low-Dose Biplanar Imaging

The EOS system is a revolutionary imaging technology that provides low-dose, biplanar X-ray imaging for detailed 3D reconstructions of the spine. One of the main advantages of the EOS system is that it delivers significantly lower radiation exposure compared to traditional CT scans, making it ideal for regular monitoring, particularly in pediatric scoliosis cases. Recent studies have shown the benefits of EOS imaging in providing accurate measurements of spinal

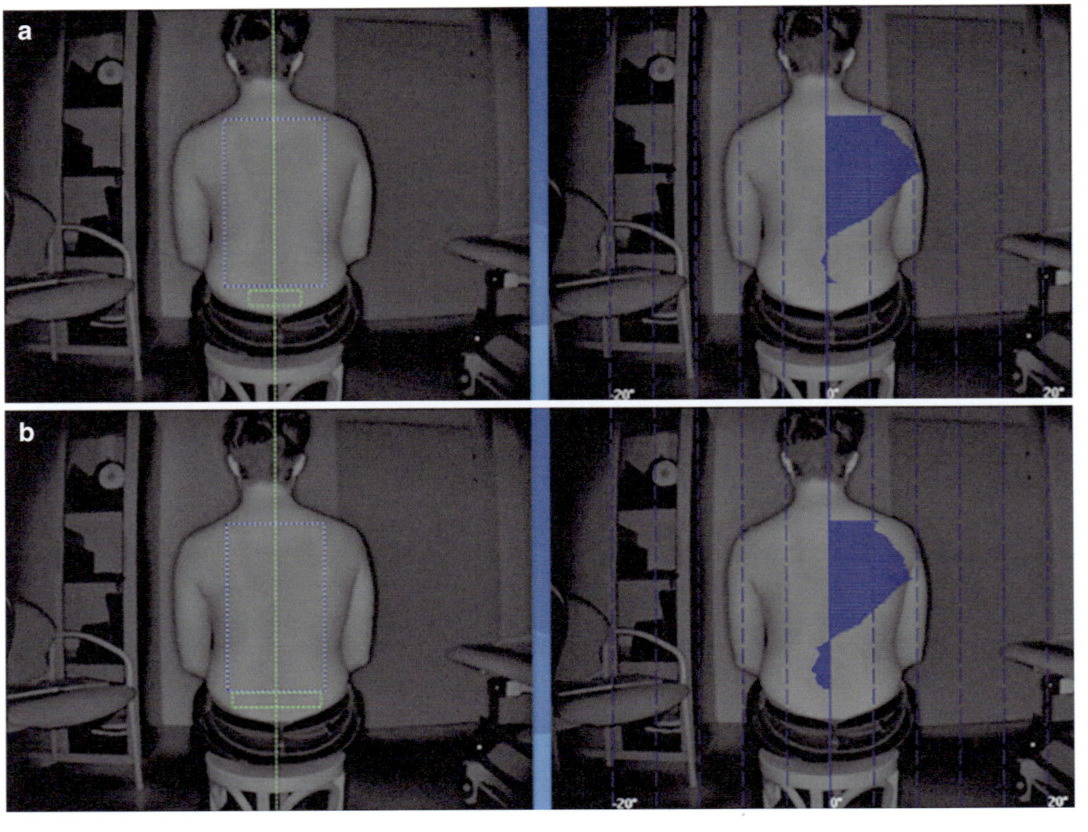

Fig. 5 3D Back analysis and identification of dissymmetry and gibbosity by using TOF cameras

alignment and deformities, as well as its application in tracking the progression of scoliosis or other spinal conditions over time [43, 44]. EOS imaging is increasingly being used in conjunction with other diagnostic tools to provide a more comprehensive analysis of the spine. Its use in assessing sagittal balance and spinal alignment in standing positions makes it indispensable for planning corrective surgeries and evaluating postoperative outcomes.

4.6 Motion Analysis and Quantified Gait Using Optoelectronic Devices

Optoelectronic motion capture systems, such as Vicon or Qualisys, have long been used for analyzing spinal motion during dynamic activities such as walking. These systems use infrared cameras to track the movement of reflective markers placed on the patient's body, enabling highly detailed 3D analysis of spinal and limb motion. This data is invaluable for assessing gait abnormalities caused by spinal pathologies and for planning corrective interventions.

Recent advances in motion capture technology have made it possible to integrate optoelectronic data with finite element models to simulate the forces acting on the spine during dynamic activities. This approach has proven useful for evaluating the effects of different spinal conditions on gait and for optimizing rehabilitation protocols.

5 In Vitro Testing

Anatomical spinal segments are commonly used in in vitro studies to simulate real-life loading conditions. These tests provide critical data on how individual vertebrae and intervertebral discs respond to various forces. Cadaveric testing is often used to simulate real-world activities, such as standing, bending, and lifting, offering insights into spinal load distribution and movement patterns [45, 46].

Until recently, loading systems were designed to apply pure moments along a single physiological axis, limiting their ability to simulate complex, combined movements (Fig. 6). However, recent advancements in the development of opti-

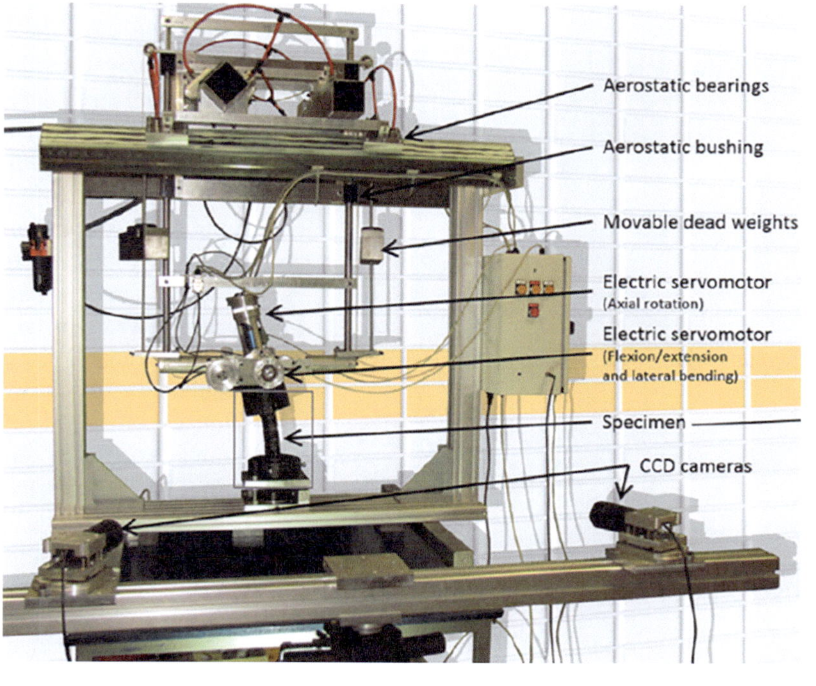

Fig. 6 Spine testing setup to apply pure couple for flexion–extension, lateral flexion, and axial rotation [46]

mized medical devices have underscored the need to focus on intricate, coupled movements. These studies highlight the significance of integrating imposed kinematics with precise measurements of the resulting forces to better replicate the complexities of physiological motion and improve device performance.

Recent innovations have allowed for more realistic simulations using robotic systems that replicate human motion, adding dynamic elements to in vitro tests.

When combined with real cadaveric spinal segments (Fig. 7), these robotic simulations enable researchers to recreate complex loading scenarios that mimic the forces experienced during dynamic activities such as walking, running, or lifting. This helps in understanding how different regions of the spine react under strain, providing essential data for improving surgical procedures and designing spinal implants [47].

In vitro data is vital for improving spinal implants and validating biomechanical models. These data allow for the precise calibration of finite element models, which are increasingly used in spinal surgery planning and implant design. The integration of in vitro data into these models has further enhanced the ability to predict postoperative outcomes, resulting in more personalized and effective treatments for spinal pathologies and also helped to improve medical devices such as spinal implants and surgical tools [48, 49].

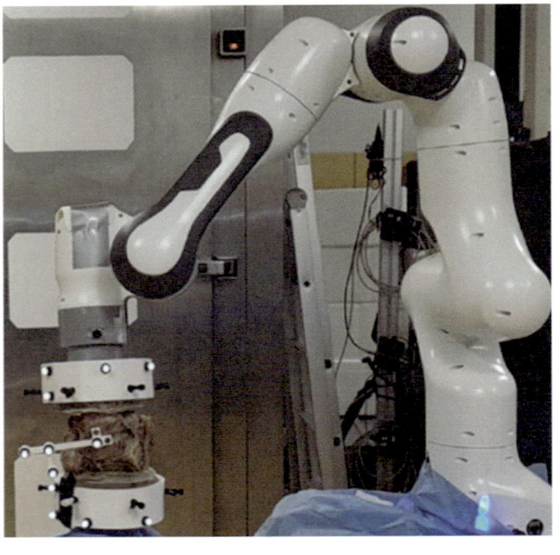

Fig. 7 Spine testing setup using a robotic arm device

The insights gained from in vitro testing are essential for understanding how specific spinal segments react under various loads, leading to the development of safer surgical techniques and more durable spinal implants.

6 Validation of Numerical Models

Numerical models, particularly finite element models (FEM), have become essential tools for simulating spinal biomechanics. However, to ensure their accuracy, these models must be validated against real-world experimental data obtained through in vitro testing. In vitro data on spinal material properties, segmental kinematics, and tissue behavior provides critical reference points for refining these models and ensuring that they accurately represent the mechanical responses of the spine.

Recent studies have focused on improving the accuracy of FEM models by incorporating more detailed in vitro data, such as patient-specific material properties derived from imaging techniques such as CT and MRI.

One of the key advancements has been the integration of real-time mechanical data from in vitro tests into FEM, allowing for dynamic simulations of spinal movement. This has proven particularly valuable in predicting the outcomes of spinal surgeries and evaluating the long-term performance of spinal implants.

These models are also increasingly used to simulate complex loading scenarios that are difficult to replicate in vivo, such as high-impact trauma or extreme spinal deformation. By comparing model predictions with in vitro data, researchers can adjust the parameters of FEM to better predict spinal behavior under a variety of clinical conditions.

6.1 Contribution of Numerical Simulations in Spinal Biomechanics

Numerical simulations, particularly those based on finite element models (FEM), have become indispensable in spinal biomechanics. FEM enables detailed simulations of how the spine responds to different mechanical forces and movements, providing insights that are difficult to obtain in vivo (Fig. 8).

FEM models are used to simulate a wide range of clinical scenarios, such as the effects of spinal fusion, the insertion of implants, or the impact of trauma on the vertebrae. These simulations help clinicians and researchers to predict spinal load distribution, identify potential failure points, and assess the overall mechanical integrity of the spine.

One of the major advancements in FEM is the ability to integrate patient-specific data, such as bone density from CT scans and tissue properties from MRI, into the models. This makes it possible to simulate how individual anatomical variations influence the outcomes of spinal surgeries or other interventions.

Furthermore, FEM simulations can now account for complex loading conditions, including dynamic forces such as those encountered during walking or lifting. This enables a more comprehensive understanding of how the spine behaves under real-life conditions.

6.2 Clinical Applications of FEM Models

FEM models have found widespread application in clinical practice, particularly for preoperative planning and implant design. By simulating various surgical approaches, clinicians can evaluate the biomechanical impact of different interventions, ensuring that the chosen procedure maximizes stability while minimizing risks such as adjacent segment degeneration or implant failure. For example, FEM models are commonly used to simulate the mechanical behavior of the spine following spinal fusion surgery. These simulations help to predict how load distribution will change across the spine and which segments are at risk of post-surgery degeneration [50] (Fig. 9).

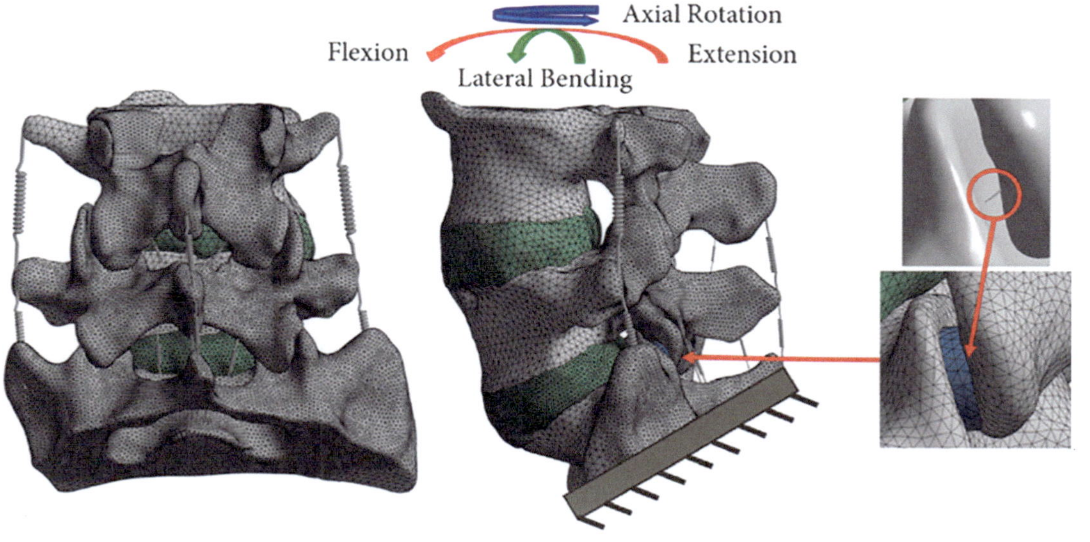

Fig. 8 Finite element model based on a lumbosacral specimen from various loading conditions and with modeling of ligaments and cartilaginous bodies. (Adapted from [50])

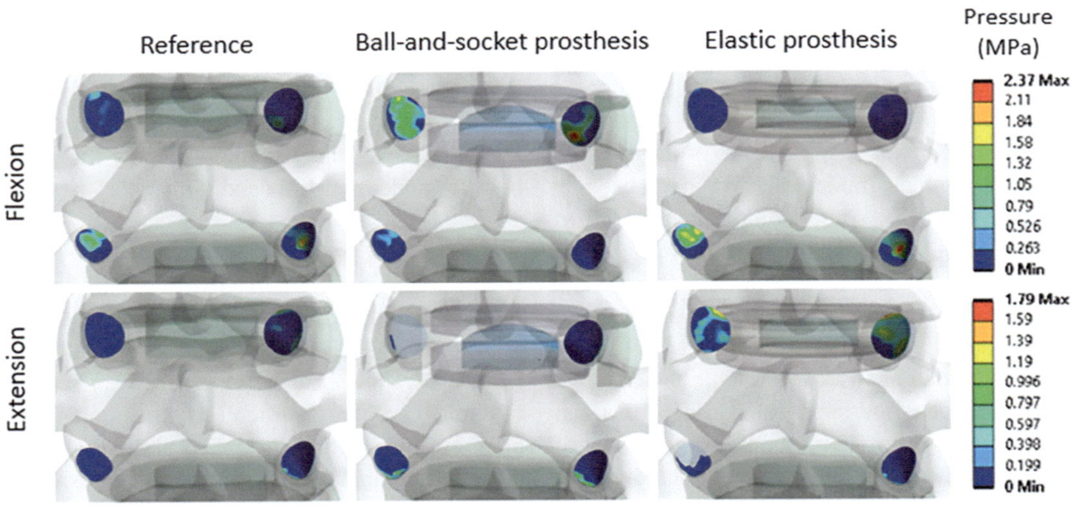

Fig. 9 Example of results provided by a specific FEM model for preoperative planning: prediction of pressure distribution in the facet joints according to the type of prosthesis (adapted from [50])

In addition, FEM is increasingly being used to design and test spinal implants, such as intervertebral cages, pedicle screws, and dynamic stabilization devices. By simulating the interaction between the implant and the surrounding tissues, FEM helps optimize implant design and to enhance durability and reduce failure rates [51, 52].

6.3 Artificial Intelligence and Biomechanical Modeling

Artificial intelligence (AI), particularly machine learning, has significantly transformed spinal biomechanics by enabling the processing and analysis of large datasets. AI algorithms can identify complex patterns within biomechanical data, allowing for more accurate predictions of spinal behavior and improving the personalization of treatment strategies [53].

Machine learning techniques are now being integrated into FEM simulations to refine the prediction of mechanical responses based on individual patient data. By training AI models on large datasets of spinal images and in vitro data, these systems can predict how a patient's spine will respond to specific surgical interventions or rehabilitation protocols [54].

AI has also proven valuable in helping clinicians to manage large datasets from imaging studies and biomechanical tests, streamlining the process of analyzing and interpreting complex information. For example, AI-based segmentation tools can automatically identify anatomical structures in MRI and CT images, reducing the time and effort required to create personalized FEM models.

AI's ability to integrate diverse data sources—from medical imaging to biomechanical tests—makes it a powerful tool for creating comprehensive, patient-specific models of the spine. These models can then be used to optimize treatment planning, predict surgical outcomes, and improve patient safety.

6.4 AI for Managing Missing Data

In spinal biomechanics, obtaining complete datasets for each patient is often challenging due to limitations in imaging techniques or clinical data collection. Artificial intelligence is increasingly being used to address this issue by filling in missing data points based on existing information, ensuring more complete and accurate biomechanical models [55]. Machine learning algorithms can extrapolate missing values from incomplete datasets by analyzing patterns in similar patients or by using transfer learning techniques, which leverage data from other related domains. This is particularly useful in cases where imaging data is only partially available, or when specific biomechanical measurements are missing [56].

These AI-powered methods enable researchers and clinicians to build more robust models, even when faced with incomplete data, ensuring that the predictions are as accurate as possible. This has led to improved outcomes in surgical planning and rehabilitation, as well as more reliable predictions of long-term spinal health.

6.5 Patient-Specific Models and Practical Applications

Patient-specific biomechanical models, created using AI and numerical simulations, have modified how clinicians approach spinal surgery. These models incorporate individual anatomical details, such as bone density, disc stiffness, and ligament elasticity, to simulate how a particular patient's spine will respond to different interventions. Using these models, surgeons can simulate various treatment options, such as spinal fusion or disc replacement, and evaluate their mechanical impact on the spine before performing surgery. This has greatly improved the ability to select the most appropriate intervention for each patient, minimizing the risk of complications and optimizing long-term outcomes. Patient-specific models are also valuable in postoperative care, where they can be used to design customized rehabilitation programs that take into account the specific biomechanical challenges a patient may face during recovery [57]. The integration of numerical simulations, artificial intelligence, and advanced data management techniques has drastically enhanced the field of spinal biomechanics. FEM models, combined with AI-based predictions, provide powerful tools for simulating spinal behavior under various conditions, optimizing surgical interventions, and personalizing treatment plans [58, 59]. These technologies have significantly improved both clinical outcomes and the ability to predict long-term spinal health, paving the way for more effective, patient-specific care.

7 Conclusion and Future Perspectives

The advancements in spinal biomechanics have significantly deepened our understanding of the spine's mechanical behavior, contributing to better diagnosis, treatment planning, and surgical outcomes. This chapter has explored how innovations in imaging, in vitro testing, numerical simulations, and artificial intelligence (AI) have transformed both research and clinical applications.

1. **Advances in Imaging and Modeling**

New imaging techniques, such as EOS and high-resolution MRI, combined with segmentation methods, have improved 3D modeling of spinal structures. These models, when integrated with finite element simulations (FEM), enable personalized treatment planning by predicting the mechanical response of each patient's spine under various conditions.

2. **In Vitro Testing and Validation**

In vitro testing continues to play a crucial role in validating numerical models and refining spinal implants. Recent innovations, such as robotic testing systems, have allowed more accurate reproduction of physiological conditions, leading to improvements in implant design and surgical techniques.

3. **Artificial Intelligence and Personalization**

AI and machine learning are revolutionizing spinal biomechanics by processing large datasets and refining FEM simulations. These tools enhance predictive modeling, automate image segmentation, and allow for more tailored treatment strategies based on individual patient data.

Future Perspectives

The field of spinal biomechanics is poised for continued growth, driven by ongoing technological innovations and an ever-increasing demand for personalized medicine. Several key areas are likely to shape the future of this discipline:

1. *Increased use of AI in decision-support systems*: As AI algorithms become more sophisticated, their integration into clinical workflows will become more seamless. In the near future, AI-powered systems could provide real-time, data-driven recommendations during surgeries, optimizing implant placement or surgical technique based on patient-specific biomechanical data. These systems could also be used to continuously monitor patients after surgery, alerting clinicians to potential complications before they become symptomatic.
2. *Enhanced imaging techniques*: The development of novel imaging technologies, such as high-resolution, dynamic imaging systems, will provide even greater insights into spinal biomechanics. Real-time imaging that captures spinal motion during activities could help identify mechanical deficiencies that contribute to chronic pain or degenerative conditions, leading to earlier interventions and more effective treatments.
3. *Integration of big data and predictive analytics*: As more biomechanical data is collected from in vitro tests, FEM simulations, and clinical studies, there will be increasing opportunities to apply big data analytics to uncover new insights into spinal health. Predictive analytics could be used to identify patterns and risk factors for spinal disorders, leading to more targeted prevention strategies and early interventions.
4. *Development of biomechanically superior implants*: Advances in biomaterials and biomechanics will lead to the creation of next-generation spinal implants that are better at mimicking the natural motion of the spine. Motion-preserving devices, such as artificial discs, will likely see improvements in both durability and functionality, providing long-term solutions for patients with degenerative disc disease.
5. *Personalized regenerative medicine*: As our understanding of spinal biomechanics deepens, there may be opportunities to combine biomechanical models with regenerative medicine approaches, such as stem cell therapy or tissue engineering, to develop personalized treatments that not only stabilize the spine but also promote the regeneration of damaged tissues.

Final Thoughts

In conclusion, spinal biomechanics is undergoing a transformation fueled by advances in technology, AI, and personalized medicine. The integration of these disciplines promises to improve patient outcomes, reduce recovery times, and enhance the precision of spinal surgery. As these tools continue to evolve, the potential for further breakthroughs in spinal health is vast, offering hope for better treatments and improved quality of life for patients with spinal disorders.

Acknowledgments We thank Mr. Jeffrey Arsham, an American translator, for rereading and correction of the original English-language manuscript.

Bibliography

1. Oxland TR. Fundamental biomechanics of the spine—what we have learned in the past 25 years and future directions. J Biomech. 2016;49(6):817–32.
2. Adams MA, Dolan P. Spine biomechanics. J Biomech. 2005;38(10):1972–83.
3. Izzo R, Guarnieri G, Guglielmi G, Muto M. Biomechanics of the spine. Part I: spinal stability. Eur J Radiol. 2013;82(1):118–26.
4. Keller TS, Harrison DE, Colloca CJ, Harrison DD, Janik TJ. Prediction of osteoporotic spinal deformity. Spine. 2003;28(5):455.
5. Christiansen BA, Bouxsein ML. Biomechanics of vertebral fractures and the vertebral fracture Cascade. Curr Osteoporos Rep. 2010;8(4):198–204.
6. Yuan HA, Brown CW, Phillips FM. Osteoporotic spinal deformity: a biomechanical rationale for the clinical consequences and treatment of vertebral body compression fractures. Clin Spine Surg. 2004;17(3):236.

7. Keller TS, Colloca CJ, Harrison DE, Harrison DD, Janik TJ. Influence of spine morphology on intervertebral disc loads and stresses in asymptomatic adults: implications for the ideal spine. Spine J. 2005;5(3):297–309.
8. Adams MA, McNally DS, Dolan P. 'Stress' distributions inside intervertebral discs: the effects of age and degeneration. J Bone Joint Surg. 1996;78-B(6):965–72.
9. Solomonow M, Zhou B-H, Harris M, Lu Y, Baratta RV. The Ligamento-muscular stabilizing system of the spine. Spine. 1998;23(23):2552.
10. Panjabi MM, Oxland TR, Yamamoto I, Crisco JJ. Mechanical behavior of the human lumbar and lumbosacral spine as shown by three-dimensional load-displacement curves. J Bone Joint Surg Am. 1994;76(3):413.
11. Thompson RE, Pearcy MJ, Downing KJW, Manthey BA, Parkinson IH, Fazzalari NL. Disc lesions and the mechanics of the intervertebral joint complex. Spine. 2000;25(23):3026.
12. Desmoulin GT, Pradhan V, Milner TE. Mechanical aspects of intervertebral disc injury and implications on biomechanics. Spine. 2020;45(8):E457.
13. Januszewski J, Vivas AC, Uribe JS. Limitations and complications of minimally invasive spinal surgery in adult deformity. Ann Transl Med. 2018;6(6):109.
14. Ailon T, Smith JS, Shaffrey CI, Lenke LG, Brodke D, Harrop JS, et al. Degenerative spinal deformity. Neurosurgery. 2015;77:S75.
15. Bowden A. Finite element modeling of the spine. In: Spine technology handbook; 2006.
16. Naoum S, Vasiliadis AV, Koutserimpas C, Mylonakis N, Kotsapas M, Katakalos K. Finite element method for the evaluation of the human spine: a literature overview. J Funct Biomater. 2021;12(3):43.
17. Zhao. Biomechanical effects of multi-segment fixation on lumbar spine and sacroiliac joints: a finite element analysis – Zhao – Orthopaedic Surgery – Wiley Online Library.
18. Leventon ME. Statistical models in medical image analysis [Internet] [Thesis]. Massachusetts Institute of Technology. 2000.
19. Strickland CG, Aguiar DE, Nauman EA, Talavage TM. Development of subject-specific geometric spine model through use of automated active contour segmentation and kinematic constraint-limited registration. J Digit Imaging. 2011;24(5):926–42.
20. Haq R, Aras R, Besachio DA, Borgie RC, Audette MA. 3D lumbar spine intervertebral disc segmentation and compression simulation from MRI using shape-aware models. Int J CARS. 2015;10(1):45–54.
21. Kim C, Park S-M, Lee S, Lee D. A deep learning harmonization of multi-vendor MRI for robust intervertebral disc segmentation. IEEE Access. 2024;12:19482.
22. Walter BA, Mageswaran P, Mo X, Boulter DJ, Mashaly H, Nguyen XV, et al. MR elastography–derived stiffness: a biomarker for intervertebral disc degeneration. Radiology. 2017;285(1):167–75.
23. Chan A, Coutts B, Parent E, Lou E. Development and evaluation of CT-to-3D ultrasound image registration algorithm in vertebral phantoms for spine surgery. Ann Biomed Eng. 2021;49(1):310–21.
24. Zhang J, Liu T, Wang Y, Jiang W, Yang K, Jin H, et al. Self-adaptive ultrasound scanning system for imaging human spine. IEEE Trans Ind Electron. 2021;69(1):570–81.
25. Pinto EM, Neves JR, Teixeira A, Frada R, Atilano P, Oliveira F, et al. Efficacy of Hounsfield units measured by lumbar computer tomography on bone density assessment: a systematic review. Spine. 2022;47(9):702–10.
26. Batawil N, Sabiq S. Hounsfield unit for the diagnosis of bone mineral density disease: a proof of concept study. Radiography. 2016;22(2):e93–8.
27. Sapin de Brosses E, Briot K, Kolta S, Skalli W, Roux C, Mitton D. Subject-specific mechanical properties of vertebral cancellous bone assessed using a low-dose X-ray device. IRBM. 2010;31(3):148–53.
28. Allaire BT, Lu D, Johannesdottir F, Kopperdahl D, Keaveny TM, Jarraya M, et al. Prediction of incident vertebral fracture using CT-based finite element analysis. Osteoporos Int. 2019;30(2):323–31.
29. Can TS, Yilmaz BK, Ozdemir S. Multifidus muscle stiffness in single-level unilateral lumbar disc herniation: comparison of two shear-wave elastography methods. Medical Bulletin of Haseki/Haseki Tip Bulteni. 2022.
30. Winn N, Balain B, Ockendon M, Cassar-Pullicino V, Lalam R. Sonographic assessment of human lumbar intervertebral disks: a cadaveric study. J Diagn Med Sonogr. 2021;37(5):427–39.
31. Ghosh N. Semi-automated generation of personalised finite element lumbar spine models: a step towards a pre-surgery planning tool for spinal fusion. Auckland; 2024.
32. Sensale M. Computational models for the preoperative planning of spinal surgeries [Internet] [PhD Thesis]. University of Sheffield. 2021.
33. Abstracts of the International Research Society on Spinal Deformities (IRSSD) Meeting 2018: Utrecht, the Netherlands. 14–16 June 2018. Scoliosis. 2018;13(S1):8, s13013-018-0154-2.
34. Keenan BE. Medical imaging and biomechanical analysis of scoliosis progression in the growing adolescent spine. Queensland University of Technology; 2015.
35. Chang Y-C, Detchev I, Habib AA. Photogrammetric system for 3D reconstruction of a scoliotic torso. In: Proceedings of the ASPRS 2009 annual conference; 2008.
36. Lukovic T, Cukovic S, Lukovic V, Devedzic G, Djordjevic D. Towards a new protocol of scoliosis assessments and monitoring in clinical practice: a pilot study. J Back Musculoskelet Rehabil. 2015;28(4):721–30.
37. Schroeder J, Reer R, Braumann KM. Video raster stereography back shape reconstruction: a reliabil-

ity study for sagittal, frontal, and transversal plane parameters. Eur Spine J. 2015;24(2):262–9.
38. Shitoev ID, Muravev SV, Karakulova YV, Pecherskiy VI, Nikitin VN, Kloyan GZ. Evolution of optical diagnosis of spinal deformity. In: Methods and future development (literature review); 2024.
39. Glinkowski W, Michonski J, Sitnik R, Witkowski M. 3D diagnostic system for anatomical structures detection based on a parameterized method of body surface analysis. In: Piętka E, Kawa J, editors. Information technologies in biomedicine. Berlin/Heidelberg: Springer; 2010.
40. Hocquelet A, Cornelis F, Jirot A, Castaings L, de Sèze M, Hauger O. Patient-specific 3D models created by 3D imaging system or bi-planar imaging coupled with Moiré–Fringe projections: a comparative study of accuracy and reliability on spinal curvatures and vertebral rotation data. Eur Spine J. 2016;25(10):3154–61.
41. Nikkhoo M, Cheng C-H, Wang J-L, Niu C-C, Parnianpour M, Khalaf K. The biomechanical response of the lower cervical spine post laminectomy: geometrically-parametric patient-specific finite element analyses. J Med Biol Eng. 2021;41(1):59–70.
42. Silvernagel MP, Ling AS. Nuyujukian P, for the brain interfacing laboratory. A markerless platform for ambulatory systems neuroscience. Sci Robot. 2021;6(58):eabj7045.
43. Melhem E, Assi A, El Rachkidi R, Ghanem I. EOS ® biplanar X-ray imaging: concept, developments, benefits, and limitations. J Child Orthop. 2016;10(1):1–14.
44. Glaser DA, Doan J, Newton PO. Comparison of 3-dimensional spinal reconstruction accuracy: biplanar radiographs with EOS versus computed tomography. Spine. 2012;37(16):1391–7.
45. Busscher I, van Dieen JH, Kingma I, van der Veen AJ, Verkerke GJ, Veldhuizen AG. Biomechanical characteristics of different regions of the human spine an *in vitro* study on multilevel spinal segments. Spine. 2009;34(26):2858–64.
46. Germaneau A, Vendeuvre T, Saget M, Doumalin P, Dupré JC, Brémand F, et al. A novel approach for biomechanical spine analysis: mechanical response of vertebral bone augmentation by kyphoplasty to stabilise thoracolumbar burst fractures. J Mech Behav Biomed Mater. 2016;59:291–303.
47. Wang W, Kong C, Pan F, Wang W, Wu X, Pei B, et al. Influence of sagittal Lumbopelvic morphotypes on the range of motion of human lumbar spine: an in vitro cadaveric study. Bioengineering. 2022;9(5):224.
48. Leszczynski A, Meyer F, Charles Y-P, Deck C, Willinger R. Development of a flexible instrumented lumbar spine finite element model and comparison with in-vitro experiments. Comput Methods Biomech Biomed Engin. 2022;25(2):221–37.
49. Lafage V, Gangnet N, Sénégas J, Lavaste F, Skalli W. New interspinous implant evaluation using an in vitro biomechanical study combined with a finite-element analysis. Spine. 2007;32(16):1706–13.
50. Zot F, Ben-Brahim E, Severyns M, Ledoux Y, Mesnard M, Caillé L, et al. Study of mechanical effects of lumbar disc arthroplasty on facet joints at the index level/adjacent levels by using a validated finite element analysis. Front Bioeng Biotechnol. 2023;11:1287197.
51. Wu Y, Ma J, Dai J, Wang Y, Bai H, Lu B, et al. Design and biomechanical evaluation of a bidirectional expandable cage for oblique lateral Interbody fusion. World Neurosurg. 2023;180:e644–52.
52. Bereczki F, Turbucz M, Pokorni AJ, Hajnal B, Ronai M, Klemencsics I, et al. The effect of polymethylmethacrylate augmentation on the primary stability of stand-alone implant construct versus posterior stabilization in oblique lumbar interbody fusion with osteoporotic bone quality— a finite element study. Spine J. 2024;24(7):1323–33.
53. Phellan Aro R, Hachem B, Clin J, Mac-Thiong J-M, Duong L. Real-time prediction of postoperative spinal shape with machine learning models trained on finite element biomechanical simulations. Int J CARS. 2024;19:1983.
54. Phellan R, Hachem B, Clin J, Mac-Thiong J, Duong L. Real-time biomechanics using the finite element method and machine learning: review and perspective. Medical Physics. 2021;48(1):7–18.
55. Cui Y, Zhu J, Duan Z, Liao Z, Wang S, Liu W. Artificial intelligence in spinal imaging: current status and future directions. Int J Environ Res Public Health. 2022;19(18):11708.
56. Siemionow KB, Forsthoefel CW, Foy MP, Gawel D, Luciano CJ. Autonomous lumbar spine pedicle screw planning using machine learning: a validation study. J Craniovertebr Junction Spine. 2021;12(3):223–7.
57. Eremina GM, Smolin AY. Effect of patient-specific factors on regeneration in lumbar spine at healthy disc and total disc replacement. Computer simulation. Comput Methods Prog Biomed. 2024;250:108172.
58. D'Andrea CR, Samdani AF, Balasubramanian S. Patient-specific finite element modeling of scoliotic curve progression using region-specific stress-modulated vertebral growth. Spine Deform. 2023;11(3):525–34.
59. Nikkhoo M, Khoz Z, Cheng C-H, Niu C-C, El-Rich M, Khalaf K. Development of a novel geometrically-parametric patient-specific finite element model to investigate the effects of the lumbar lordosis angle on fusion surgery. J Biomech. 2020;102:109722.

Biology of Spinal Fusion

Cédric Y. Barrey, Alexis Morgado, Wassim Baasssiri, and Théo Broussolle

1 Part 1: Fundamentals and Terminology

The bone is a dense material, one of the most resistant of the human body. It is made of water, cells, organic matter (mainly collagen), and minerals (sodium, calcium, phosphorus, magnesium, etc.). Bone cells include osteoprogenitors, osteoblasts, osteocytes, and osteoclasts. Macroscopically, the bone can be divided into cortical bone, organized in osteons and lamellae, and spongious bone, also called "trabecular," composed of a spans system and containing the bone marrow (Fig. 1).

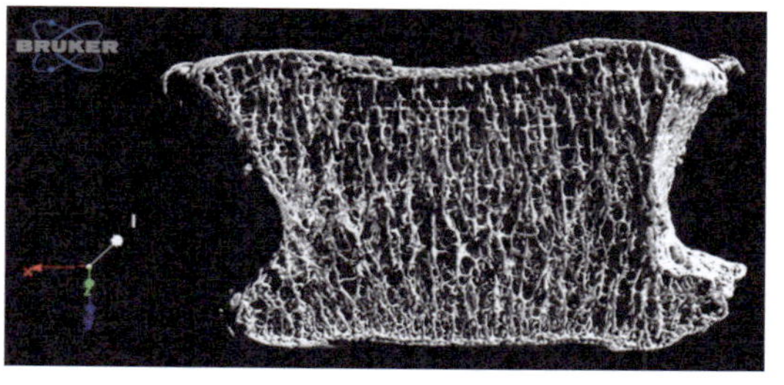

Fig. 1 Three-dimensional reconstruction of lumbar vertebra demonstrating the cortical, subchondral and cancellous bone. (Courtesy of H. Follet, Mateis acquisition, Lyon, with permission)

Cortical bone offers greater mechanical resistance compared to cancellous bone, but it is less effective from a graft material perspective. Cancellous bone has superior osteogenic properties. Indeed, cancellous bone contains larger number of viable cells in the marrow and offers via its trabecular structure a perfect scaffold for vascular ingrowth and exposure to inductive cytokines (Figs. 2 and 3).

Functions of bone are multiple [1]: supporting the weight of the body, permitting the movements of the limbs and the different segments of the trunk and product some blood stem cells via the bone marrow hematopoiesis process. It may also serve as a protection for internal organs such as brain, spinal cord, lungs, and heart. Finally, it constitutes a massive reserve of minerals such as phosphate or calcium.

C. Y. Barrey (✉)
Department of Spine and Spinal Cord Surgery, Hôpital P. Wertheimer, GHE, Hospices Civils de Lyon (HCL), and University Claude Bernard of Lyon 1, Lyon, France
e-mail: cedric.barrey@chu-lyon.fr

A. Morgado · W. Baasssiri · T. Broussolle
Department of Spine and Spinal Cord Surgery, Hôpital P. Wertheimer, GHE, Hospices Civils de Lyon (HCL), Bron-Lyon, France

Université Claude Bernard Lyon 1, Villeurbanne, France
e-mail: alexis.morgado@chu-lyon.fr; wassim.baassiri@chu-lyon.fr; theo.broussolle@chu-lyon.fr

C. Y. Barrey (ed.), *Spine Surgery*, SFCR Experts Series 1,
https://doi.org/10.1007/978-3-031-85446-0_5

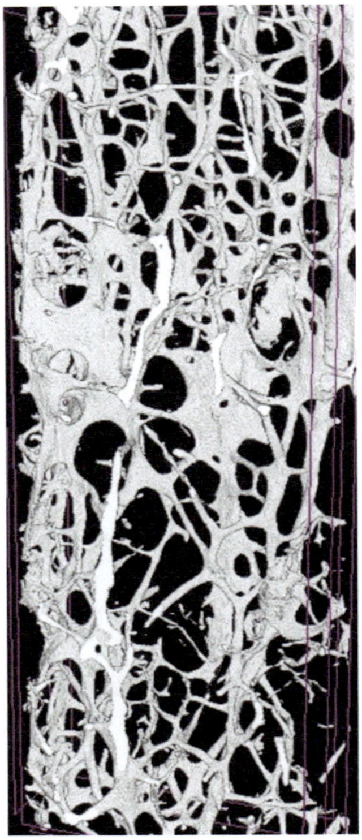

Fig. 2 Three-dimensional reconstruction of trabecular structure. (Courtesy of H. Follet, Mateis acquisition, Lyon, with permission). Although cancellous bone is less resistant compared to cortical, its trabecular structure is very favorable to vascular ingrowth, and to fluids and proteins circulation

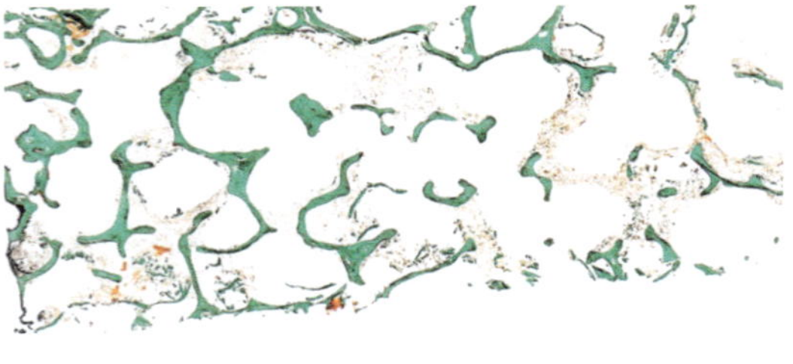

Fig. 3 Photomicrograph showing trabecular bone with Goldner coloration originating from L2 vertebra in a 79-year-old male. The mineralized (green) and osteoid (orange) matrix are well-individualized. (Courtesy from H. Follet, INSERM, Lyon, with permission)

Vertebrae belong to load-bearing bones such as tibias, femurs, pelvis, and so on, as well as their mechanical role is in the foreground. They are exposed not only to gravity but also to muscles action. Cortico-trabecular structure of vertebrae is unique and represent their most important physiological feature. Mechanical properties of cortical and cancellous bone have been extensively reported in the literature with significant variability subject-to-subject (**see** Table 1).

1.1 Osteoconductivity

Osteoconductivity refers to the ability of a geometrical structure to promote new bone formation by permitting adhesion, migration, and proliferation of bone cells, as well as formation of extracellular matrix on its surface and pores [1, 2]. It represents a passive process mainly based on physical and mechanical properties. Chemical nature of the physical structure and geometry, in particular the size and density of its porosity, may have an impact on his osteoconductivity capacity.

1.2 Scaffold

In regenerative medicine, a scaffold consists of a geometrical structure capable of supporting tissue development [1, 3]. In the orthopedical field, by permitting attachment, proliferation, and migration of bone cells, as well as fluid flow and diffusion, a scaffold allows for the formation of new bone. Indeed, porous scaffold creates a favorable environment for the proliferation of bone cells and for the circulation of fluids, oxygen, and nutriments.

Table 1 Comparison of mechanical properties for cortical versus cancellous bone [1]

Mechanical property	Cortical bone	Cancellous bone
Compressive strength (MPa)	150–200	2–10
Tensile resistance (MPa)	50–150	10–100
Young's modulus	15–40	0.02–0.5
Elastic modulus	5–20	10

1.3 Porosity

Porosity refers to the proportion of voids/cavities within the material over the total volume of the structure [1–4]. Porosity permits the circulation of bone cells (including osteoblasts and osteoclasts) and/or fluids through the structure according to the pores size. Macroporosity corresponds to pores size >100 μm and < 400 μm, allowing the circulation of bone cells when microporosity corresponds to pores size <10 μm, permitting the circulation of fluids and proteins [5]. It has been suggested that the optimal ratio of porous volume for bone ingrowth was around 75–80% [5]. In addition, structure and geometry of the channels similar to the native bone appeared to be most successful to promote new bone formation. Compared to surface porosity, i.e., when the pores are present only on surface area, interconnective porosity, i.e., when the pores exist throughout the entire structure, appeared to be less resistant and seemed to degrade more rapidly. Porosity may be provided by the existence of pores within the material (i.e., synthetic ceramics) or by the inter-granules' spaces (i.e., bioactive glass). Inadequate porosity will affect the ingrowing bone and will delay the normal rate of bone healing and remodeling process.

1.4 Osteoinductivity

Osteoinductivity represents an active molecular process referring to the ability to induce new bone formation by recruiting and allowing for differentiation of bone cells, i.e., differentiation of osteoprogenitors and stem cells into osteoblastic lineage. A biomaterial that is osteoinductive contains cytokines capable of inducing differentiation of osteoprogenitor stem cells or osteogenic cells. Osteoinductive potential has been reported in demineralized bone matrix (DBM) and various morphogenetic proteins (BMP, TGF-β, EGF, etc.) [6].

1.5 Osteostimulation

Osteostimulation refers to the capability to promote bone growth and bone remodeling [7].

1.6 Osteogenesis

Osteogenesis refers to the ability of living bone cells, i.e., osteoblasts coming from the living bone tissue, to generate new bone. It therefore represents a cellular process. A biomaterial that is osteogenic contains viable cells (mature osteoblasts and/or osteogenic precursor cells) capable of directly forming new bone.

1.7 Osteointegration

Osteointegration is the property of a material to develop and establish a solid, direct, and durable bond with the surrounding bone tissue without the presence of intervening fibrous tissue [8]. Even if osteointegration was originally introduced to describe a biologic fixation of the titanium dental implants, it is now largely accepted to describe the attachment of other biomaterials used for dental and orthopedic applications as well [8, 9].

1.8 Biocompatibility

Biocompatibility implies that a material can be implanted in close contact with a living biological tissue without generating any undesirable local or systemic negative effect but producing the most appropriate response from the host tissue [8–10]. A highly biocompatible material limits the inflammation response from the host and its adverse effects.

2 Part 2: Bone Remodeling and Bone Healing

The bone is a living tissue with the ability for self-repair. In fact, the bone is continuously being produced as a consequence of the balance between osteoblasts activity responsible for new bone formation and osteoclasts action in charge of bony resorption. This permanent production–resorption process is called "bone remodeling" [1–12].

Bone healing, after fracture, osteotomy, or arthrodesis, is the result of sequential events that

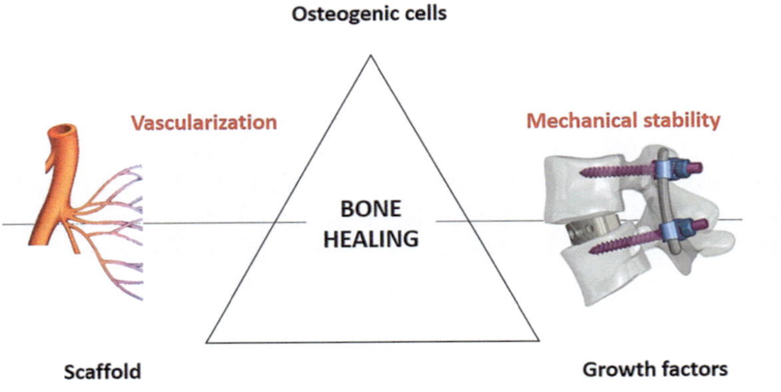

Fig. 4 The diamond concept, introduced in 2007 by Giannoudis et al. [15, 16], supporting the multidimensional process for bone healing

take place successively consisting of recruitment and proliferation of osteoprogenitor cells, coming from surrounding tissues, followed by osteoblastic differentiation, matrix formation, and finally mineralization [13–14]. It is important to note that osteogenic precursor cells participate from the beginning during the early phases of the healing process [13–14].

Bone healing therefore represents a complex process requiring different elements regrouping under the diamond concept [15–16] (Fig. 4):

- Cells specialized for osteogenesis.
- Scaffold with osteoconductive properties.
- Growth factors inducing osteostimulation and signals for osteoinductivity.
- Adequate environment in terms of local vascularization and mechanical stability.

What is important to understand from the diamond concept is that in parallel to biological factors, the mechanical support is highly influencing the capacity for bone healing. As a consequence, at the end of the procedure, the spine surgeon must leave the spine in the optimal mechanical conditions to promote bony consolidation.

Biomechanically, according to Wolff's laws [17], bone formation is conditioned by stresses under which it is loaded. Indeed, in 1892, Julius Wolff reported that mechanical loads may influence bone architecture in living persons [13, 14, 17]. Absence of mechanical stresses will result in bony resorption, whereas excessive stresses will induce osteonecrosis. Wolff's law suggests that a certain amount of loads is therefore desirable to promote bone remodeling and enhance spinal fusion. Otherwise, supporting the concept, it has been shown that, new lamellar bone, during bone healing after fracture or arthrodesis, will develop parallel to the largest, compressive or tension, local loads [5, 13, 14].

Optimal biomechanical environment with adequate control of 3D motion is thus crucial to promote the fusion. On one side, instability has shown to be not compatible with bony healing, compromising the formation of the bone callus. On the other side, excessive rigidity with complete unload of the bone graft is not desirable and may result in graft resorption. In addition, if bone substitutes are utilized and implanted, mechanical properties of these materials should be as close as possible to the native bone, i.e., mechanical compatibility, in order to limit the risk of bone resorption, osteopenia, and/or biomaterial impaction.

During spine fusion surgery, the ultimate objective is to obtain permanent bony bridges between two adjacent vertebras (in order to control pain and/or spinal instability). In this perspective, the surgeon initially stabilizes the spinal segment using hardware ("primary stability" given from the osteosynthesis) and achieve bone grafting in the surgical site in order to get to term permanent and definitive spinal fusion. The bone graft will consolidate progressively following the surgery and will completely fuse at the end within a few months. During this process, also called "creeping substitution," there is the gradual replacement of the dead bone (i.e., morselized bone graft pieces), progressively resorbed by the osteoclasts, by a new living bone, produced by the osteoblasts [1] (Fig. 5).

Prior to the implantation of any graft materials, the surgeon must absolutely prepare and develop the ideal biological environment for bone healing [18]. Indeed, the graft site is where molecular and physiological processes will evolve, facilitating a rapid and successful osteogenesis and leading to bone continuity and bone consolidation according to the concept of optimal "biological chamber" [15, 16, 18].

Different factors may therefore affect bone healing [5, 7, 19]:

- *Local biological factors*: vascularization, preparation of graft bed, local pathological process (tumor/infection/radiation).
- *Local mechanical factors*: biomechanical stability, distribution of loads.
- *Systemic factors*: smoking, nutrition, drugs, inflammatory disease, osteoporosis.

In the case of bone healing failure, instead of new bone formation, interposing fibrous tissue will develop at fusion site, leading to chronic pseudarthrosis (Fig. 6).

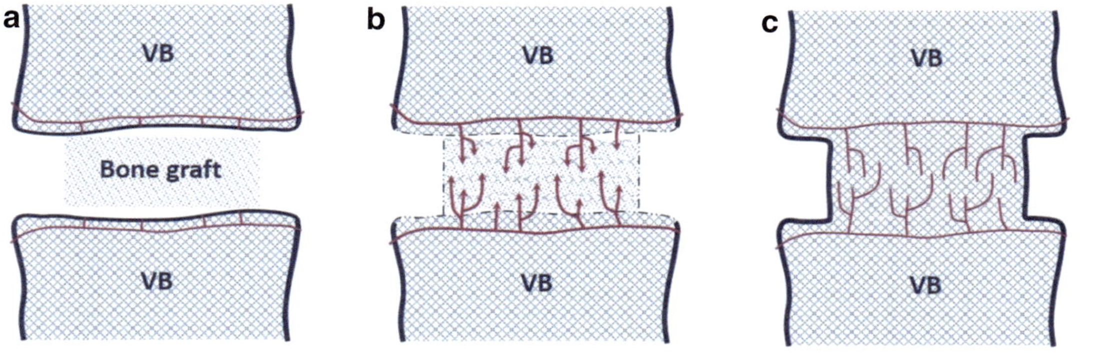

Fig. 5 Process of bone graft consolidation and remodeling from A to C. At the end of the process, the graft is completely remodeled with total continuity of peripheric cortical and central cancellous bone from one vertebra to another. VB, vertebral body

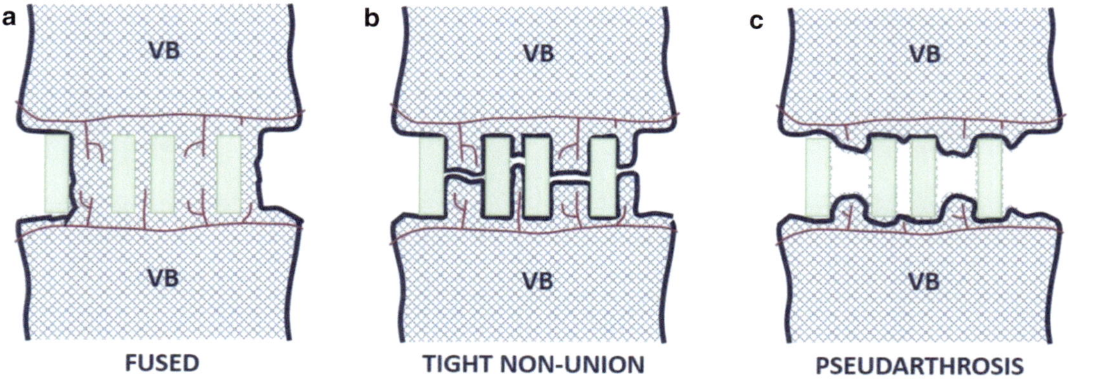

Fig. 6 Graft inserted inside interbody cages (PLIF/TLIF cages) may result in fusion, full bony bridges, and remodeling (**a**), tight nonunion with only partial growth of the bone inside the implants and interposition of a fibrocartilaginous gap zone (**b**), or pseudarthrosis characterized by the resorption of the graft, absence of any bony continuity between the two adjacent vertebras but the presence of fibrous tissue filling the fusion site rather than new bone (**c**)

3 Part 3: Graft Materials

During spinal fusion, bone grafting is performed quasi-systematically and rely on different graft materials [1–4, 6, 12, 20] (see Table 2). The ultimate objective is the graft material being progressively replaced by the own-bone of the patient itself. These graft materials belong to biomaterials, i.e., materials suitable and compatible to be integrated into living tissue. Biomaterial(s) consist of substance(s) that, by interacting with components of living systems, may promote the natural course of healing process [21]. Once implanted in the surgical site, these bone graft materials will progressively get resorbed, more or less matching the rate at which new bone is formed. They will be replaced by own host bone through a biological process called "creeping substitution."

The different material for bone grafting will be presented in details and discuss in the chapter "Bones Substitutes" by T. Broussolle and C. Barrey. Until now, there is no one perfect and ideal bone substitute. Each present with their own advantages and limitations seeing the great variations in term of composition, mechanical resistance, and biological properties [12, 20, 22]. The bone substitute has to be chosen according to many different criteria including the type of the surgery, the surgical site, the expected role for the graft, the patient's characteristics, and the surgeon's preference.

We therefore summarize below only briefly the different options for bone grafting during spinal fusion.

Autologous Graft It is considered as the gold standard compared to all other graft materials [1–5, 12, 20, 22]. Autologous bone can be harvested from the surgical site (facets, lamina, spinous process) or from another site (iliac crest). The utilization of local bone from the posterior elements during posterior spine fusion surgery is the rules (Fig. 7). One must be informed that the

Table 2 The different biomaterials for bone grafting [1–4, 6, 12, 20]

Biomaterial	Autograft	Allograft		Synthetic bone substitute	
Subcategory	Local bone/iliac crest	DBM	Bone bank	Ca-P ceramics	Bioactive glass
Characteristic	Bone originating from the patient	Demineralized bone matrix containing growth factors	Mineral structure of the bone originating from a human (living donor or cadaver)	Variable proportion of HA and TCP	Composed of minerals naturally present in the human body

DBM demineralized bone matrix; *HA* hydroxyapatite; *TCP* tricalcium phosphate

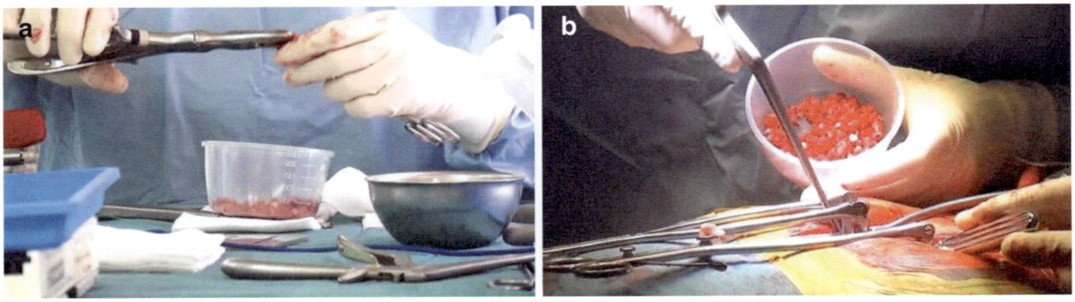

Fig. 7 In spine surgery, autologous graft come typically from the surgical site being harvested from the posterior vertebral elements (lamina/facets). This bone needs then to be meticulously cleaned in order to remove all the surrounding soft tissue (**a**). At the end of the procedure, the cleaned bone is replaced on the surgical site against the decorticated elements after adequate preparation of the "graft bed" (**b**). It has been reported that spine surgery became, since the 1990s, the first reason for autologous bone grafting [5]

bone harvested from the local host must be meticulously cleaned by removing all the soft tissues attached on its surface in order to promote bony fusion. During anterior surgery, local bone is typically not available even if the local osteophytes coming from the endplates may be resected and used to fill the cage. Due to its high osteogenic potential, fresh autologous graft is considered as the best graft material. It combines the three fundamental biological properties that are needed to promote bone formation: osteogenic, osteoinductive, and osteoconductive. In addition, it gets the advantage of being nonpathogenic and nonimmunogenic. Their drawback is limited supply and the potential for donor-site morbidity. In addition, the bone quality declines with age and patient comorbidities such as smoking, making the autograft less efficient in these populations.

Allograft It corresponds to human bone but originates from another human person (living donor or cadaver), provided by bone banks [1–5]. The preparation and fabric process result in destruction of cells and most of bone growth factors. Allograft is therefore highly osteoconductive, partially osteoinductive but not osteogenic (do not contain viable cells). Preservation and conditioning of femoral heads during hip prosthesis surgery represent the main source for allograft in spine fusion surgery. Compared to autografts, it has been reported that allografts were associated with a lower rate of fusion success in spinal procedures for both interbody and posterolateral arthrodesis [22]. The advantages of allografts are their relative abundance, avoidance of donor-site related complications, and availability of various shapes and sizes that can be adapted to the utilization (Fig. 8).

Demineralized Bone Matrix (DBM) Initially discovered by Marshall Urist in 1965 [23], DBM corresponds to an allograft bone that has had the inorganic mineral removed from cortical bone leaving after all only the organic "collagen" matrix, which contains the osteoinductive factors and type 1 collagen. DBM became available in clinical use in 1991. The removal of the bone mineral scaffold exposes more biologically active bone morphogenetic proteins making this biomaterial osteoinductive, favoring the differentiation of osteoprogenitors cells into osteoblasts, but with limited osteoconductivity and reduced mechanical properties [20, 22, 24]. In clinical studies, DBM demonstrated promising results as a bone graft extender. For instance, through a prospective multicenter controlled study, Cammisa et al. reported similar fusion rates in posterolateral fusion comparing DBM + autograft (52%) versus autologous graft alone (54%) [25].

Xenograft It corresponds to nonhuman bone, typically coming from bovine animals. Its utilization is limited regarding the risk for virus transmission, even if probably minimal.

Bone substitutes: A bone substitute is a biomaterial that aims to replace the autologous bone graft with the ultimate objective to reach similar rates of fusion. Historically, the first substance utilized to fill bony defects in patients was reported by a Parisian plasterer, Dresmann, in 1892 [26]. He observed some evidence of bone ingrowth in close contact to this calcium sulfate-based substance. Calcium phosphate ceramics represent nowadays one of the most used bone substitutes in clinical practice (see below). Although the use of collagen alone has been unsuccessful to promote spinal fusion, it may contribute efficiently in forming new bone as a carrier for growth factors and ceramics [1–4, 6, 12]. Among synthetic bone substitutes, bioactive glass, which osteostimulative property, was discovered initially in the 1960–1970s [27], represents an interesting alternative option (Fig. 9). Barrey et al., using bioactive glass as bone extender, reported promising results in adult cervical and thoracolumbar posterior spinal surgery [28].

Crystallinity It refers to the geometrical structure of a biomaterial more or less ordered and geometrically organized [1]. Crystallinity is associated with mechanical resistance, delayed degradability, and osteoconductive properties.

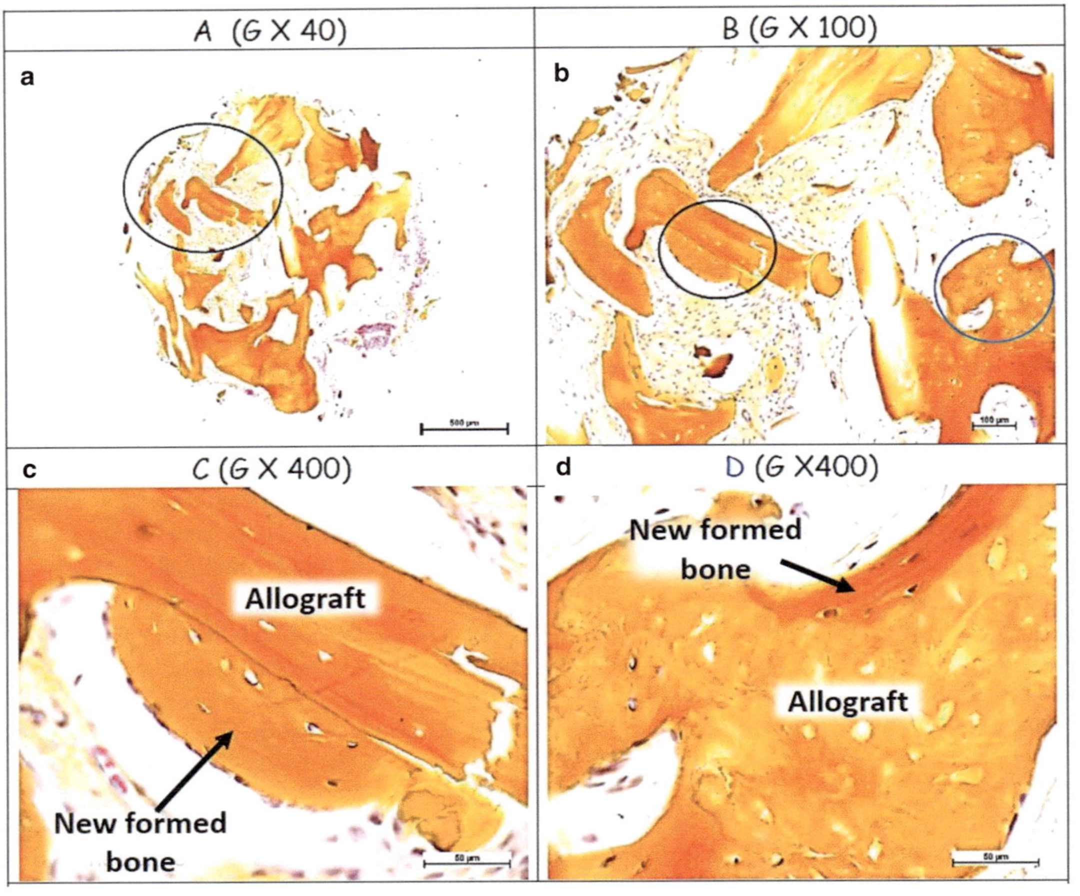

Fig. 8 Micro-granule (Ø 800 μm) of human trabecular bone (**a**) at 5 months after dental implantation (histological sample obtained from bone coring and drilling). On magnification images ×100 (**b**) and ×400 (**c** and **d**), new bone formation with the presence of osteocytes may be visualized in close contact to human allograft. Hematoxylin and Eosin Safran coloration. (From OST™ Development, Saint-Beauzire, France, with permission)

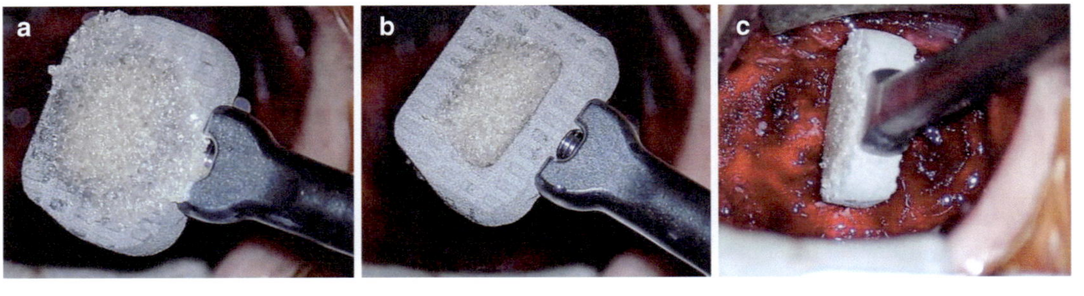

Fig. 9 Bone substitutes (hereby putty of bioactive glass) are frequently used during cervical fusion surgery to fill the interbody cage. View of the superior (**a**) and inferior (**b**) surface of the carbon titanium-coated cervical cage prior cage insertion (**c**) during ACDF procedure

Growth Factors They include "BMP" for bone morphogenic protein, which activity was first discovered by Urist in the 1960s [23]. BMPs are multifunctional growth factors belonging to the transforming growth factor beta (TGF-beta) superfamily, playing a positive role for bone formation [12, 29]. These specific cytokines have demonstrated to be active in stimulating bone cells activities including proliferation and differentiation. To date, around 20 BMP family members have been identified and characterized [12, 29]. Recent progresses in pharmacological technologies and recombinant techniques permit to isolate BMP in adequate quantities for clinical use, contrary to demineralization method in which >10 kg of animal cortical bone was necessary to extract a few μg of osteoinductive factors. Through these modern technological processes, recombinant human BMPs (rh-BMPs) may be produced in unlimited quantities and standard concentrations. Preclinical and clinical studies have shown that BMP-2 (or rh-BMP2), i.e., dibotermin alfa, can be utilized in various therapeutic orthopedical surgeries such as bone defects, nonunion fractures, and spinal fusion [29–32]. One limitation is that BMPs are soluble factors with the risk of migration away from the fusion site and the need to combine them with a carrier.

Bone Marrow Aspirate (BMA) BMA represents an attractive option to obtain osteoprogenitor cells and growth factors. In order to potentialize the advantages of graft material and to compensate the absence of osteoconductivity and mechanical support, BMA is typically combined with an appropriate carrier. In addition, to be effective, and because of low progenitor cells concentration, various techniques, based on centrifugation, have been developed in order to concentrate the BMA.

Graft Extender and Graft Enhancer Bone graft materials can be classified on the whole under three major groups: bone graft extenders, bone graft enhancers, and bone graft substitutes [5, 20, 33]. As suggested by the term, an extender is used to add to available autograft in order to expand both volume and efficacy of the limited autograft. The ultimate objective using graft extender/autograft combination is to reach equivalent rates of fusion compared to autograft alone. On the contrary, a bone graft enhancer, combined with autograft, aims to improve the successful rate of fusion in comparison to that observed with autograft alone. Finally, bone substitutes may be used alone, thus replacing autologous bone graft and leading to similar rates of fusion.

Calcium-phosphate (Ca-P) ceramics represent one of the most frequent biomaterials used for bone healing in clinical practice [20, 34]. The term "ceramics" derives from the ancient Greek "Keramos," which means pottery. These Ca-P ceramics are made of nonorganic matter and produced according to the sintering process (heating at >800 °C temperature but avoiding liquefaction), leading to a crystalline structure. They present different hardness and porosity and are mainly osteoconductive, serving as a scaffold structure for new bone formation. Their compressive resistance is very variable, approximately 20–200% of the resistance of the cortical bone, making them more or less vulnerable to compressive loads. Ca-P ceramics are typically "biphasics" [34–36] containing two basic components:

- Hydroxyapatite (HA).
- Tricalcium phosphate (TCP).

Both contains calcium and phosphate with a Ca/P ratio a little bit higher for HA (Ca/P = 1.67 for HA vs. Ca/P = 1.5 for TCP). Increase of Ca/P ratio is associated with more mechanical resistance and slower resorption. The proportion (respective percentage) of these two components have an impact of chemical and mechanical properties of the biomaterial [34–36]. Compared to HA, TCP is more resistant but more rapidly degraded by osteoclast (12–18 months vs. >2 years for HA). For instance, in the animal model study by Eggi et al. [36], histological analysis found that up to 85.4% of the originally implanted TCP was degraded after 6 months, whereas the volume reduction of HA was only 5.4% after the same period. Absence and/or too slow degradation of the ceramic may be a concern, considering that persistent residue of bone substitute in the long term may induce variations of stress distribution within the fusion mass, thereby compromising it mechanically [37]. On the other hand, too rapid resorption of the substitute is undesirable with the risk that fibrous tissue ingrowth occurs first instead of bone formation, therefore preventing the creeping substitution by the host bone.

Following implantation, the biomaterial will progressively get resorbed in the next months or years, i.e., degradation process (Fig. 10). This biodegradation consists of a chemical process (hydrolysis/oxidation) due to the action by chemical agents (enzymes and/or cells) and resulting into changes of physical properties of the material with modification of volume, shape, and/or mechanical resistance [36, 37]. The process has to be slow enough in order to permit that the bio-

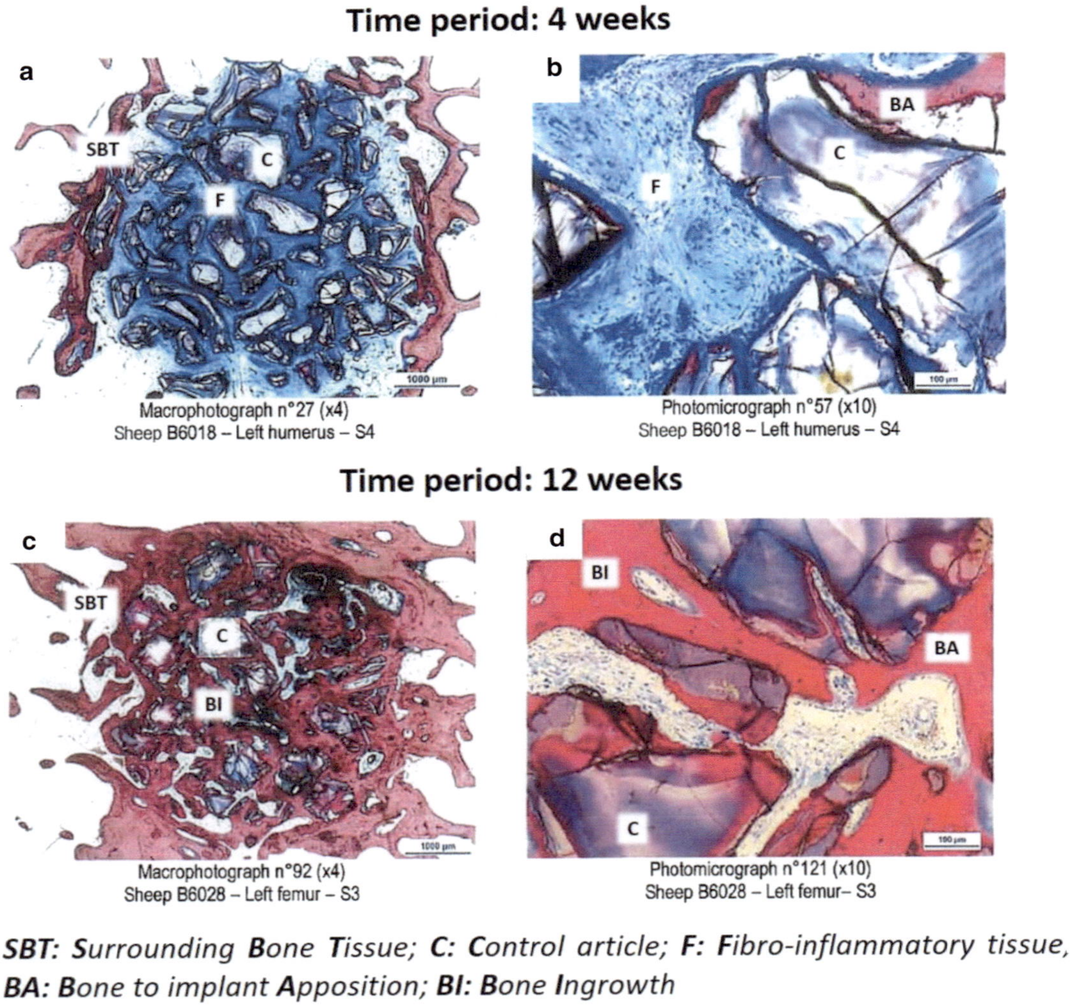

Fig. 10 Biodegradation of synthetic bone granules (bioactive glass) in a sheep animal model (drill defect). At 4 weeks, the synthetic biomaterial (in blue color) is still clearly individualized on macro (**a**) and micro (**b**) histological views. At 12 weeks, it has been progressively resorbed and replaced by new formed bone (in pink color) as demonstrated on macro (**c**) and micro (**d**) view. From 1 to 3 months, the biomaterial volume decreased from 52% to 33%. (From NORAKER™ data—study number 215396, Lyon, France, with permission)

material stay intact long enough to allow for bone proliferation. Too rapid biodegradation should be prevented to limit the deterioration of the biomaterial prior to bone healing is totally achieved.

The different graft material may be combined together to cumulate the advantages of each of them and increase the volume of graft material implanted, i.e., "composite grafts." For instance, it has been reported, though randomized study, that mixture of autologous graft and Ca-P ceramic during spinal deformity surgery, according to the concept of "graft extender," resulted in very positive results in term of fusion [38]. This strategy permits to supplement the local bone that is typically limited in terms of quantity and volume. Another attractive option may be to associate a synthetic bioceramic with blood or, better still, bone marrow harvested from the iliac crest.

The choice considerations for biomaterial depends on many variable factors including [1, 4, 20, 22, 34]:

- The expected role for the graft: mechanical stability versus filling graft.
- The biological host environment into which it is placed: availability of stem cells/vascularization/growth factors.
- The volume necessary and surface of bone host to be covered.
- The surgical site: availability of local autologous bone.
- The patient: age/comorbidity making the local bone more or less good quality.
- The surgeon's preference: related to experience, literature data, training and education.

Overall, the choice for the optimal bone substitute is not an easy one and depends on many different factors including first of all the surgical site and the expected role for the graft. Until now the ideal bone generator for clinical use in spinal surgery is still under investigation.

4 Part 4: Spinal Fusion

Spinal fusion represents nowadays a very common surgical procedure permitting to treat a larger variety of spinal disorders [39]. It has been estimated that several tens of thousands in France and several hundred thousand in the United Staes of fusion surgeries are performed each year [39]. Mechanical complications including pseudarthrosis represent one of the most frequent complications after spinal arthrodesis, estimated to around 10–15% and up to 30% [5, 39–40], and have been reported as one of the main causes for reoperation [22, 39–40]. The frequency of pseudarthrosis is notably high, up to 30–40%, in multilevel fusion surgery and adult spinal deformity surgery [39–40].

4.1 Arthrodesis

It refers to the surgical procedure whose aim is to fuse permanently two adjacent vertebras together. It is also called "joint fusion surgery." Arthrodesis may be instrumented or non-instrumented.

4.2 Fusion

It refers to the biological process that makes two adjacent joint bones (or vertebras) definitely connected together. After fusion, the two vertebras (or more) will present with bony continuity (bony bridges) and will form only one continuous bone.

4.3 Instrumentation

It refers to the osteosynthesis, i.e., screws, rods, cages, and all metallic internal devices whose aim is to immobilize the spinal segment to be fused. In recent years, significant progresses in the technology of spinal instrumentation have maximalized the efficiency of mechanical stabilization and control of 3D motion.

During spinal arthrodesis, the goal is not only to stabilize the spinal segment with the instrumentation but also to bring graft material in order to obtain bony fusion along the spinal segment (Fig. 11). This bony fusion is generally obtained during the 3–months following the surgery and ensure the long-term stability of the construct. This process implies the transformation of the morselized graft into a solid and homogenous cancellous bone corresponding to remodeling phenomenon. In fact, the process of spinal fusion is considered similarly as a process of bone healing in which specialized cells, molecular factors, and minerals are progressively incorporated into a rigid framework.

4.4 SPINAL FUSION

The spinal fusion represents a complex and slow process of cellular and molecular events that take place in the next weeks and months following the surgical procedure and that can be divided into three main phases [41–42] (Fig. 12):

- *Inflammatory phase*: It starts immediately in the next hours just after decortication and lasts around 2–3 weeks. Decortication releases the osteoprogenitor cells from the bone marrow, allowing them for colonizing the fusion site. In addition, a large variety of inflammatory cells are recruited in the fusion site with massive secretion of cytokines and growth factors. At this stage, NSAI drugs may compromise this process and should be avoided during this early period.
- *Reparative phase*: This phase, which may last around 4–6 weeks, includes neovascularization, resorption of necrotic tissue, differentiation of osteoprogenitor cells into osteoblasts, and formation of bone callus. This callus progressively embeds and welds the bone graft fragments in the fusion site, leading to cohesion of the morselized graft, which becomes more and more compact.
- *Remodeling phase*: During the last phase, the morselized graft is progressively transformed into a solid, mineralized, mature, and homogenous cancellous bone. It may last up to 10 months depending on systemic and local factors. In animal models, it has been demonstrated that both types of bone formation, membranous and enchondral, were observed to occur during fusion process [5]. Mature fusion mass will be composed by peripheric cortical bone and central trabecular bone and marrow.

Meticulous preparation of graft bed and optimization of the local biological environment at the fusion site is of importance. As a consequence, during posterior surgery, this implies to clean adequately the bony surfaces of the posterior elements (posterior arches/facets/transvers process) by removing all the soft tissue, articular capsules, and cartilages. Decortication is also advised in order to expose the local host cancellous, thus permitting to the osteoprogenitor cells to escape from the bone marrow and to colonize the fusion area [5]. Also, it is advised to place the graft material in close contact to the decorticated bony surfaces, as seen in Fig. 11. In fact, through animal models, it has been reported that absence of decortication during posterolateral arthrodesis could result in fusion failure [41]. Similarly, during interbody fusion surgery, cleaning properly the endplates with removal of cartilage endplates and disc debris is strongly advised. Indeed, it has been shown that the presence of nucleus mixed with bone graft during anterior fusion surgery could delay and/or decrease the bone formation inside the cage, thus influencing the final fusion [43]. To promote the fusion process, regardless of the surgical approach, any interposing tissue between the local host bone and the graft material must be eliminated.

Even if autograft represents the best graft material, combining osteogenic, osteoinductive, and osteoconductive properties, local autologous bone, harvested during posterior approach (from posterior bony structures: lamina, facets, spinous process), presents some limitations mainly due to its predominant cortical nature. Indeed, because of limited porosity of the cortical bone, the capacity for bone cells migration and vascular ingrowth is reduced. As a consequence, it may be profitable to mix this local bone with synthetic bone substitutes, as shown in Fig. 11.

According to the surgical approach, the biomechanical environment and the forces applied to the spine will significantly differ [44]. During posterior techniques, the bone graft will be predominantly exposed to tensile forces. On the contrary, in anterior procedures, the graft will be placed under compressive loads, requiring utilization of resistant graft material capable of supporting the loads and/or placement of the graft inside a cage.

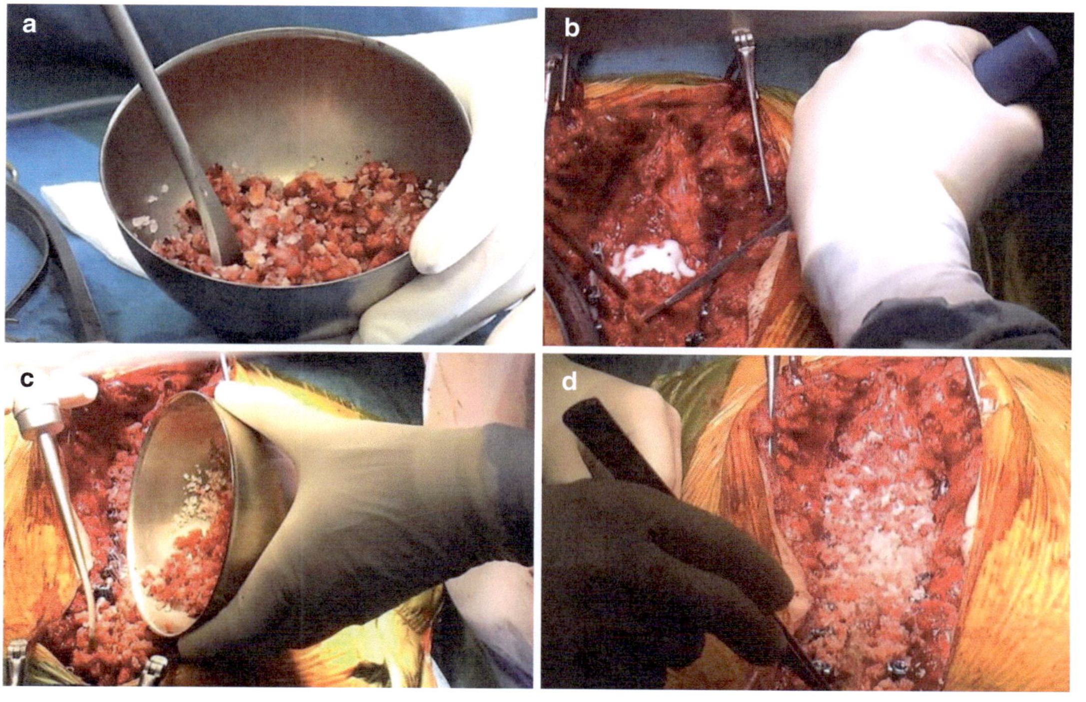

Fig. 11 Combination of autologous graft and bone substitute during spinal deformity surgery. The graft material is prepared by mixing meticulously the autologous graft with the biomaterial, respecting more or less 50/50 of volume for each, and with a few millimeters of saline serum (**a**). After decortication and preparation of the "graft bed" (**b**), the mixture is placed against the decorticated posterior elements (**c**) and therefore covers at the end all the instrumented spinal levels (**d**)

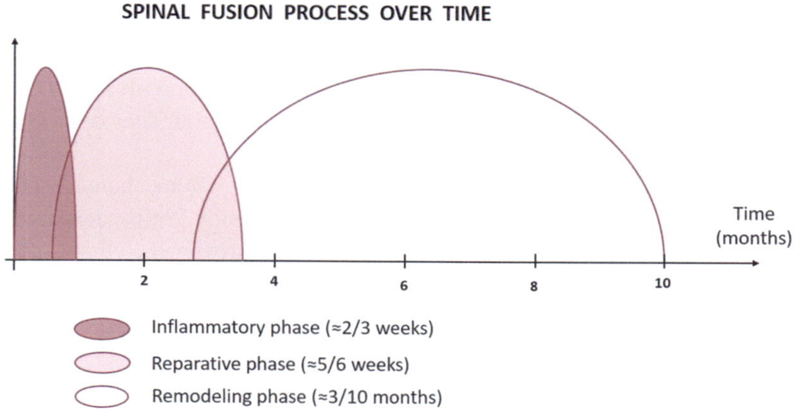

Fig. 12 Natural history of spinal fusion process that can be divided into three main phases: inflammatory, reparative, and remodeling [41, 42]

When spinal fusion is attempted, optimal stabilization with perfect control of 3D motion is mandatory, as excessive micro-motion will hamper the bony consolidation. Initial stability is provided by the spinal instrumentation and most authors considered that bone substitutes and growth factors will not be able to compensate insufficient fusion techniques. Stabilization techniques for the spine are presented in details in the chapter "Instrumentation of the Spine" by E. Ferrero. Instrumentation relies on cages and plating systems for anterior surgery and screws and rods for posterior surgery. Many different systems and strategies are reported according to the spinal disorder, patient's characteristics, and surgeon's preference [44]. The spine surgeon has to understand the biomechanics and the fundamental concepts for spinal instrumentation in order to leave the instrumented spine after surgery in the optimal mechanical conditions for bone fusion.

Main factors that may affect the primary stability of the instrumented spine segment are [44]:

- The nature of the instrumentation (screws/hooks/bands/anterior cages/combined surgery).
- The patient's bone quality.
- The area of the spine involved, more or less mobile naturally (cervical/lumbar/thoracic/junctions).

The efficacy of spine stabilization at the end of the surgery (related to the placement of the instrumentation/number and size of implants/surgical technique/quality of bone/corrective maneuvers).

Bony fusion after spinal arthrodesis is generally obtained during the first 3–12 months and most authors considered that fusion not acquired at 12 months is highly suggestive of pseudarthrosis. Risk factors for pseudarthrosis are well-know and extensively reported in the spine literature [42–45]:

- Age
- Osteoporosis
- Smoking
- Chronic inflammatory diseases
- Surgery-related factors: long constructs, extension to pelvis

Some of these risk factors (nicotine exposure, NSAI, excessive postoperative physical activity) have been investigated though animal models and have been associated with the decrease in the rate of spinal fusion [45–46]. For instance, Keller et al. observed that administration of indomethacin resulted in reduction of blood flow and inhibition of inflammatory response, causing delay of bone healing [46]. Different sites for spinal fusion may be used:

- Posterior arthrodesis with the graft placed against the posterior elements. The surface of posterior elements (lamina, spinous process) is typically decorticated associated with partial facetectomy in order to open the facets joints and thus promote intra-facet fusion.
- Posterolateral arthrodesis between the transverse processes necessitating extensive exposure with the risk for muscle devascularization and denervation.
- Interbody arthrodesis in which the graft is performed between the two vertebral bodies at the place of the intervertebral disc. Interbody fusion is considered as the gold standard at least for short constructs. In the case of long constructs, especially for spinal deformities surgery, interbody fusion is not an option at each instrumented level. Interbody fusion is typically recommended to treat degenerative lumbar conditions and may be achieved through different approach: posterior (PLIF/lateral-PLIF), transforaminal (TLIF), lateral (XLIF/OLIF), and anterior (ALIF).
- Circumferential with the combination of the graft sites described above [47].

Biomechanically, as discussed above, interbody graft material will be exposed to compressive loads, which may have a positive influence on spinal fusion process, according to Wolff's laws. On the contrary, posterior grafts are less mechanically solicited, mainly exposed to tensile forces only. There is a clear impact on the arthrodesis site on fusion rates [47–48], with combined AP surgery providing the higher rates (Figs. 13 and 14).

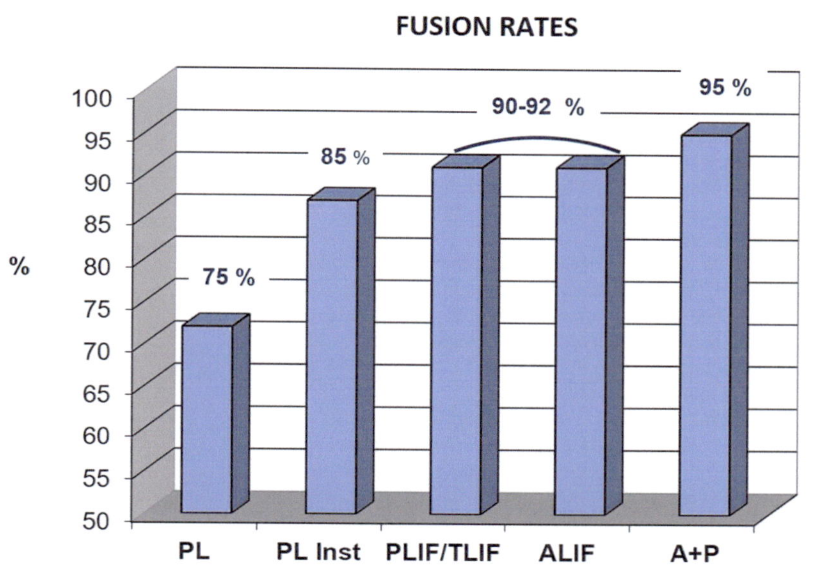

Fig. 13 Fusion rates according to the arthrodesis technique from the literature [48]. PL, posterolateral graft alone; PL Inst, posterolateral graft + pedicle screws; PLIF, posterior lumbar interbody fusion; TLIF, transforaminal lumbar interbody fusion; ALIF, anterior lumbar interbody fusion; A + P, combined arthrodesis by anterior plus posterior approach (ALIF + pedicle screws)

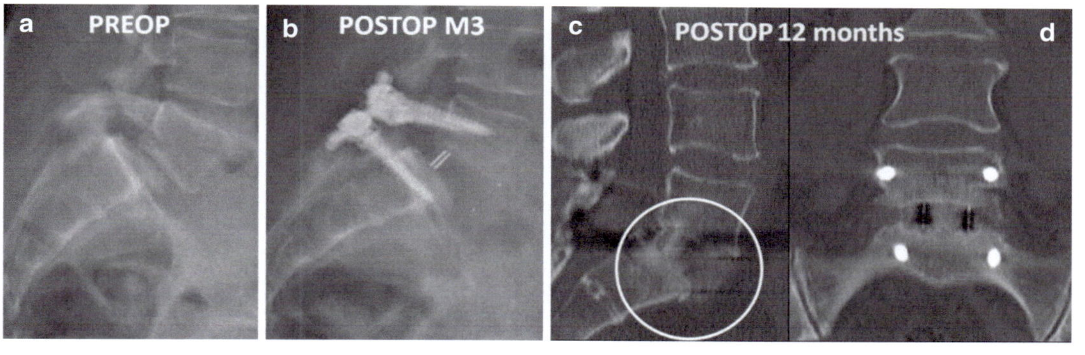

Fig. 14 Spinal fusion observed at 1 year following circumferential stabilization by ALIF cage and pedicle screws. Low-grade isthmic spondylolisthesis (**a**) was stabilized using a combination of anterior then posterior approach (**b**). CT scan at 1 year demonstrates the complete bone healing inside the cage, with bony continuity endplate to endplate, on both sagittal (**c**) and frontal (**d**) view

5 Conclusion

A clear understanding of the biology of spinal fusion is mandatory to help the clinician in his clinical practice. The biological and mechanical factors that may affect bone healing and fusion rates must be fully integrated regarding the bone grafting strategy. Many different graft materials are now available and the choice must be guided according to the expected role for the graft, host site, local biological environment, mechanical conditions, and finally patients' characteristics. The technique is also of importance, especially the preparation of the graft bed, application of the graft material, and performing proper spinal stabilization. Undoubtfully, advances in pharmacology and tissue engineering will optimize the osteogenic potential of bone graft substitutes in the future. Also, even if complex and challenging, gene therapy with implantation of genetically modified cells at fusion site demonstrated very promising results.

References

1. Arts C. Calcium-phosphate biomaterials for bone healing. Practical guideline for implementation in clinical practice. In: J.J.C. Arts. Maastricht, the Netherlands; 2019.
2. LeGeros RZ. Properties of osteoconductive biomaterials: calcium phosphates. Clin Orthop Relat Res. 2002;395:81–98.
3. Berven S, Tay BK, Kleinstueck FS, Bradford DS. Clinical applications of bone graft substitutes in spine surgery: consideration of mineralized and demineralized preparations and growth factor supplementation. Eur Spine J. 2001;10 Suppl 2(Suppl 2):S169–77.
4. Hannink G, Arts C. Bioresorbability, porosity and mechanical strength of bone substitutes: what is optimal for bone regeneration? Injury. 2011;42(Suppl 2):S22–5.
5. Boatright KC, Boden SD. Biology of spine fusion. Biology and clinical applications. In: Bone regeneration and repair: Biology and clinical applications. Humana Press Inc.; 2005. p. 225–39.
6. Ludwig SC, Boden SD. Osteoinductive bone graft substitutes for spinal fusion: a basic science summary. Orthop Clin North Am. 1999;30(4):635–45.
7. Lind M, Bunger C. Factors stimulating bone formation. Eur Spine J. 2001;10(Suppl 2):S102–9.
8. LeGeros RZ, Craig RG. Strategies to affect bone remodeling: osteointegration. J Bone Miner Res. 1993;8(Suppl 2):S583–96.
9. Lavik E, Ranger L. Tissue engineering: current state and perspectives. Appl Microbiol Biotechnol. 2004;65(1):1–8.
10. Williams DF. On the mechanisms of biocompatibility. Biomaterials. 2008;29(20):2941–53.
11. Boden SD. The biology of posterolateral lumbar spine fusion. Orthop Clin North Am. 1998;29(4):603–19.
12. Boos N, Marchesi D. Biology of the spine. Biology of fusion with one and bone substitutes. In: AO-spine manual, principles and techniques, vol. 1. Thieme; 2007.
13. Frost HM. Wolff's law and bone's structural adaptation to mechanical usage: an overview for clinicians. Angle Orthod. 1994;64:187–212.
14. Frost HM. A 2003 update of bone physiology and Wolff's law for clinicians. Angle Orthod. 2004;74(1):1–15.
15. Giannoudis PV, Einhorn TA, Marsh D. Fracture healing: the diamond concept. Injury. 2007;38(Suppl 4):S3–6.
16. Giannoudis PV, Einhorn TA, Schmidmaier G, Marsh D. The diamond concept–open questions. Injury. 2008;39(Suppl 2):S5–8.
17. Wolff J. The Law of Bone Remodeling. Berlin/Heidelberg/New York: Springer; 1986. (translation of the German 1892 edition)
18. Calori GM, Giannoudis PV. Enhancement of fracture healing with the diamond concept: the role of the biological chamber. Injury. 2011;42(11):1191–3.
19. Sandhu HS, Boden SD. Biologic enhancement of spinal fusion. Orthop Clin North Am. 1998;29(4):621–31.
20. Gunzburg R, Szpalski M, Passuti N, Aebi M. The use of bone substitutes in spine surgery, 2002A state of the art review. Springer-Verlag; 2002.
21. Shin H, Jo S, Mikos AG. Biomimetic materials for tissue engineering. Biomaterials. 2003;24(24):4353–64.
22. Buser Z, Jakoi A, Katbamna B, Basho R, Wang JC. Bone grafting and spinal fusion options. In: Holly L, Anderson P, editors. Essentials of spinal stabilization. Cham: Springer; 2017.
23. Urist MR. Bone: formation by autoinduction. Science. 1965;150(3698):893–9.
24. Shepard NA, Rush AJ, Scarborough NL, Carter AJ, Phillips F. Demineralized bone matrix in spine surgery: a review of current applications and future trends. Int J Spine Surg. 2021;15(Suppl 1):113–9.
25. Cammisa FP, Lowery G, Garfin SR, Geisler FH, Klara PM, McGuire RA, Sassard WR, Stubbs H, Block JE. Two-year fusion rate equivalency between Grafton DBM gel and autograft in posterolateral spine fusion: a prospective controlled trial employing a side-by-side comparison in the same patient. Spine (Phila Pa 1976). 2004;29(6):660–6.
26. Peltier LF, Bickel EY, Lillo R, Thein MS. The use of plaster of Paris to fill defects in bone. Ann Surg. 1957;146(1):61–9.
27. Hench LL. The story of Bioglass. J Matter Sci: Matter Med. Springer Science. 2006;17:967–78.
28. Barrey C, Broussolle T. Clinical and radiographic evaluation of bioactive glass in posterior cervical and lumbar spinal fusion. Eur J Orthop Surg Traumatol. 2019;29(8):1623–9.
29. Chen D, Zhao M, Mundy GR. Bone morphogenetic proteins. Growth Factors. 2004;22(4):233–41.
30. Boden SD, Schimandle JH, Hutton WC, Chen MI. 1995 Volvo Award in basic sciences. The use of an osteoinductive growth factor for lumbar spinal fusion Part I: Biology of spinal fusion. Spine (Phila Pa 1976). 1995;20(24):2626–32.
31. Burkus JK, Sandhu HS, Gornet MF, Longley MC. Use of rhBMP-2 in combination with structural cortical allografts: clinical and radiographic outcomes in anterior lumbar spinal surgery. J Bone Joint Surg Am. 2005;87(6):1205–12.
32. Mroz TE, Wang JC, Hashimoto R, Norvell DC. Complications related to osteobiologics use in spine surgery: a systematic review. Spine (Phila Pa 1976). 2010;35(9 Suppl):S86–104.
33. Cornell CN. Osteoconductive materials and their role as substitutes for autogenous bone grafts. Orthop Clin North Am. 1999;30(4):591–8.
34. LeGeros RZ, Lin S, Rohanizadeh R, Mijares D, LeGeros JP. Biphasic calcium phosphate bioceramics: preparation, properties and applications. J Mater Sci Mater Med. 2003;14(3):201–9.
35. Tay BK, Patel VV, Bradford DS. Calcium sulfate- and calcium phosphate-based bone substitutes. Mimicry of the mineral phase of bone. Orthop Clin North Am. 1999;30(4):615–23.

36. Eggi PS, Muller W, Schenk RK. Porous hydroxyapatite and tricalcium phosphate cylinders with two different pore size ranges implanted in the cancellous bone of rabbits A comparative histomorphometric and histologic study of bony ingrowth and implant substitution. Clin Orthop Relat Res. 1988;232:127–38.
37. Jarcho M. Calcium phosphate ceramics as hard tissue prosthetics. Clin Orthop Relat Res. 1981;157:259–78.
38. Delecrin J, Takahashi S, Gouin F, Passuti N. A synthetic porous ceramic as a bone graft substitute in the surgical management of scoliosis: a prospective, randomized study. Spine (Phila Pa 1976). 2000;25(5):563–9.
39. Reisener MJ, Pumberger M, Shue J, Girardi FP, Hughes AP. Trends in lumbar spinal fusion—a literature review. J Spine Surg. 2020;6(4):752–61.
40. Mummaneni PV, Meyer SA, Wu JC. Biological approaches to spinal instrumentation and fusion in spinal deformity surgery. Clin Neurosurg. 2011;5B(14):110–6.
41. Boden SD, Schimandle JH, Hutton WC. An experimental lumbar intertransverse process spinal fusion model. Radiographic, histologic, and biomechanical healing characteristics. Spine (Phila Pa 1976). 1995;20(4):412–20.
42. Toribatake Y, Hutton WC, Tomita K, Boden SD. Vascularization of the fusion mass in a posterolateral intertransverse process fusion. Spine (Phila Pa 1976). 1998;23(10):1149–54.
43. Li H, Zou X, Laursen M, Egund N, Lind M, Bunger C. The influence of intervertebral disc tissue on anterior spinal interbody fusion: an experimental study on pigs. Eur Spine J. 2002;11(5):476–81.
44. Arlet V. Spinal instrumentation. In: AOspine manual, principles and techniques, vol. 1. Thieme; 2007.
45. Silcox DH, Daftari T, Boden SD, Schimandle JH, Hutton WC, Whitesides TE. The effect of nicotine on spinal fusion. Spine (Phila Pa 1976). 1995;20(14):1549–53.
46. Keller J, Bunger C, Andreassen T, Bak B, Lucht U. Bone repair inhibited by indomethacin. Effects on bone metabolism and strength of rabbit osteotomies. Acta Orthop Scand. 1987;58(4):379–83.
47. Barrey CY, Boissiere L, D'Acunzi G, Perrin G. One-stage combined lumbo-sacral fusion, by anterior then posterior approach: clinical and radiological results. Eur Spine J. 2013;22(Suppl 6):S957–64.
48. Fritzell P, Hagg O, Wessberg P, Nordwall A, The Swedish Lumbar Spine Study Group. Chronic low back pain and fusion: a comparison of three surgical techniques: a prospective multicenter randomized study from the Swedish lumbar spine study group. Spine (Phila Pa 1976). 2002;27(11):1131–41.

Principles of Spinal Instrumentation

Emmanuelle Ferrero, Leonard Chatelain, and Marc Khalife

1 Cervical Spine

1.1 Posterior Cervical Instrumentation

Different types of implants are available for posterior instrumentation of the cervical spine; they vary according to the cervical level and the anatomical structure requiring fixation.

1.1.1 Screws

Cervical screws are commonly used for stabilization and fusion in degenerative, deformity, or trauma cases. Usually, in the lower cervical spine (from C3 to C7), articular screws are inserted according to Magerl technique: ascendant and divergent (Fig. 1). In case of revision surgery, without good bone surface in the facet, pedicle screws can be used [1, 2]. Nevertheless, cervical pedicles are very small and it is recommended to use navigation to implant pedicle screws (Fig. 2) [3]. For cervicothoracic fixation, C7 pedicle screws may also be very useful to use as the screws head will have a better alignment with T1 screw head.

In the upper cervical spine, screw fixation is different. In C1, lateral mass screws are used. As the lateral mass may be short, it is important to analyze the anatomy on a preoperative CT scan and/or to use navigation, at least fluoroscopy. Then a partially threaded screw is inserted to avoid lesion of the venous plexus and C2 roots. A second option, if the posterior arch is thick, is to drill it and then to insert the screw from the posterior arch of C1 to the lateral mass (Fig. 3). For C2 fixation, pedicle screws are the most commonly used; they are usually ascendant and slightly convergent. If pedicle is too small, lateral mass screws or laminar screws can be inserted (Fig. 4). C1C2 fixation with C1 lateral mass and C2 pedicle screws is called Harm's technique (Fig. 5) [4, 5]. A C1C2 fixation can also be performed through a C2C1 transarticular screw, again navigation is helpful. The entry point of this screw is usually 3 mm above C2C3 joint (Fig. 6).

Occipito-cervical fixation is usually performed with rod and plates, in case of C1 fracture, occipito-cervical instability, and spinal cord compression at occipito-cervical junction. Plates are screwed on each side of the nuchal line with short screws in the occipital bone, and then plates are connected to usual cervical spine rods and inserted into C2 screws, sometimes lower. A perfect contouring of the rod is required. It is of utmost importance to assess the Mac Gregor angle when doing occipito-cervical fixation [6, 7]. This angle, measured between C2 lower endplate and the line joining hard palate and occiput

E. Ferrero (✉) · L. Chatelain · M. Khalife
Orthopedic and Spine Surgery Department, Hopital Européen Georges Pompidou, Université Paris Cité, Paris, France

C. Y. Barrey (ed.), *Spine Surgery*, SFCR Experts Series 1,
https://doi.org/10.1007/978-3-031-85446-0_6

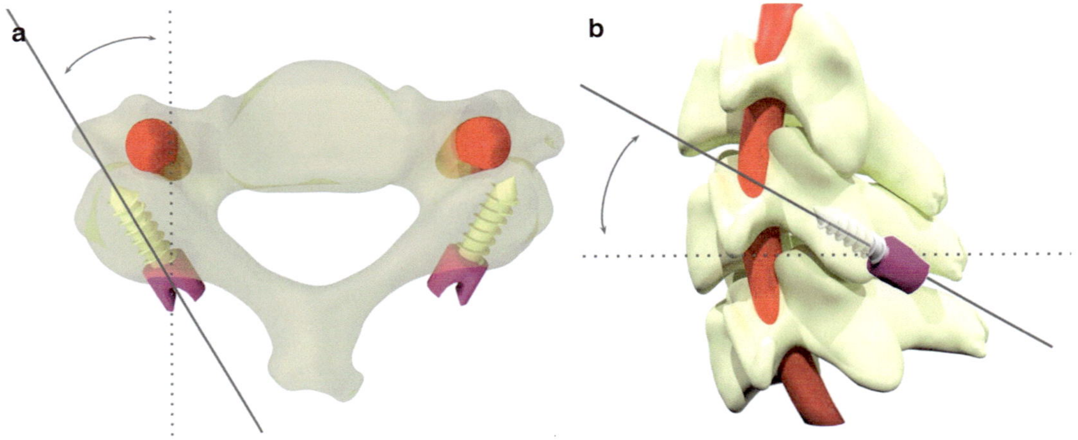

Fig. 1 Sketch of Magerl's technique for cervical screws (**a**) coronal view, (**b**) sagittal view

Fig. 2 Sketch of cervical pedicular screws (axial view)

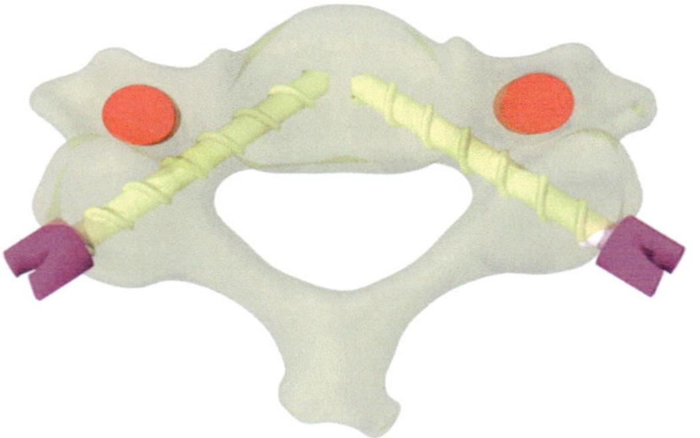

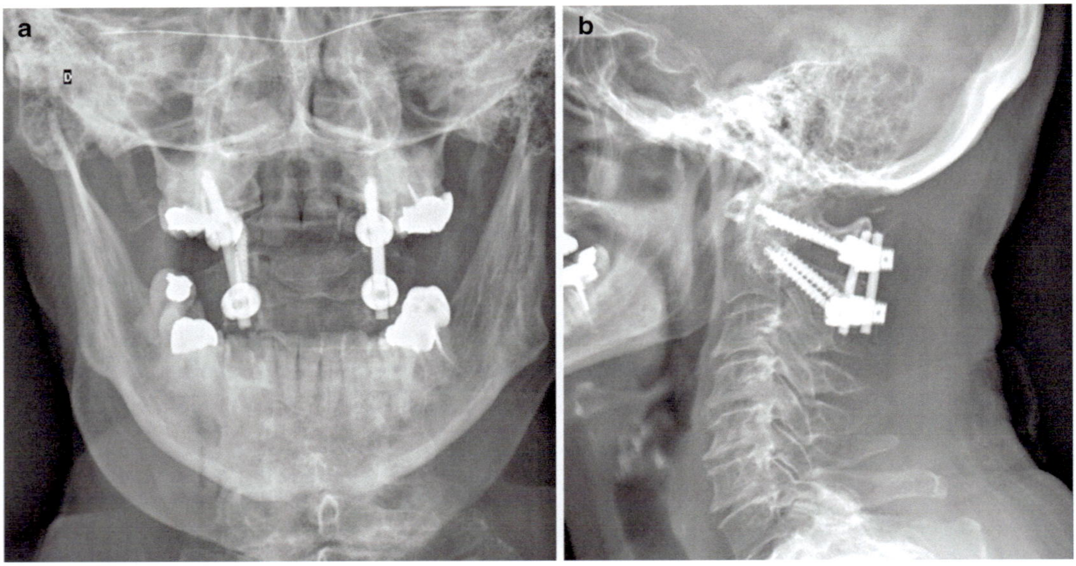

Fig. 3 C1C2 fixation with Harm's technique (**a**) coronal X-rays, (**b**) sagittal X-rays

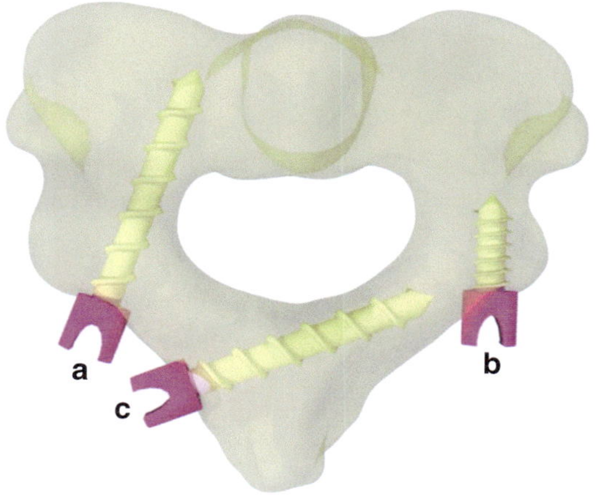

Fig. 4 Different types of C2 screws (**a**) pedicular, (**b**) facet, (**c**) laminar)

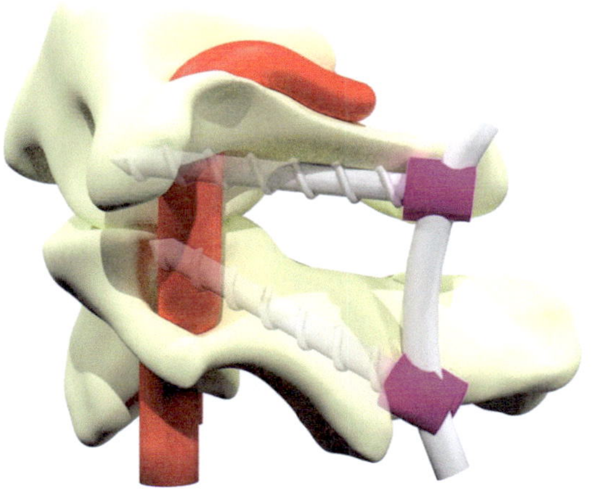

Fig. 5 Sketch of Harm's fixation (sagittal view)

base, should be between 0° and 30° to avoid gaze, breathing, or swallowing disorders (Fig. 7). Pre-contoured rods are also available including the plate and may be very useful. It is important to add some bone graft in occipito-cervical fixation to obtain fusion since this area is associated with a high risk of pseudoarthrosis (Fig. 8).

1.1.2 Hooks

If screw instrumentation cannot be performed, supra- and sub-laminar hooks may be helpful from C1 to C7. Once they are inserted, some contraction is added to stabilize the instrumentation in compression (Fig. 9). Hook construct is never-

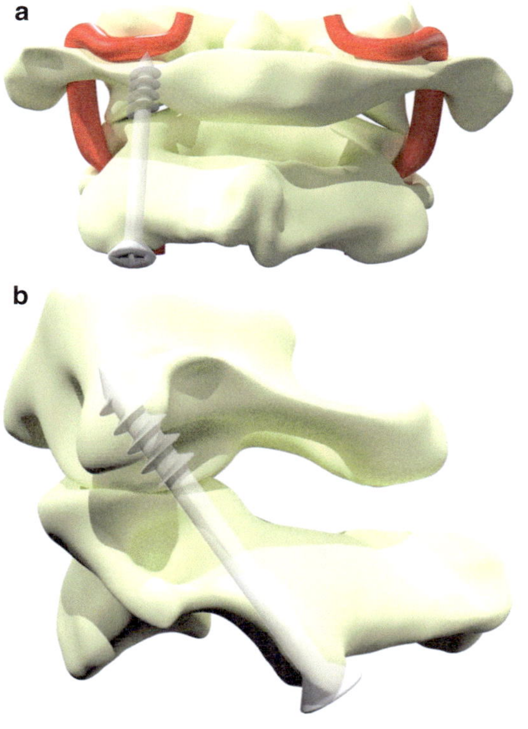

Fig. 6 Sketch of C1C2 transarticular screw (**a**) coronal view, (**b**) sagittal view)

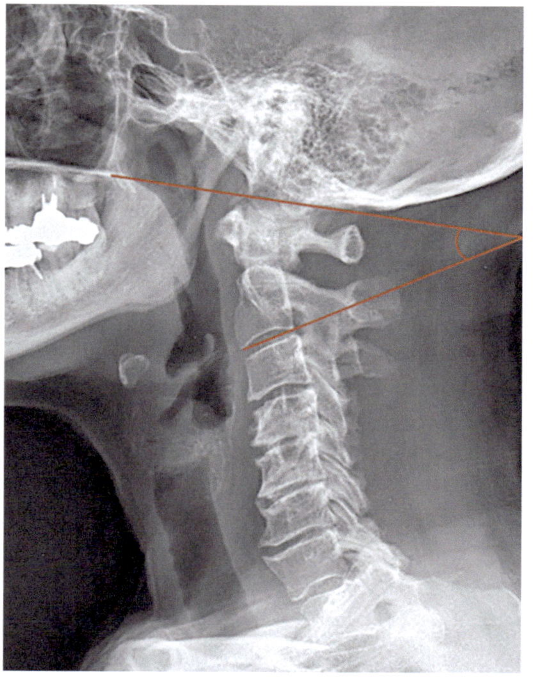

Fig. 7 Mc Gregor angle measurement (hard palate - occiput line and C2 endplate)

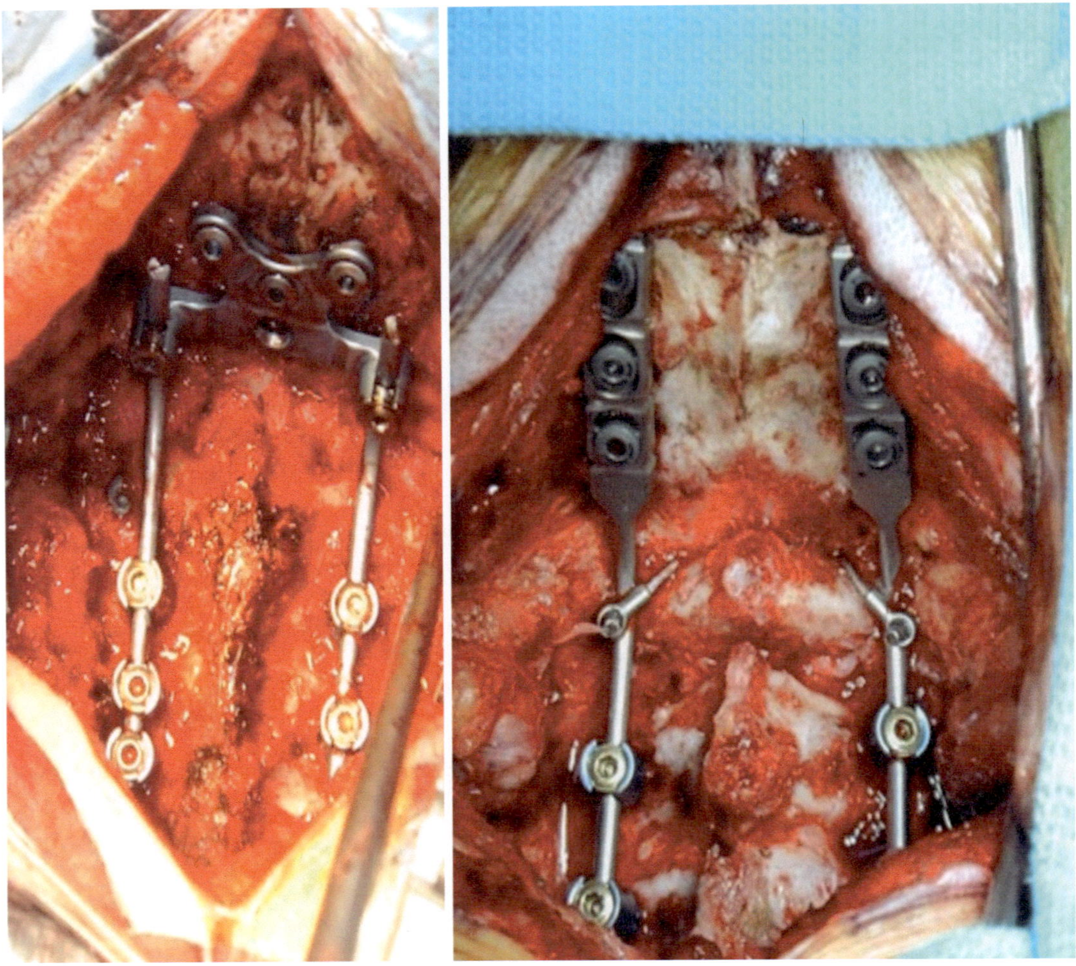

Fig. 8 Example of occipito-cervical fixation with two types of rods and plates

theless less rigid than screw fixation and cannot be achieved in case of previous laminectomy.

1.1.3 Ligament

In upper cervical spine, it is also possible to do a lacing between C1 and C2, with metallic wire or polyester band. Different lacing techniques have been described by Gallie or Brooks around lamina and spinous process. The use of ligament is impossible in case of laminectomy and is less rigid than hooks. With hooks or lacing, adding bone graft is essential (Fig. 10) [8].

1.1.4 Laminoplasty Implants

Laminoplasty encompasses different surgical procedures for cervical decompression. It roughly consists of an opening of the lamina with a burr. In the open door laminoplasty, the posterior arc is rotated on one side and fixed to the articular mass on the other side using a small plate and screws (Fig. 11) [9].

1.2 Anterior Cervical Instrumentation

Anterior cervical spine instrumentation can be performed with cage, plate, and arthroplasty implants. Anterior cervical fusion can be required in cases of disc herniation, spinal cord compression with myelopathy, or some fracture. Anterior screwing of C2 fracture is also an

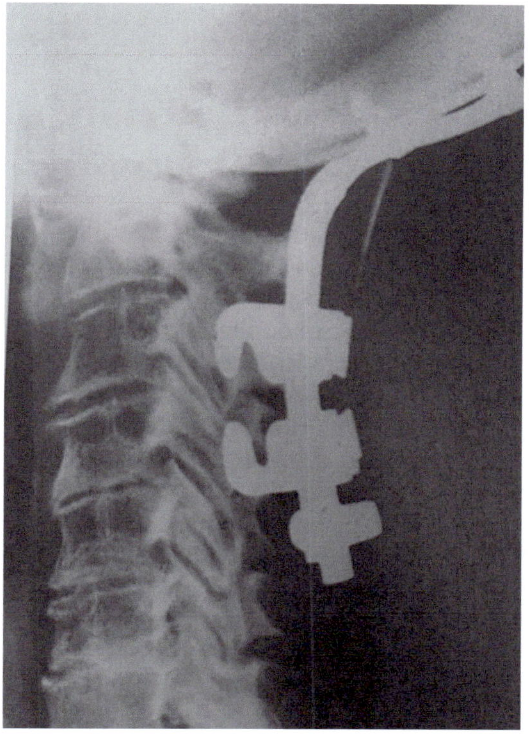

Fig. 9 Sagittal X-rays of a cervico-occipital fusion with cervical hooks

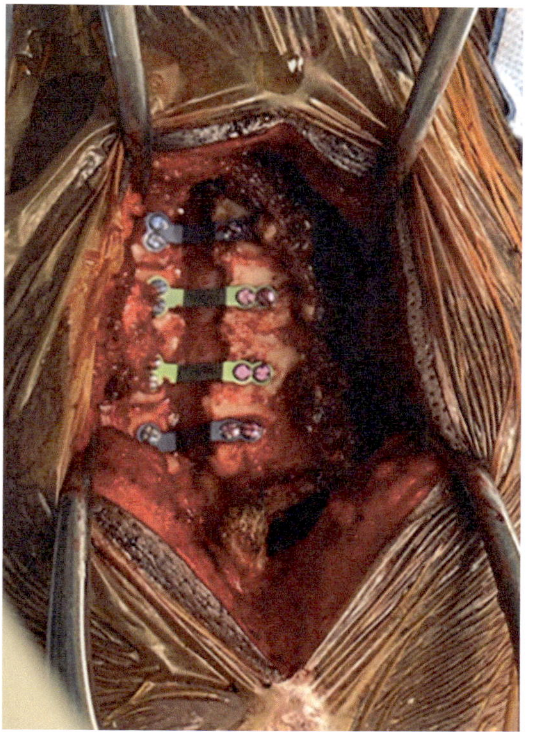

Fig. 11 Cervical laminoplasty implants (posterior view)

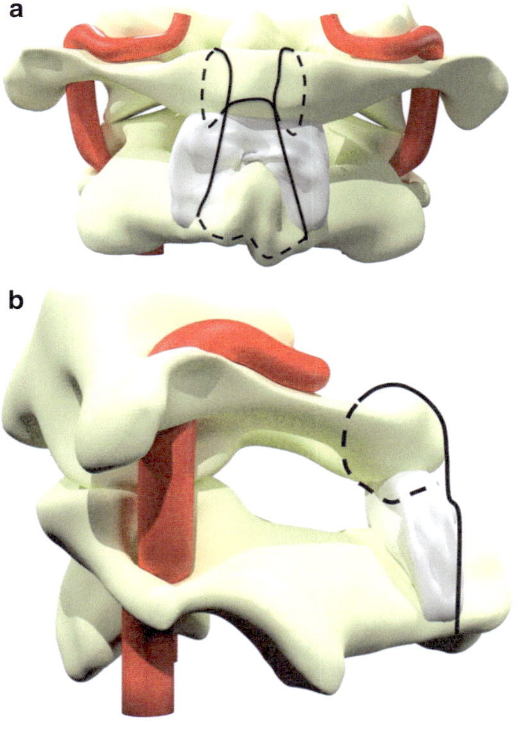

Fig. 10 Sketch of C1C2 lacing technique (**a**) coronal view, (**b**) sagittal view)

option but a little disused today due to high pseudoarthrosis rate.

1.2.1 Cage and Plate

Through an anterior approach, after disc removal and endplate preparation, anterior cage can be inserted to fix the cervical spine and increase the disc height and the foraminal height [9]. These cages are in polyetheretherketone (PEEK) or titanium. In case of decompression, it is necessary to release the posterior longitudinal ligament. Different types of cages are available: stand-alone, stabilized with anchors or with screws (Fig. 12) [9]. Cages need to be filled with autograft or synthetic bone to allow fusion. In some cases, to enhance stabilization (traumatology, multilevel fixation), a plate fixed with screws is added. It requires a wider exposure, and one must be careful not to pull too much on the laryngeal nerves, esophagus, and trachea (Fig. 13).

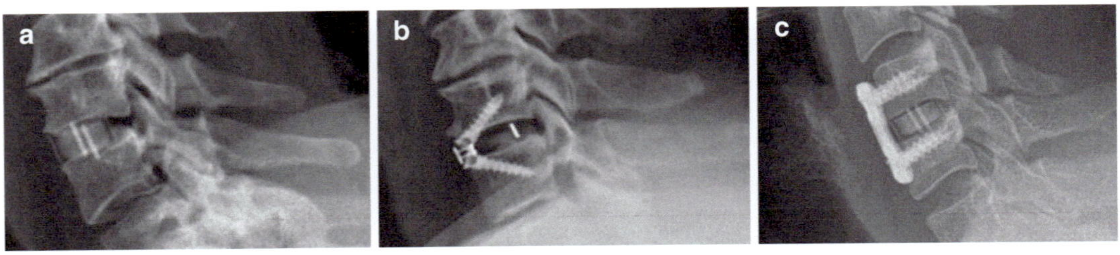

Fig. 12 Different types of anterior cervical cages (**a**) stand alone, (**b**) screwed cage, (**c**) cage and plate

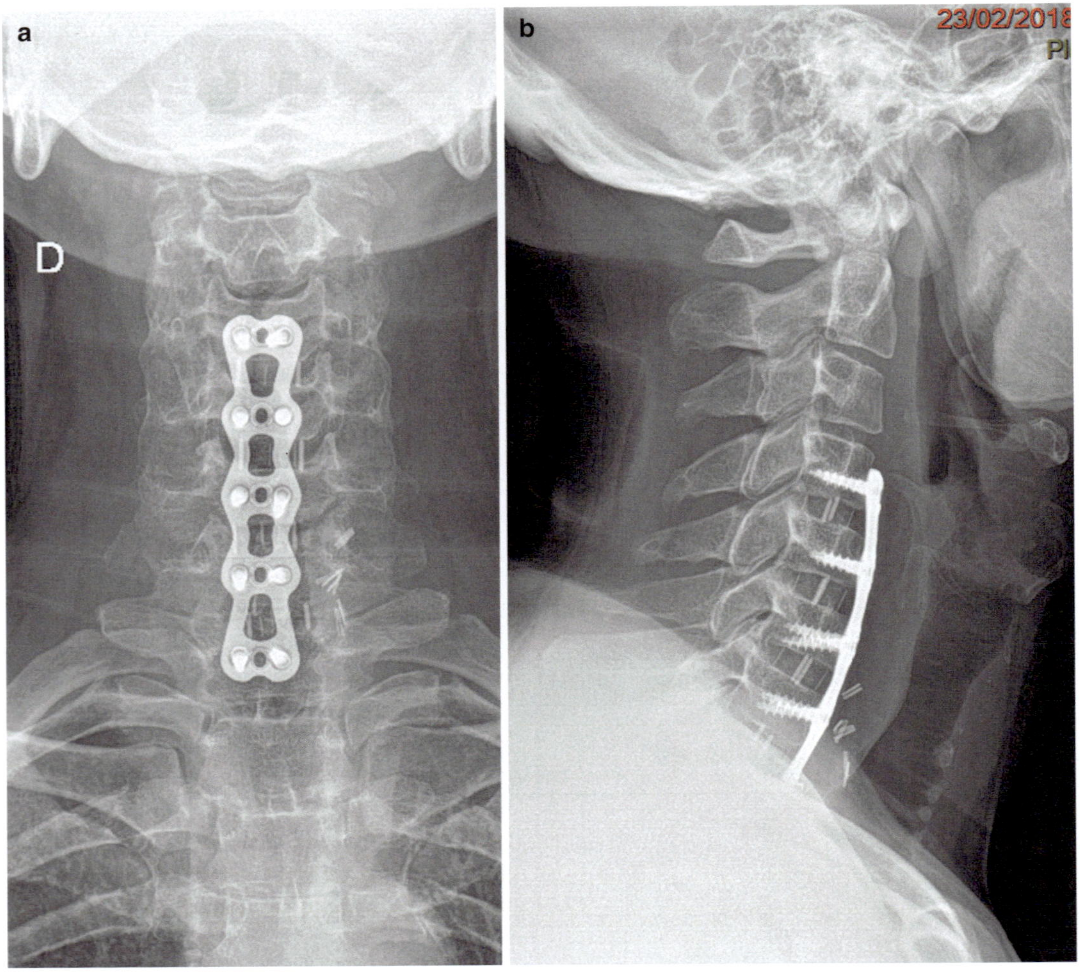

Fig. 13 Coronal (**a**) and sagittal (**b**) X-rays of anterior cages and plate

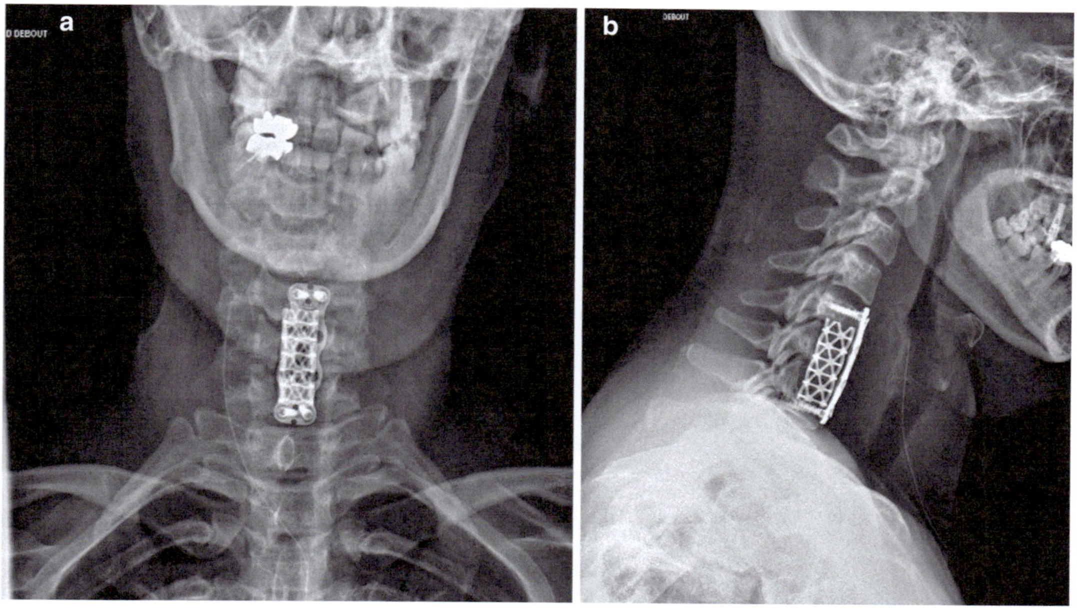

Fig. 14 Coronal (**a**) and sagittal (**b**) X-rays of anterior corpectomy with mesh cage and plate

1.2.2 Corpectomy Cage

In case of severe myelopathy with osteophytes or ossification of the posterior longitudinal ligament or fractures, vertebral body resection is required. Then a corpectomy cage is inserted between the endplates of the vertebrae above and below. The cage can be a mesh cage or an expandable cage filled with bone [10]. It should be stable between the two endplates (Fig. 14). Fixation can be improved with a plate and screws, but some cages are expandable and available with integrated plate at each end (Fig. 15). Nevertheless, there is less space to fill with bone graft in expandable cages [11].

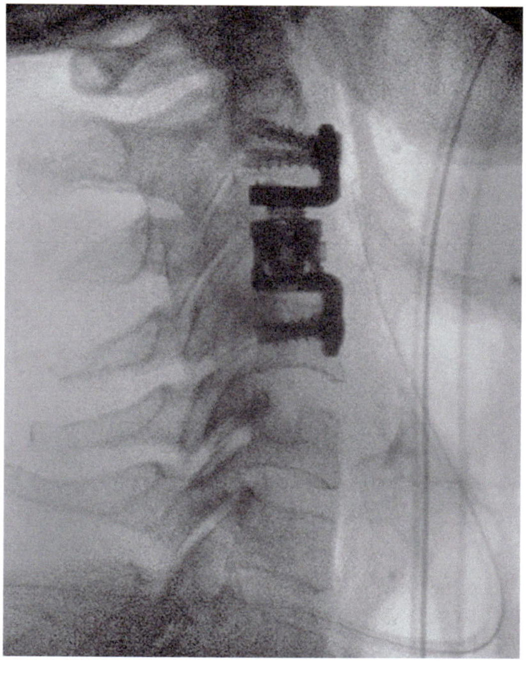

Fig. 15 Sagittal X-ray of cervical anterior corpectomy with expandable cage

1.2.3 Disc Replacement

In case of disc herniation or degeneration with inflammatory endplate Modic 1 without facet degeneration, a total disc replacement may be proposed (Fig. 16). The details of the indication and technique are developed in the cervical book.

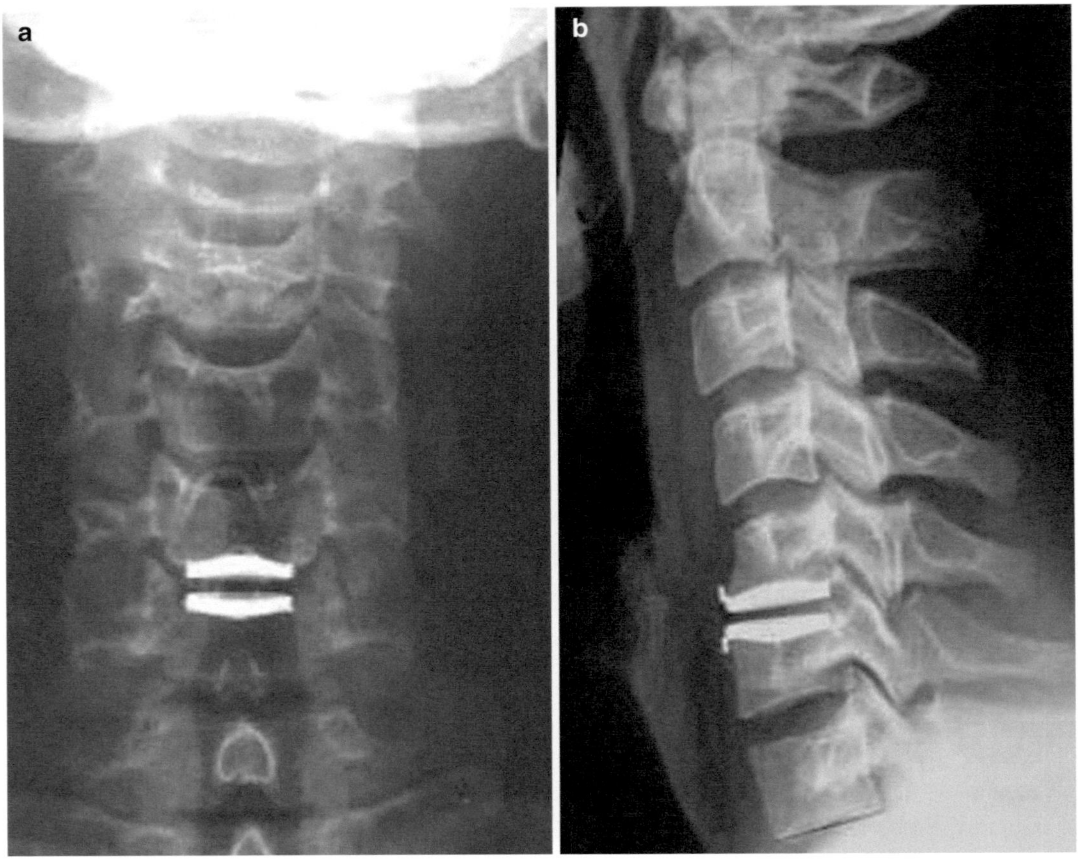

Fig. 16 Coronal (**a**) and sagittal (**b**) X-rays of cervical disc replacement

2 Thoracic Spine

2.1 Posterior Thoracic Instrumentation

2.1.1 Screws

Nowadays, pedicle screws in the thoracic spine are the most commonly used implant (Fig. 17). They are used in different pathologies of the thoracic spine: spinal cord compression, deformity, spondylodiscitis, tumor, and fracture [12]. They may be used for an osteosynthesis or a fusion. According to Roy-Camille technique, screws entry point is located at the intersection between a line in the middle of the facet joint and a horizontal line in the middle of the transverse process, 1 mm below the joint [13, 14]. This technique was developed to insert screws with Roy-Camille plates (Fig. 18). More recently, Dick described a more convergent trajectory with an entry point at the intersection between a line at the upper third of the transverse process and a line on the external third of the facet (Fig. 19) [15].

It is important to analyze pedicles' anatomy on preoperative CT scan to assess the possible length (usually between 30 and 40 mm in the thoracic spine) and the width of the screw (usually between 4.5 and 5.5 mm in the thoracic spine). Pedicles are larger in T1 and T2 and at the thoracolumbar junction. Sometimes pedicles are very small with only cortical bone; in that case a motorized drill may be useful to find the pedicle or to do an "in-out-in" trajectory (Fig. 20). Pedicle orientation is also important to assess;

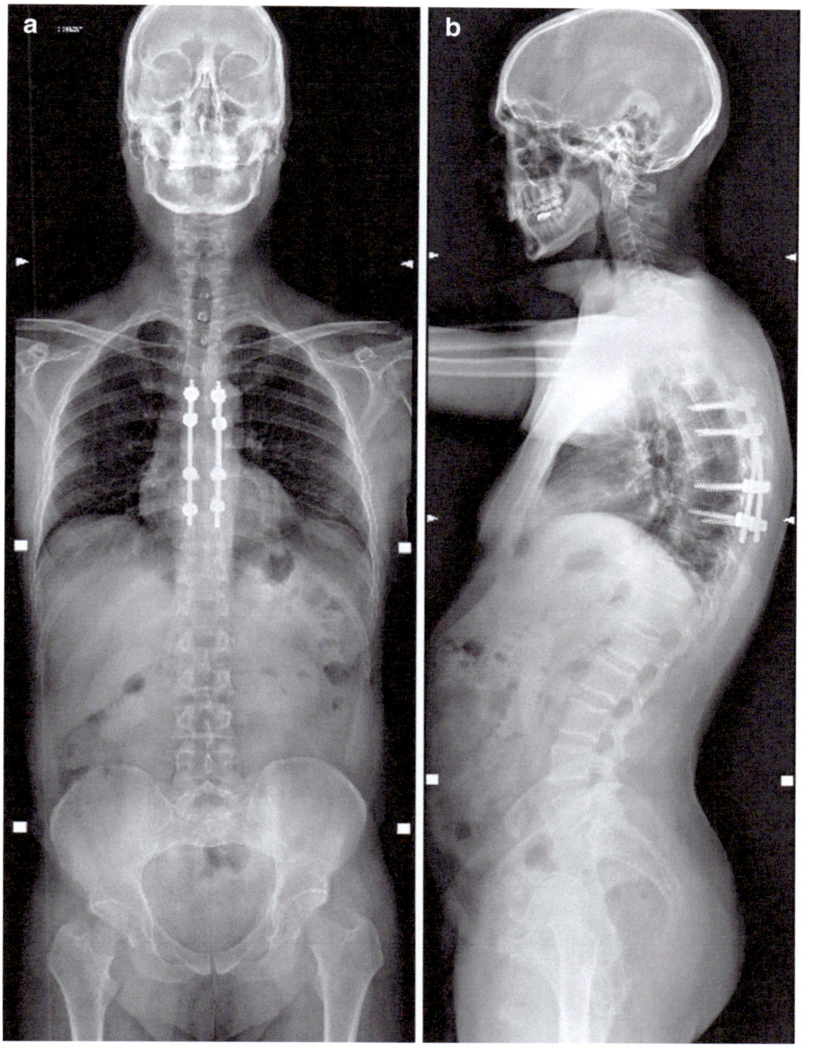

Fig. 17 Coronal (**a**) and sagittal (**b**) X-rays of posterior thoracic fixation with screws

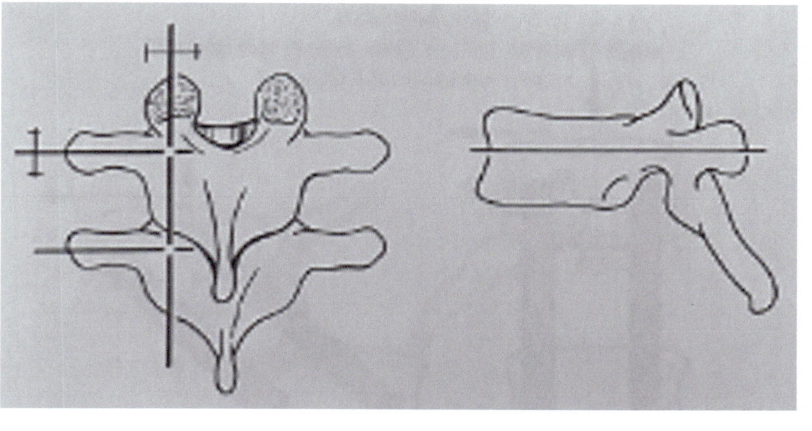

Fig. 18 Pedicular thoracic screwing—Roy-Camille's technique

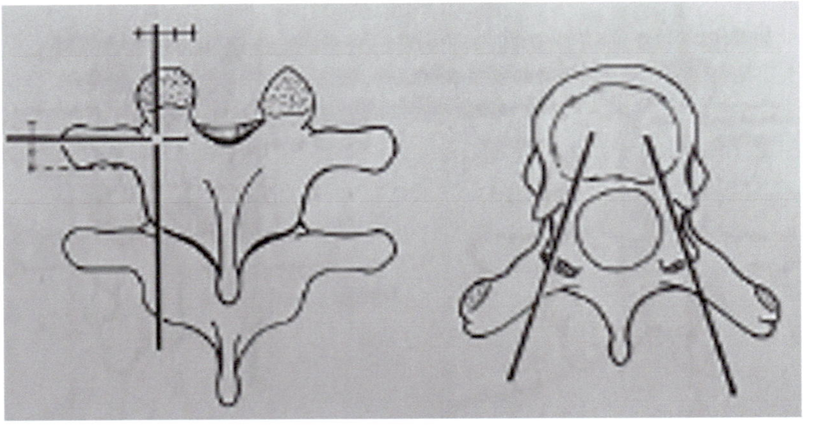

Fig. 19 Pedicular thoracic screwing—Dick's technique

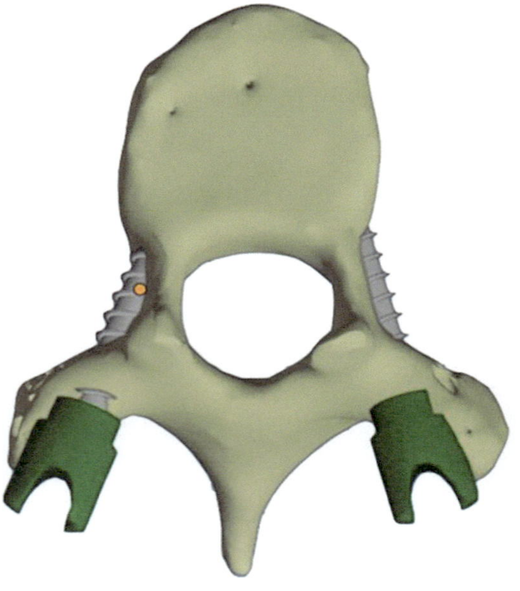

Fig. 20 Example of in-out-in fixation with tiny thoracic pedicles (axial view): author's drawing

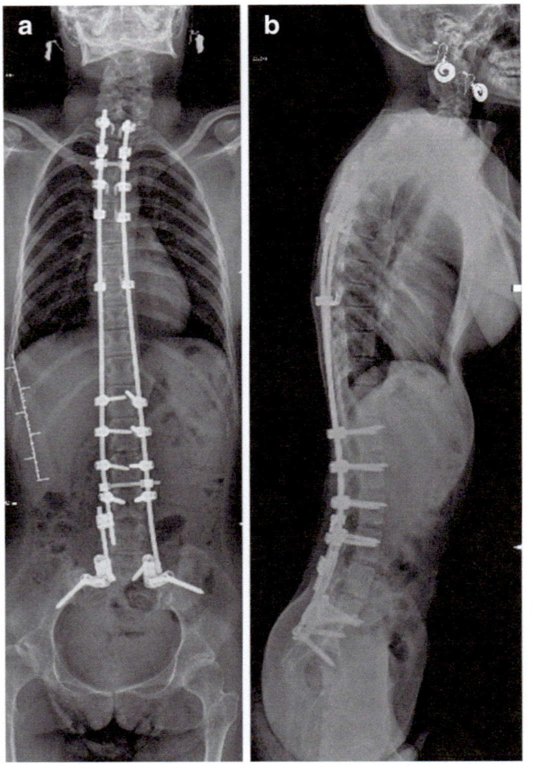

Fig. 21 Coronal (**a**) and sagittal (**b**) X-rays of a patient with thoracic hooks instrumentation

often, they are more convergent in T1 and T2 and then straighter from T4 to T10 [16].

2.1.2 Hooks

Hooks were implanted before screws in the spine, with similar indications. Different types of hooks were developed to adapt to the different anatomical structures of the vertebra and to the insertion direction depending on the expected correction (Fig. 21) [17–19].

The three main hook types are laminar, pedicle, and transverse. Hooks are made up of a blade, which is the part in contact with the vertebra and a body that unites to the rod. The blade can vary in length, width, and type of end. A clamp can be

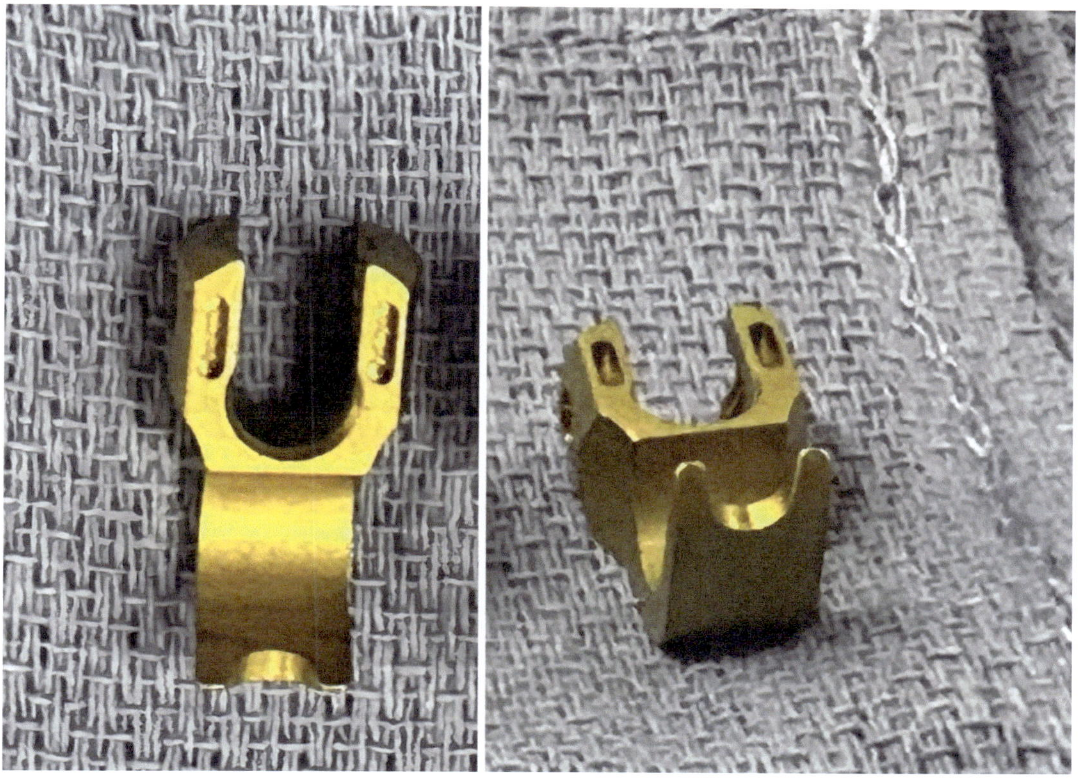

Fig. 22 Example of a pedicle hook

performed with two hooks (or a hook and a screw) facing each other and tightened in compression.

Pedicle Hook
Its blade is inserted very inclined by sliding between the articular processes until contact with lower part of the pedicle of the overlying vertebra. To be inserted, the lower facet of the upper vertebra needs to be partially resected. A pedicle rugine may be inserted before the hook. The end of the blade is bifid to hang on to the pedicle and stabilize the hook laterally (Fig. 22).

Laminar Hook
It can be inserted above (supra-) or below (sub-) the lamina. The end of the blade is rounded and inserted between the laminae into the canal (Fig. 23). The blades of the thoracic laminar hook are narrower to remain applied against the lamina and avoid its penetration into the spinal cord; they can be longer to be aligned with thoracic screw laterally.

To be inserted, a partial resection of the ligamentum flavum is usually performed as well as the medial part of the inferior facet of the upper vertebra with a Kerrison's rongeur.

Transverse Hook
It is similar to laminar hook with a smaller body height. Its blade is applied on the transverse process (Fig. 24). It realizes with the pedicle hook the pediculo-transversal clamp (Fig. 25). To prepare its insertion, a special rugine that allows removing the periosteum from the anterior face of the transverse is used. The hook is then inserted using the implant holder clamp between the transverse process and the rib.

2.1.3 Sublaminar Wires or Bands

Luque Sublaminar metallic wires were initially developed by Luque (1972), in combination with

Harrington technique, creating the Harri–Luque instrumentation for deformity correction or fracture stabilization (Fig. 26) [20, 21]. They were made of stainless steel of different diameters. Very good corrections have been reported with the use of sublaminar wiring in thoracic curves, but all of the forces that maintain the reduction and fixation of the vertebrae are concentrated in the extremely small area of contact between the sublaminar wires and the laminae, sometimes leading to rupture of the cortical bone. Moreover, original strength is important but as soon as the wires are damaged, there is a decreased resistance of 63% and only two or three iterative tightening are possible. Removal is very difficult and at risk for the spinal cord. That is the reason why they were progressively abandoned.

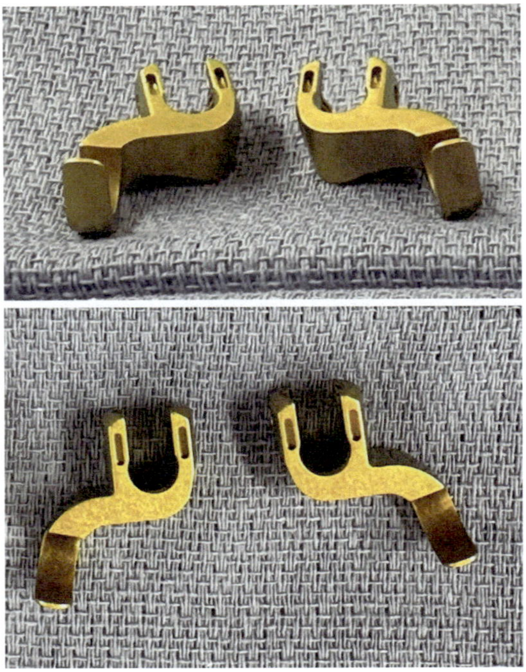

Fig. 23 Example of sublaminar lateral hooks (right and left)

Bands Sublaminar band consists of a polyester band passed under the lamina or around a lamina and transverse process and connected to the rod by a metallic clamp. With little bulk, the sublaminar band distributes forces over extensive areas of cortical bone, permitting application of increased reduction forces (Fig. 27) [22–24].

In deformity correction, the sublaminar band construct acts essentially by posteromedial translation of the vertebrae, which are applied against contoured rods with physiological sagittal curves. In scoliosis patients, hybrid constructs are commonly used combining pedicle screws at the lumbar level to perform derotation and restore

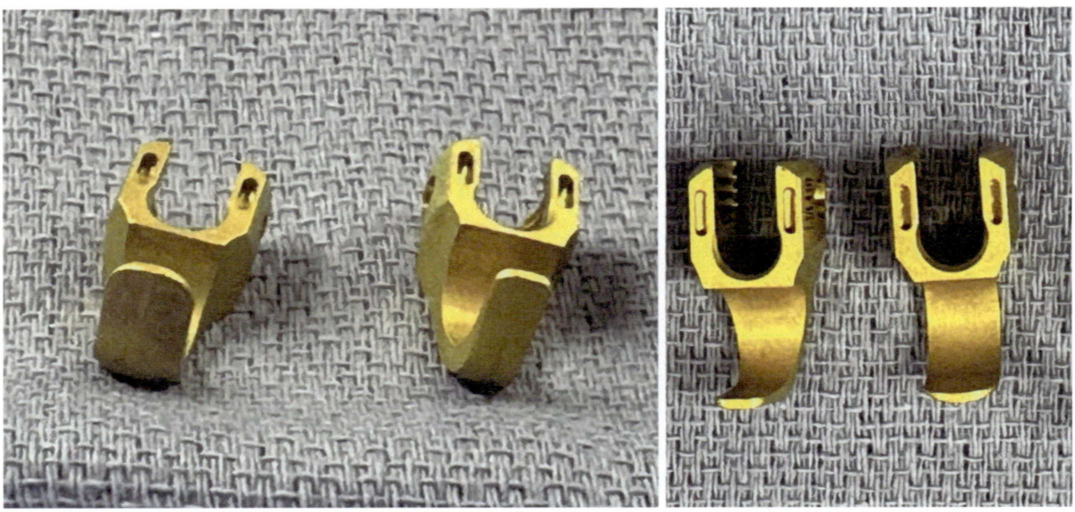

Fig. 24 Example of supra-laminar or transverse hooks

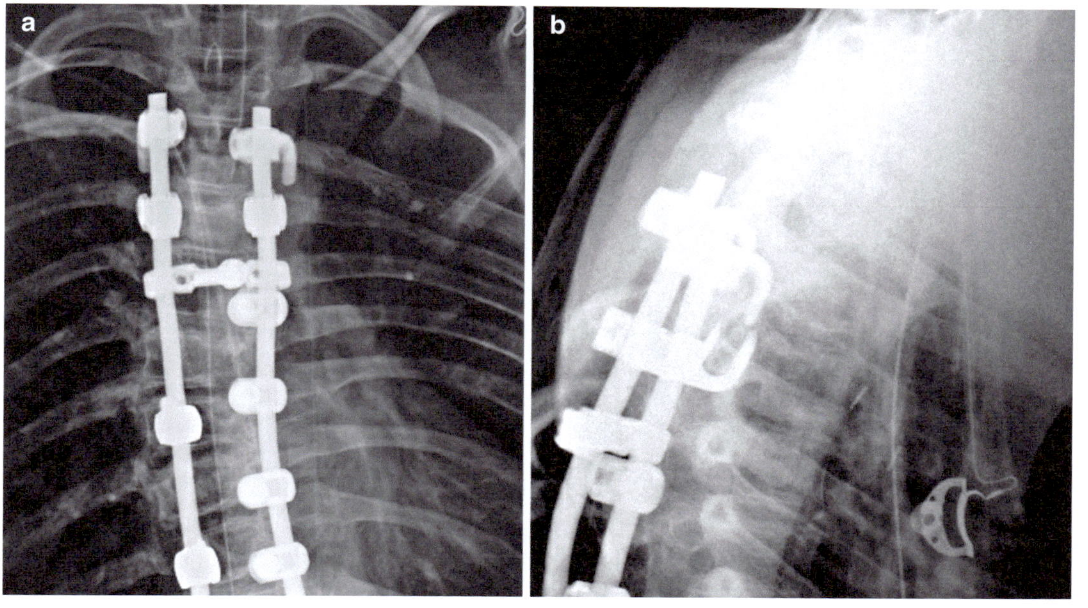

Fig. 25 Coronal (**a**) and sagittal (**b**) X-rays of a pediculo-transverse clamp in T3T4

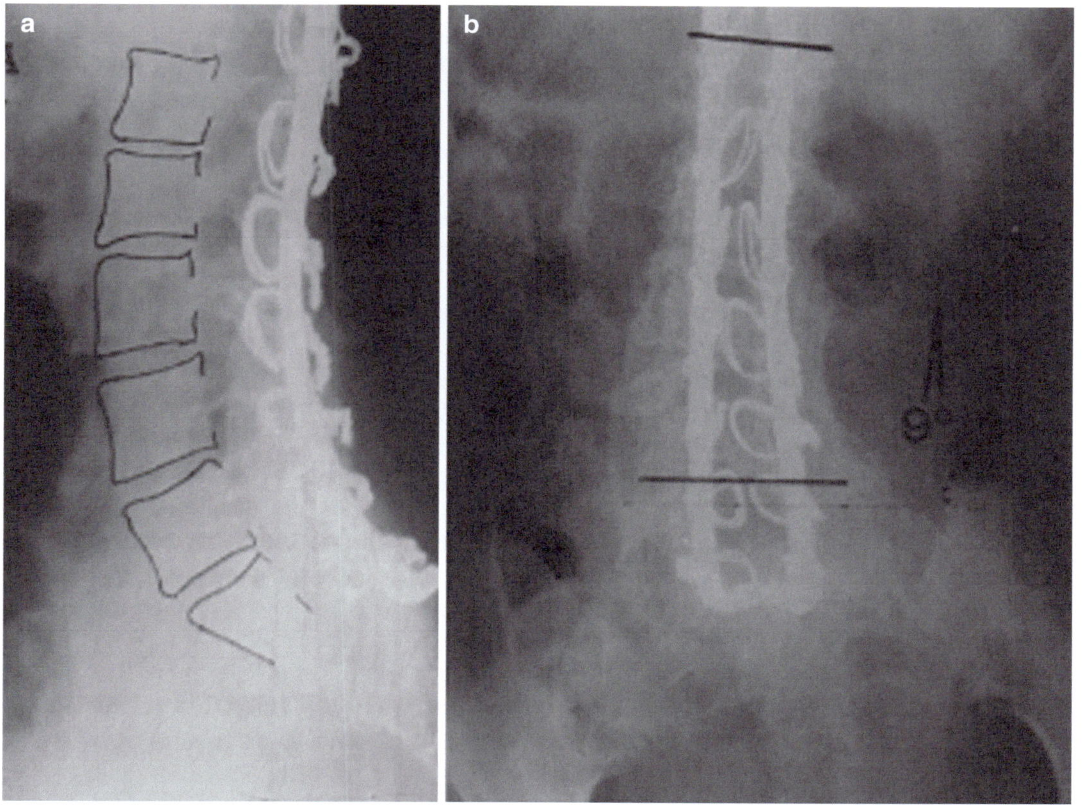

Fig. 26 Sagittal (**a**) and coronal (**b**) X-rays of a neurologic scoliosis correction with metallic wires. *(Cahiers d'enseignement de la SOFCOT n°53)*

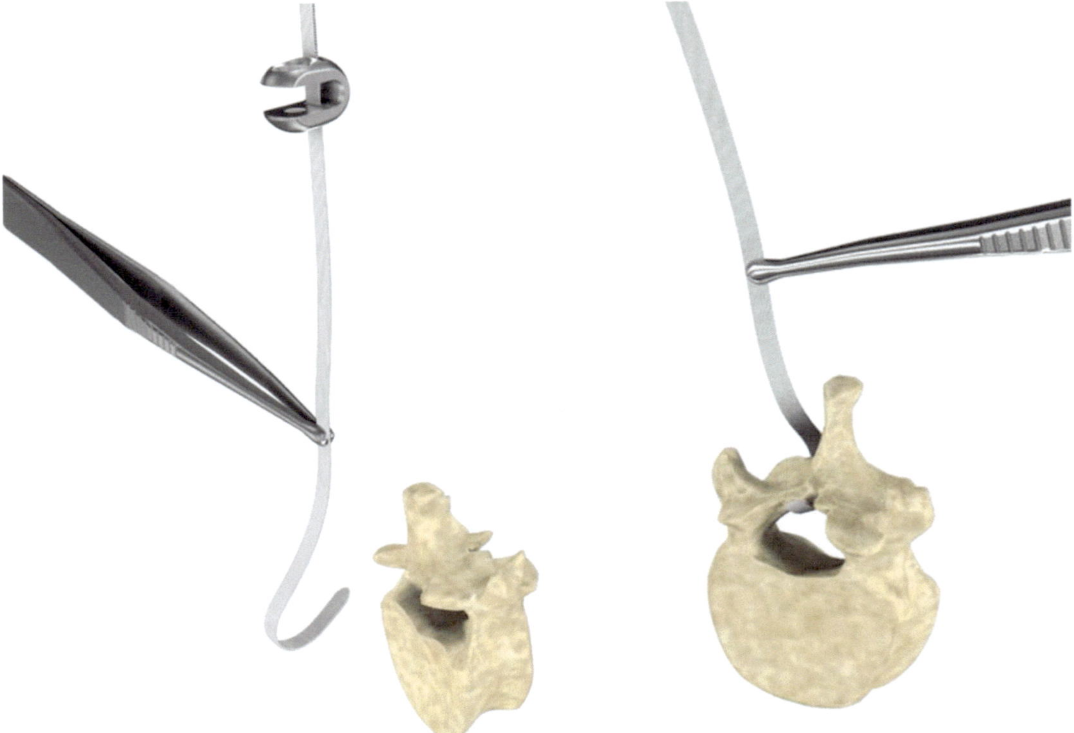

Fig. 27 Example of polyester band, passed under the lamina (Implanet©, Martillac, France)

lordosis; sublaminar bands in the concavity and apex of the thoracic deformity to correct the thoracic spine by posteromedial translation; and screws at the upper instrumented levels to balance the construct by compression and distraction (Fig. 28). In situ bending can also be used at any time during this procedure [24].

Postoperatively, imaging studies—particularly magnetic resonance imaging (MRI) of the canal—are possible because the bands are in polyester and the clamp is made of titanium, which limits artefacts.

Sublaminar bands may also be used on the lamina of the lower instrumented level to protect it from pull out. They are also more and more used on the upper instrumented vertebra (UIV) to protect from proximal junctional kyphosis (PJK). Doodkorte et al. conducted a biomechanical study of less rigid fixation techniques, including sublaminar ties and sublaminar bands and transverse hooks [25]. They demonstrated that these methods allowed a gradual transition of forces at the proximal end of the instrumentation, thus reducing the risk of PJK with a soft landing. Several techniques are available to achieve this ligament reinforcement. The oldest involves passing a band under the UIV lamina and a band under the overlying vertebra. The band is then tensioned over the rods using a suitable connector, more rarely over the screw heads (Fig. 29). A second technique consists in passing a band through the base of the spinous process, after perforating it with a drill. Some authors do this on the UIV and UIV + 1 or UIV + 2, sometimes the one below. The band is then tensioned on the rods using a connector (Fig. 30). A third, similar technique involves passing the bands through the spinous process, but this time linking it onto a crosslink positioned between the two rods (Fig. 31) [26–28].

When using an implant (hook, wire, band) inside the canal, attention must be paid to the diameter of the canal. Therefore, it is recommended to do a preoperative MRI or CT scan to detect a narrow canal or congenital abnormality.

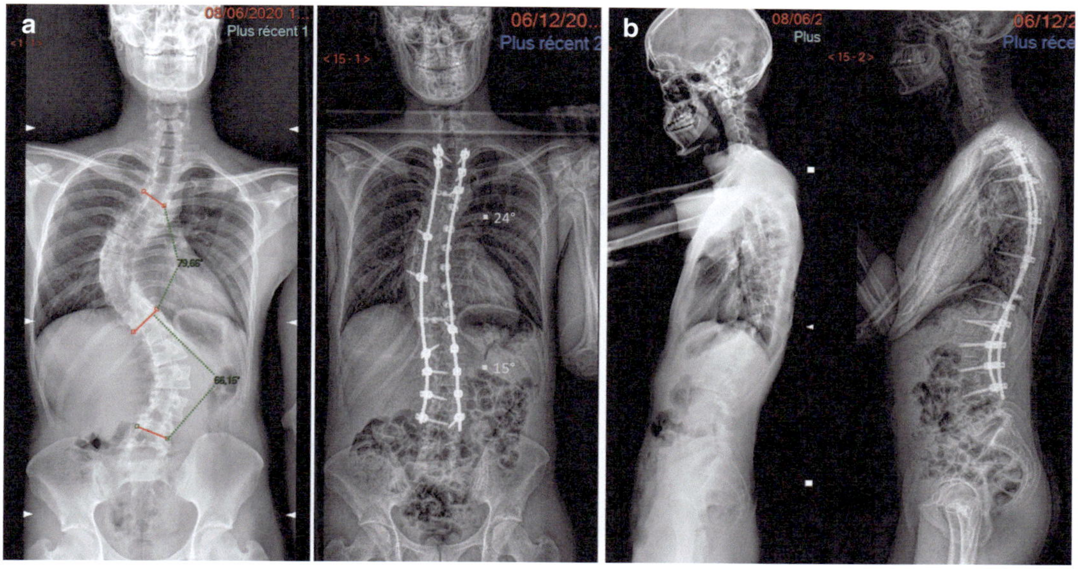

Fig. 28 Coronal (**a**) and sagittal (**b**) X-rays of an idiopathic scoliosis correction with screws and thoracic sublaminar bands

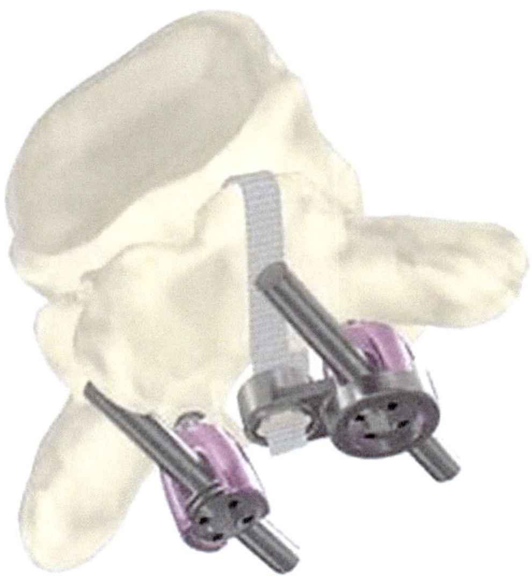

Fig. 29 Sublaminar bands fixed over the screw (Implanet©, Martillac, France)

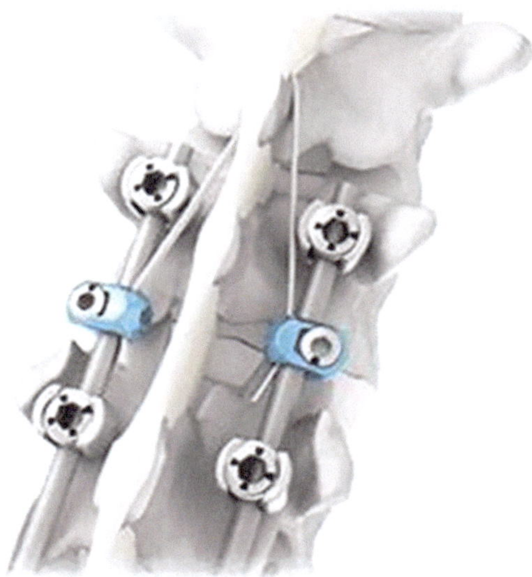

Fig. 30 Polyester band passed in the spinous process and fixed on the rods with a connector (Implanet©, Martillac, France)

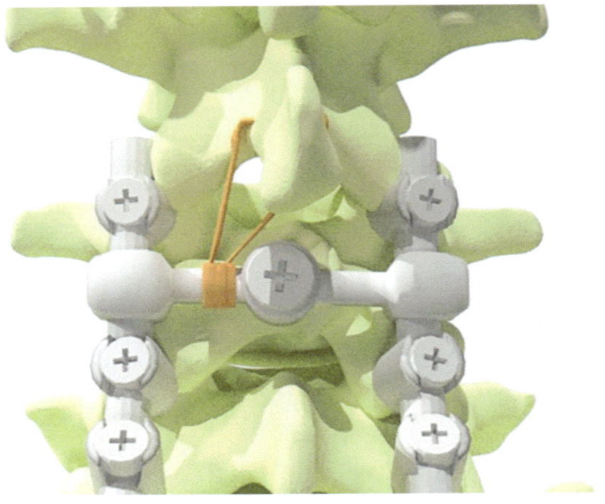

Fig. 31 Polyester band passed in the spinous process and fixed on a crosslink (*Tolga Sursal, Int J Spine Surg 2023* PMID: 37673684, PMCID: PMC10626134, https://doi.org/10.14444/8515)

2.2 Anterior Thoracic Instrumentation

2.2.1 Screws

Anterior instrumentation with screws is rarer than pedicle screws. It was mostly developed for scoliosis surgery. One of the first techniques was the one developed by Dwyer (1964) and then Zielke (1975), with the "Ventral Derotation Spondylodesis" [29, 30]. Today, the principle is similar. Through an anterior approach (a thoraco-phreno-lumbotomy approach), screws are inserted in the vertebral bodies anterior to the canal and compression or distraction is applied on the rods into the screws to correct the deformity (Fig. 32). Discectomy need to be performed at each instrumented level and bone graft is

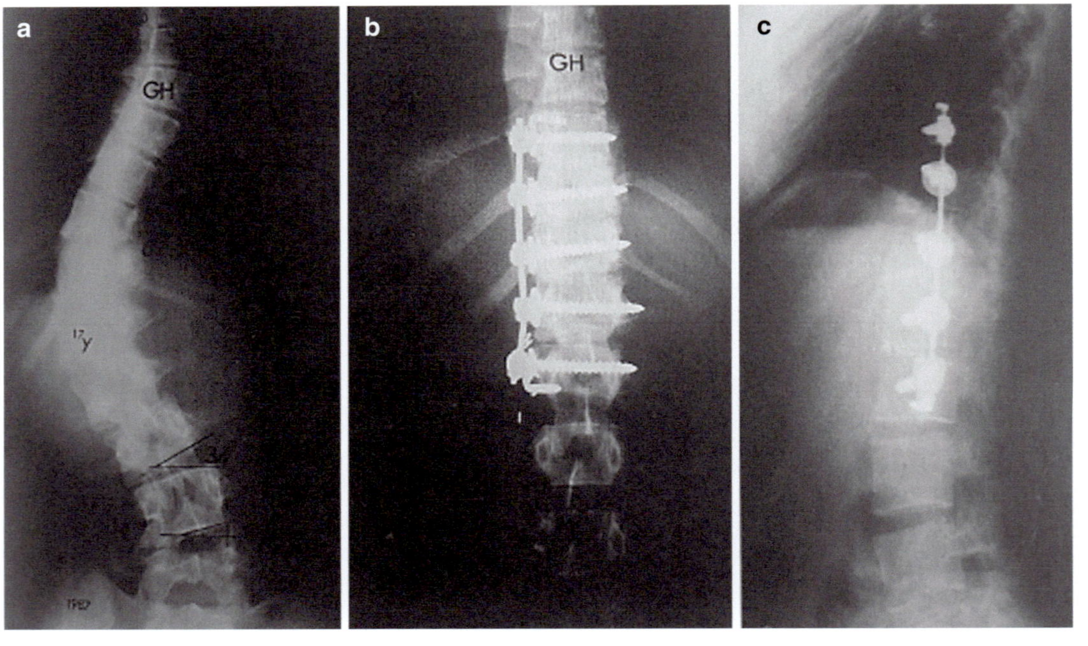

Fig. 32 Example of Zielke anterior instrumentation for a thoracolumbar scoliosis (**a**) preoperative coronal X-ray, (**b**) postoperative coronal X-ray, (**c**) postoperative sagittal X-ray) *(Cahiers d'enseignement de la SOFCOT n°53)*

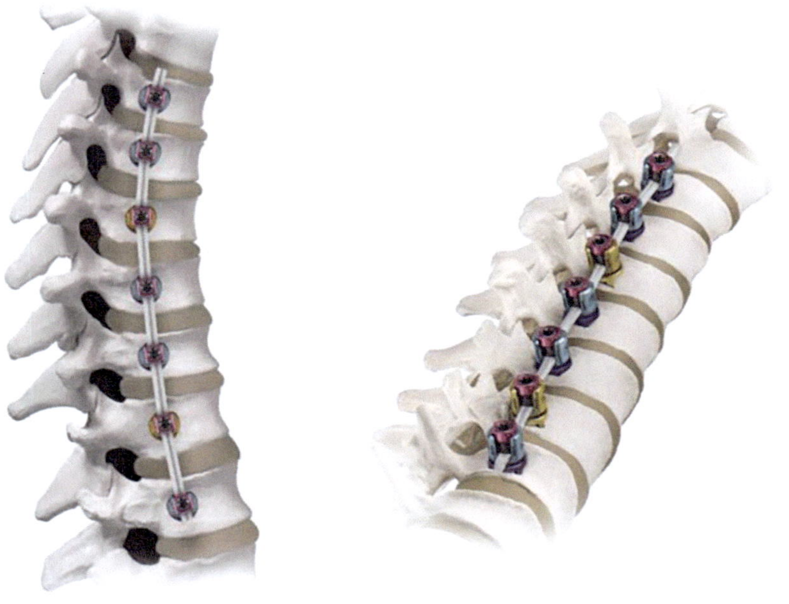

Fig. 33 Vertebral body tethering instrumentation (lateral and oblique view) (Implanet©, Martillac, France)

added into the disc spaces to perform fusion. It allows performing short selective fusion. Nevertheless, this instrumentation is not recommended in case of osteoporotic bone or very stiff curve.

A new anterior instrumentation is back in fashion since few years: the vertebral body tethering (VBT) [31, 32]. Under thoracoscopy, a polypropylene cable is tightened between a series of screws that are inserted into the vertebral bodies from the convexity of the scoliotic curvature. It allows correction for flexible adolescent idiopathic scoliosis with immature skeletons: intraoperatively with cable tension, which varies according to the patient's skeletal maturation and postoperatively with the deceleration of convex growth generated by the cable, combined with concave growth, which leads to additional correction over time (Fig. 33). However, specific indications for VBT are still debated.

2.2.2 Disc Cage and Plate

Anterior interbody fusion can be performed with disc cage in the thoracic spine through a lateral approach. It is particularly used at the thoracolumbar junction after posterior correction in case of disc opening and to improve fusion. A plate may be added to the interbody cage on the two adjacent vertebrae to improve stiffness. Anterior thoracic plate may also be used after anterior thoracic disc herniation resection (Fig. 34) [33].

2.2.3 Corpectomy Cage

They can be used in the thoracic spine through an anterior or posterior approach, associated with a posterior fusion with pedicle screws. They are inserted after an anterior corpectomy (for fracture, metastasis, spondylodiscitis) or a posterior vertebral column resection for deformity correction or tumor resection [34]. They need to be filled with bone (Fig. 35).

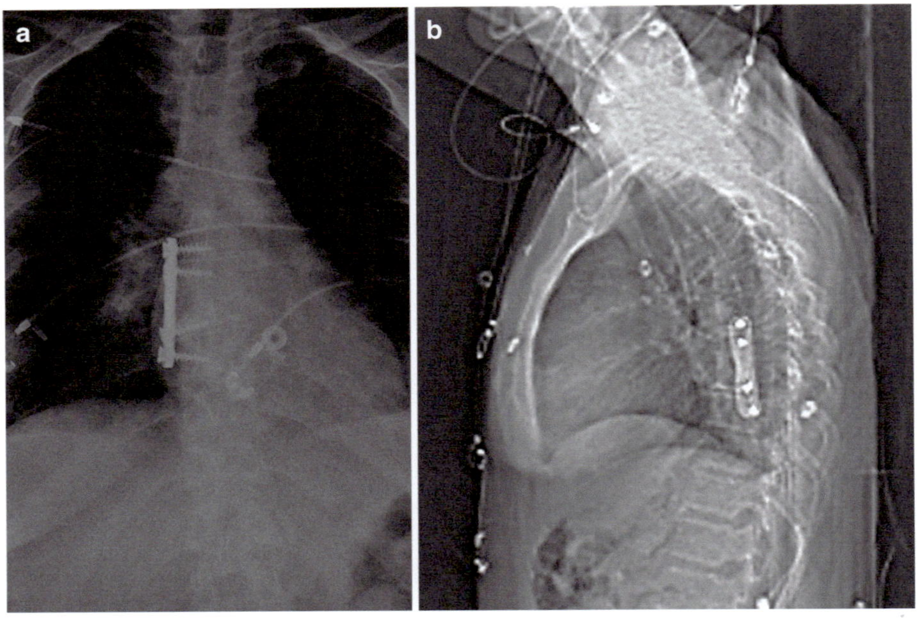

Fig. 34 Coronal (**a**) and sagittal (**b**) X-rays of a thoracic fixation with plate and screws after anterior herniated disc resection

Fig. 35 Coronal (**a**) and sagittal (**b**) X-rays of a kyphosis correction with vertebral column resection and mesh cage

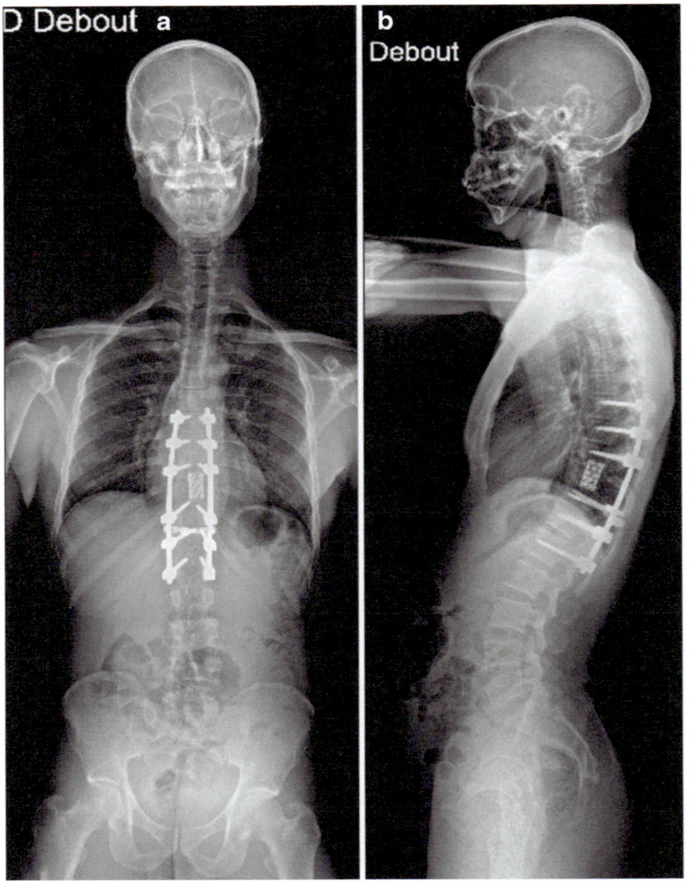

3 Lumbar Spine

3.1 Posterior Lumbar Instrumentation

3.1.1 Screws

Posterior instrumentation of the lumbar spine mainly consists of pedicle screws. A dedicated section details the different pedicle screw features in this chapter (Fig. 36).

Far less commonly used, certain surgeons use facet screws to perform lumbar spine fixation. There are a variety of implants and techniques. Thus, regular cortical screws can be used or specifically designed screws with cortical thread in the laminar part and cancellous for the articular part. These screws can cross midline with an entry point contralateral to the targeted facet or can be ipsilateral with a less diverging trajectory [35]. Certain companies also developed small cages to achieve facet fusion.

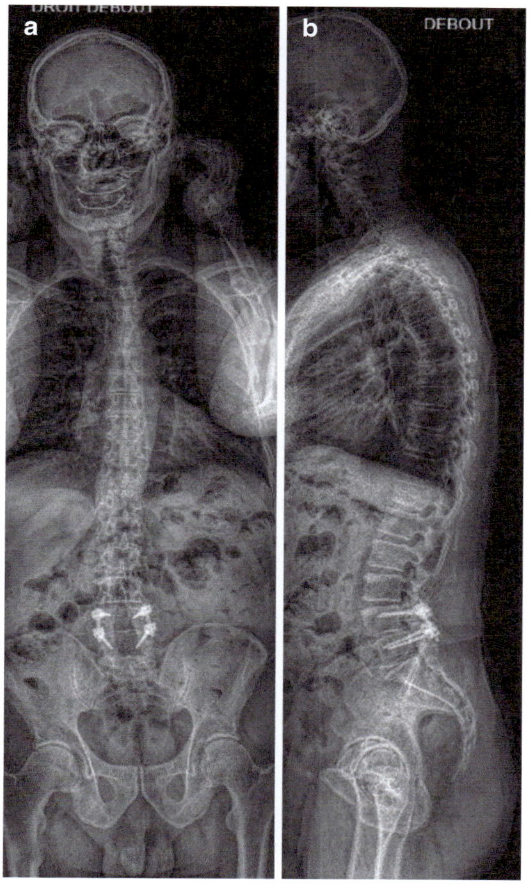

Fig. 36 Coronal (**a**) and sagittal (**b**) X-rays of lumbar pedicular screws

3.1.2 Hooks

Hooks are not used in degenerative lumbar surgery as central decompression is required in most of the cases, precluding the use of sublaminar hooks; and the use of pedicle hooks would be dangerous for the exiting nerve root and would require extensive facetectomy. However, in certain indications, sublaminar hooks can be useful implants. For instance, in lumbar fractures treated open, sublaminar hooks may be added to pedicle screws at the lower extremity of the construct to increase mechanical stability without having to extend one vertebral level lower (Fig. 37). Last, the use of sublaminar hooks can be found in indirect repairs of spondylolysis.

3.1.3 Pars Screws

Another type of screwing can be used in lumbar vertebrae to treat spondylolysis: the pars screw. Buck's technique has been described to repair pars nonunion with direct screwing of the pars, associated with bone graft of the osseous defect [35]. On each side, a 4.5 mm cortical screw is placed from the caudal part of the lamina directed toward the ipsilateral pedicle (Fig. 38). Repair techniques in spondylosis are to be indicated only if there is no or limited spondylolisthesis in young patients.

3.1.4 Interspinous Implants

Last, interspinous implants are used by certain teams to perform central stenosis decompression without the risk of neurological and dural complications associated with an intracanal surgery (Fig. 39). However, this technique induces kyphosis is the implant is too posterior as it increases the distance between the posterior arcs and may be insufficient to perform a thorough decompression, particularly in the lateral recesses and foramens. Outcome with such implants was not proven superior over conventional decompression [36, 37].

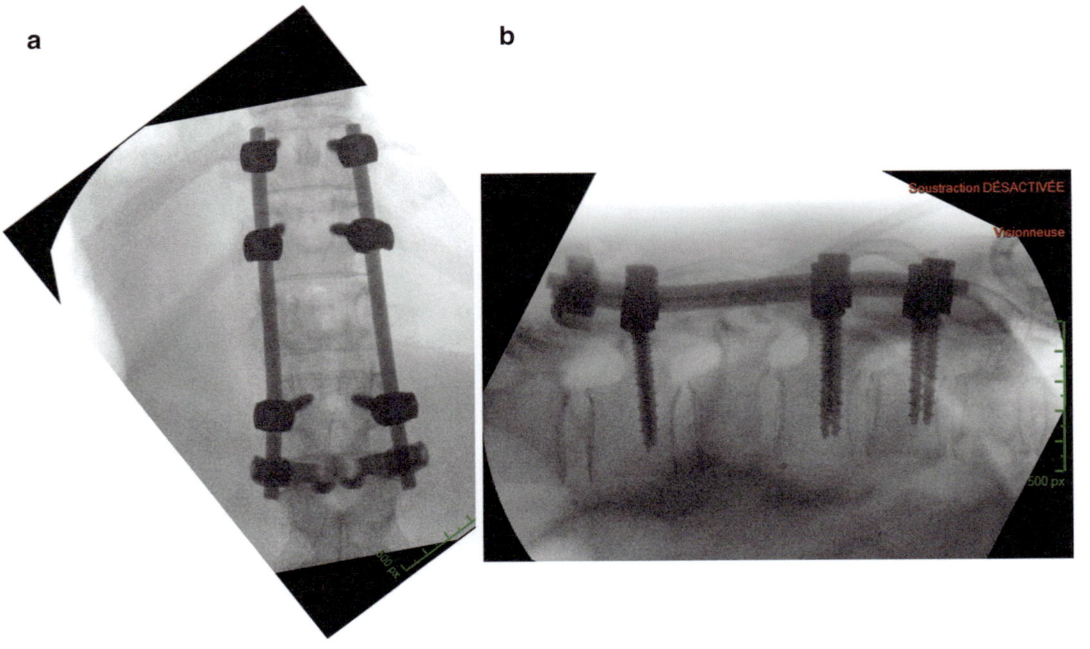

Fig. 37 Coronal (**a**) and sagittal (**b**) X-rays of T11 to L2 fixation, with hooks and screws on L2, for L1 fracture

3.2 Anterior Lumbar Instrumentation

There are various types of anterior column instrumentation: total disc replacement, anterior plates, corpectomy cages, and mainly interbody cages that can be implanted through a posterior or anterior approach. The design of interbody cages varies according to the approach, and are available in two materials: polyetheretherketone (PEEK) or titanium. To achieve fusion, these cages are filled with bone graft (autograft harvested from iliac crest or laminectomy), demineralized bone matrix, or rh-BMP2.

3.2.1 ALIF

Through an anterior approach, mainly retroperitoneal, anterior lumbar interbody fusion (ALIF) cages are implanted after disc removal and endplate preparation. These cages are fixed to the adjacent vertebral bodies by screws or blades (Fig. 40). An anterior plate can be added to increase mechanical stability. ALIF cages are the biggest cages, allowing great correction in the sagittal plane, as well as lower risk of subsidence [38]. However, there are specific complications associated with the anterior approach, particularly of vascular injury, which is why certain teams have this anterior approach performed by a vascular surgeon [39]. The vascular configuration must be assessed before undertaking this procedure. This anterior approach is used also for total disc replacement.

3.2.2 LLIF

Lateral approach has been described to implant interbody cages, with a far lower risk of vascular injury. Lumbotomy approach can be performed for levels above L5–S1, as the iliac crest is in the way otherwise. Some teams use an oblique approach for L5–S1, with an incision located in the iliac fossa (oblique lateral interbody fusion: OLIF). The lateral approach passes through the three layers of parietal muscles successively to reach the psoas. The spine can be reached either with a pre-psoatic approach by reclining the mus-

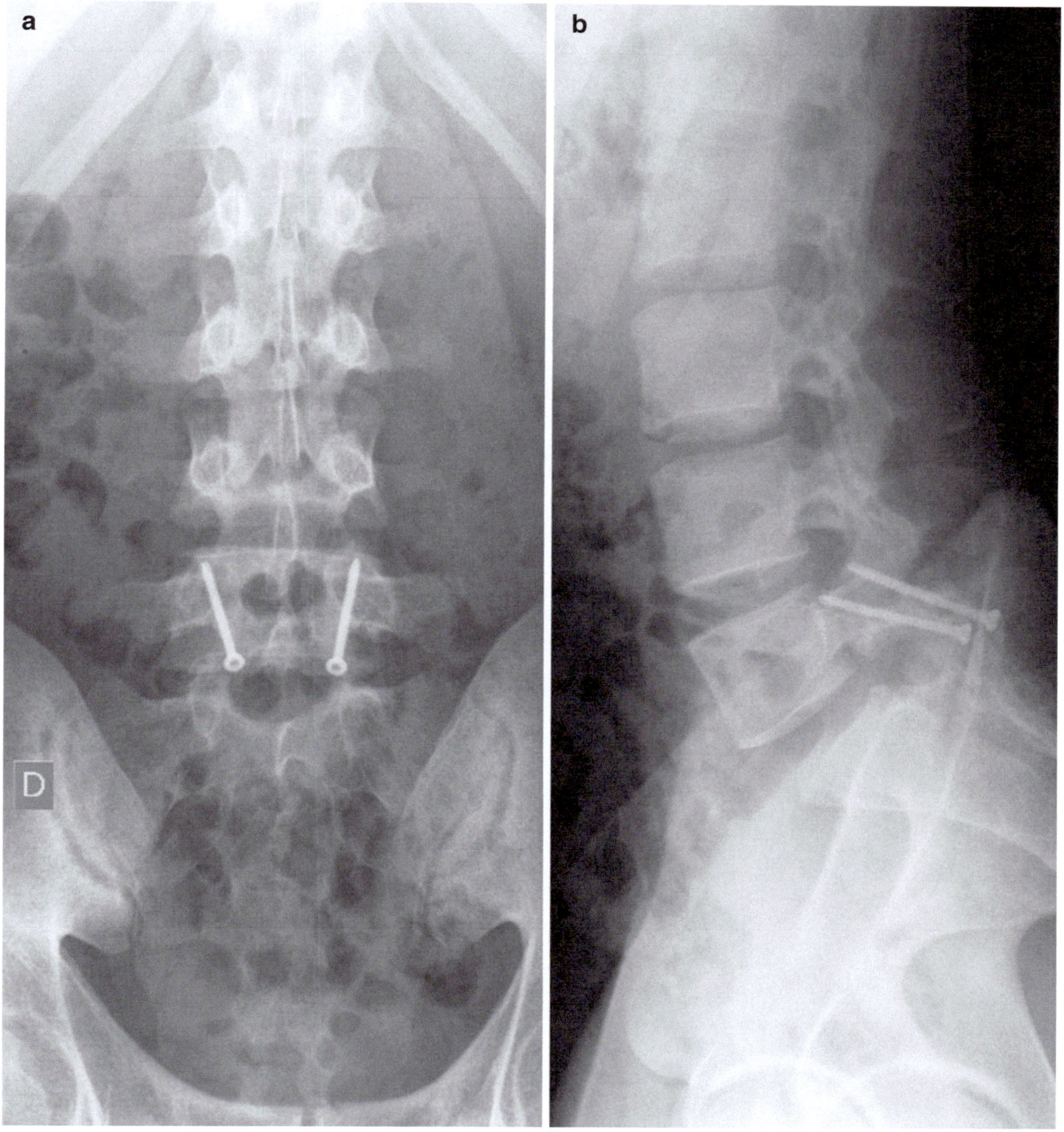

Fig. 38 Coronal (**a**) and sagittal (**b**) X-rays of pars screws

cle posteriorly, or through the psoas in which case intraoperative neuromonitoring is mandatory to locate lumbar nerve roots (Fig. 41). A higher subsidence rate has been described with this technique, requiring to implant wide cages crossing the lateral line of vertebral bodies on each side [40]. Lateral cages have the same fixation features, and a lateral plate can also be added to increase stability. This approach is also used for lumbar corpectomies above L5. To replace the vertebral body that has been totally or partially removed, a corpectomy cage is implanted, which can be in mesh, custom-made, or expandable (Fig. 42).

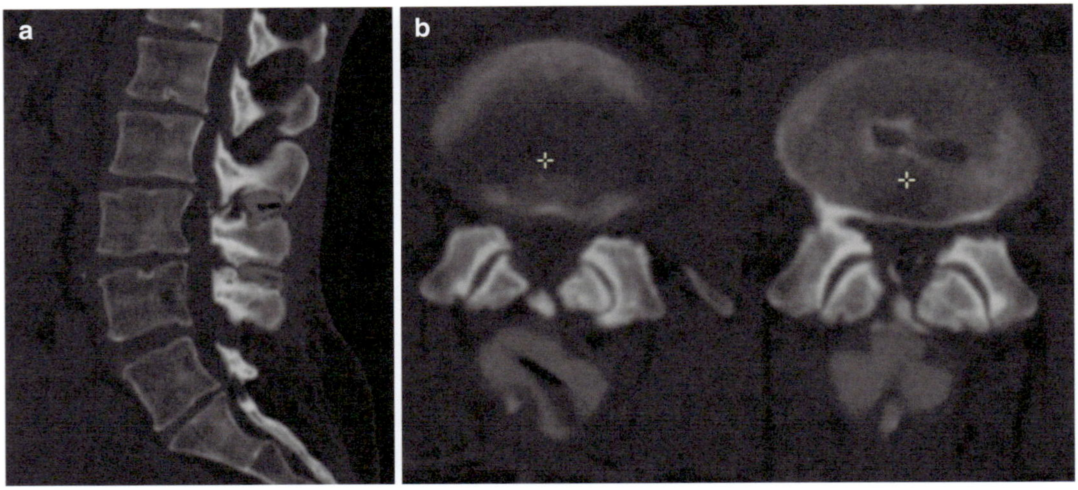

Fig. 39 Example of L2L3 and L3L4 interspinous implant with lumbar canal stenosis: sagittal (**a**) and axial (**b**) CT scan views

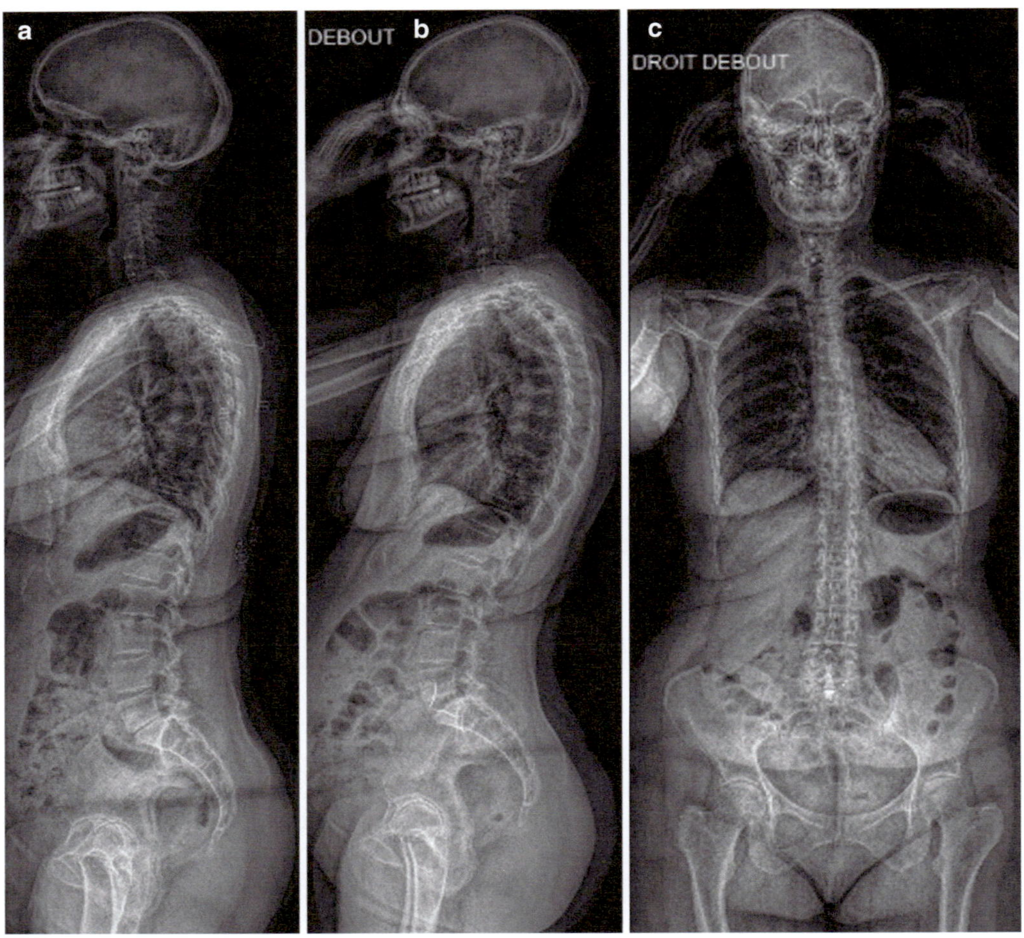

Fig. 40 Sagittal preoperative (**a**) and coronal (**c**) and sagittal (**b**) postoperative X-rays of a patient with L5S1 ALIF fixed with blades

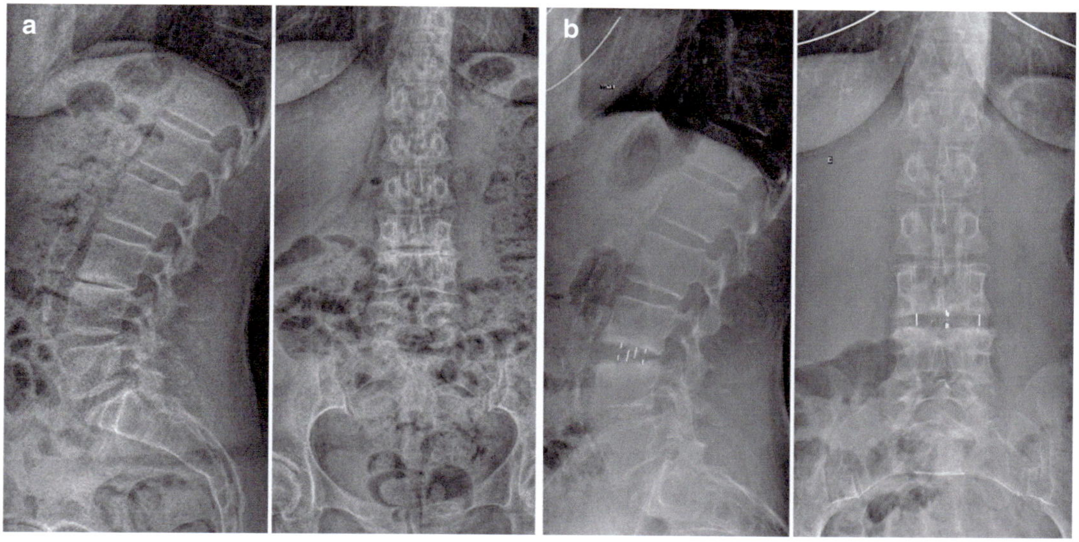

Fig. 41 Sagittal and coronal preoperative (**a**) and postoperative (**b**) X-rays of a patient with L3L4 LLIF

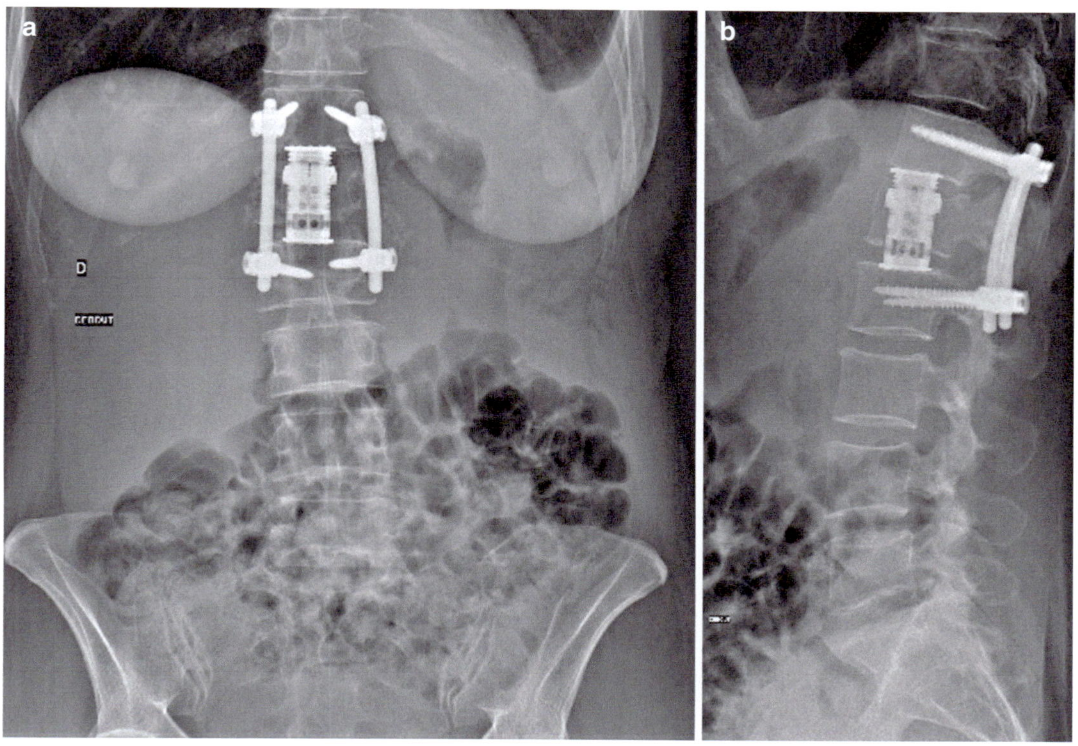

Fig. 42 Coronal (**a**) and sagittal (**b**) X-rays of L1 corpectomy with expandable cage

3.2.3 TLIF and PLIF

The two last lumbar interbody fusions are transforaminal (TLIF) and posterior (PLIF). Both procedures are performed during posterior approach, which presents the advantage of providing anterior column support without adding another procedure when a posterior has to be done, for decompression or extensive correction purposes. However, due to the presence of neurological structures, the disc is likely less thoroughly removed and the cages are smaller, thus increasing the risk of subsidence. PLIF cages are straight and are implanted on each side without extensive resection of the articular processes, unlike TLIF cages (Fig. 43). The latter ones can be banana-shaped, requiring rotation to be placed in the anterior third of the interbody space (Fig. 44). There are also straight TLIF cages that can be used asymmetrically to correct coronal deformity. The indication to implant PLIF or TLIF cages in addition to the pedicle screw construct remains debated. Although certain authors found no benefit in adding a TLIF cage, others recommend its use in kyphotic or mobile spondylolisthesis, and if an inflammatory disc disease is associated [41, 42].

3.3 Pedicle Screws

The principle of instrumenting the thoracic and lumbar spine using pedicle screws was developed by Raymond Roy-Camille in 1963, utilized with plates [13]. More than two decades later, Yves Cotrel and Jean Dubousset transformed spinal osteosynthesis with the "CD" system, allowing a segmental fixation, first using hooks, then using pedicle screws [43]. Since their creation, several generations of screws have been marketed, with features that evolved such as dual thread (Fig. 45). Pedicle screws are now widely used in spinal surgery and are available in different designs serving various purposes, as detailed hereafter.

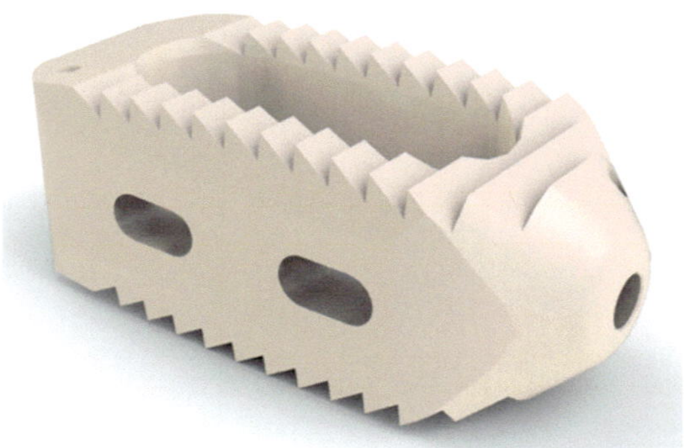

Fig. 43 Example of a PLIF cage (Novaspine©, Amiens, France)

Screws are made up of a threaded part that varies in length and diameter (different threads exist) and a screw head. Different types of screws are available: polyaxial, monoaxial, and uniplanar. The most common type of pedicle screw has a "tulip-shaped" head, with a top loading of the rod, further blocked by locking screws. In some instrumentation systems, the rod is loaded through the side using a connector or a lateral hole in the head.

Monoaxial screws feature no mobility between the head and the shank, avoiding any loss of correction in the adaptive angulation of the head during maneuvers [44]. However, this characteristic makes it more difficult to use monoaxial screws in spinal deformity cases. Hence, polyaxial screws are the most commonly used as they offer the greatest ease of use. The mobility of the head can be partially regulated by tightening the screw deeper, thus blocking head mobility on the spinal posterior arc. More recently, uniplanar screws have been marketed, offering head mobility along the craniocaudal axis but none in the coronal plane. These screws can be used in deformity cases as their partial mobility makes them easy to use, and the uniplanar feature allows a greater correction in the coronal plane and direct vertebral derotation [45].

Pedicle screws can be used for minimally invasive or percutaneous surgery. In the latter, the screw heads must have extensions in order to enable the insertion of the rod after the placement of all pedicle screws. In most cases, these screws are cannulated to allow their insertion using a Kirschner wire after having catheterized the pedicle with Jamshidi trocars. Fenestrated screws may also be used to enable cement augmentation of the vertebral body [46].

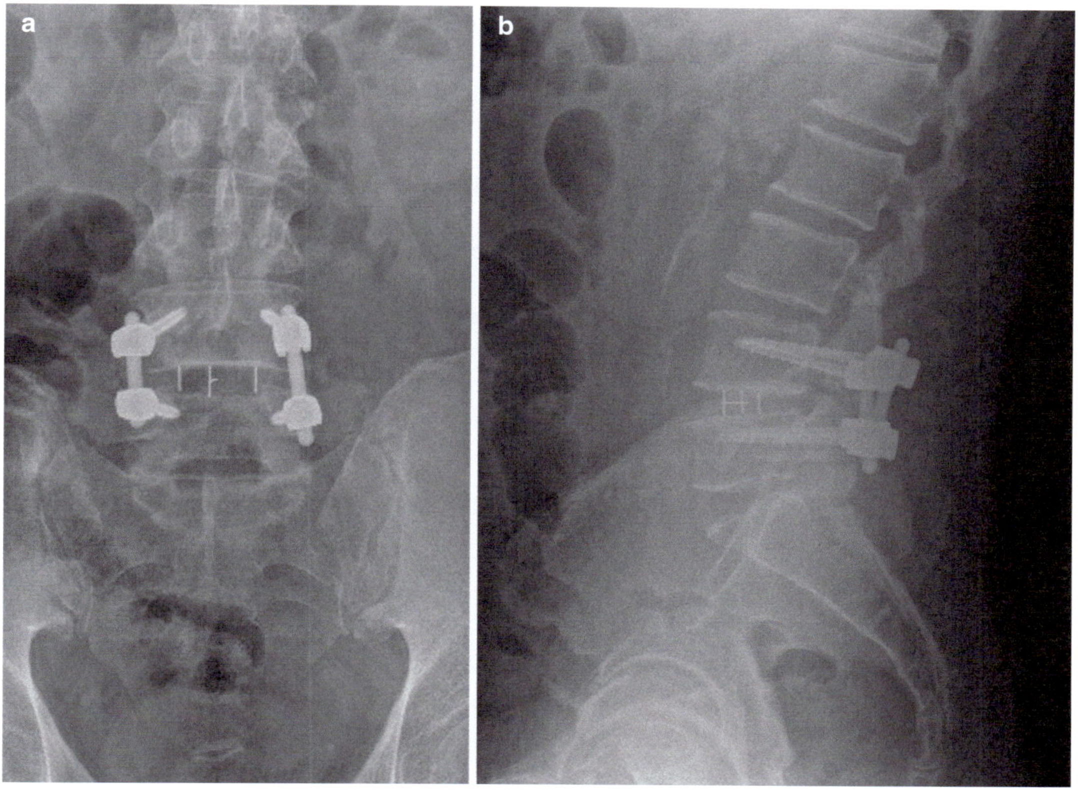

Fig. 44 Coronal (**a**) and sagittal (**b**) X-rays of L4L5 TLIF

Fig. 45 Example of a simple (**a**) and dual (**b**) thread pedicular screw

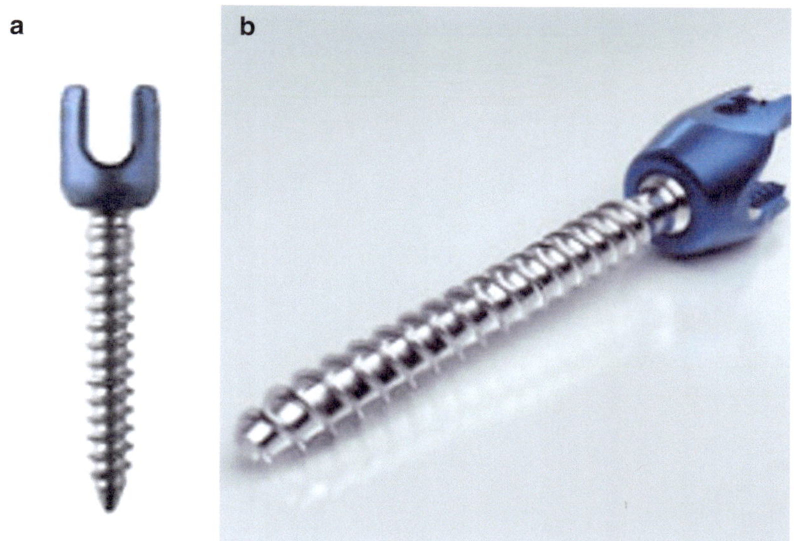

While the pedicle screws are the most frequently used, certain surgeons prefer to use cortical screws. Pedicle screws are oriented in convergence to provide better pullout strength, parallel to the upper endplate, whereas the cortical screw's trajectory is divergent toward the ipsilateral upper corner of the vertebral body. This technique would permit a positioning of the screw in a bone of greater quality [16].

Last, on top of this great variety of screws, there are various types of rods that can be used for spinal osteosynthesis. Hence, rods can differ in terms of diameter and material. The rods are usually made of, from the most to the least flexible: pure titanium, a titanium alloy, or cobalt-chrome. Increased rod diameter plus cobalt-chrome rods augment the power of correction as more flexible rods partially lose contouring during maneuvers. However, stiffer constructs may be more frequently associated with implant failure. More and more teams also increase the number of rods, reaching up to six rods, to decrease the stress on the primary rods [47]. Conversely, other teams use flexible rods to provide a dynamic stabilization of the spine (Fig. 46). Even though motion is preserved, instrumented

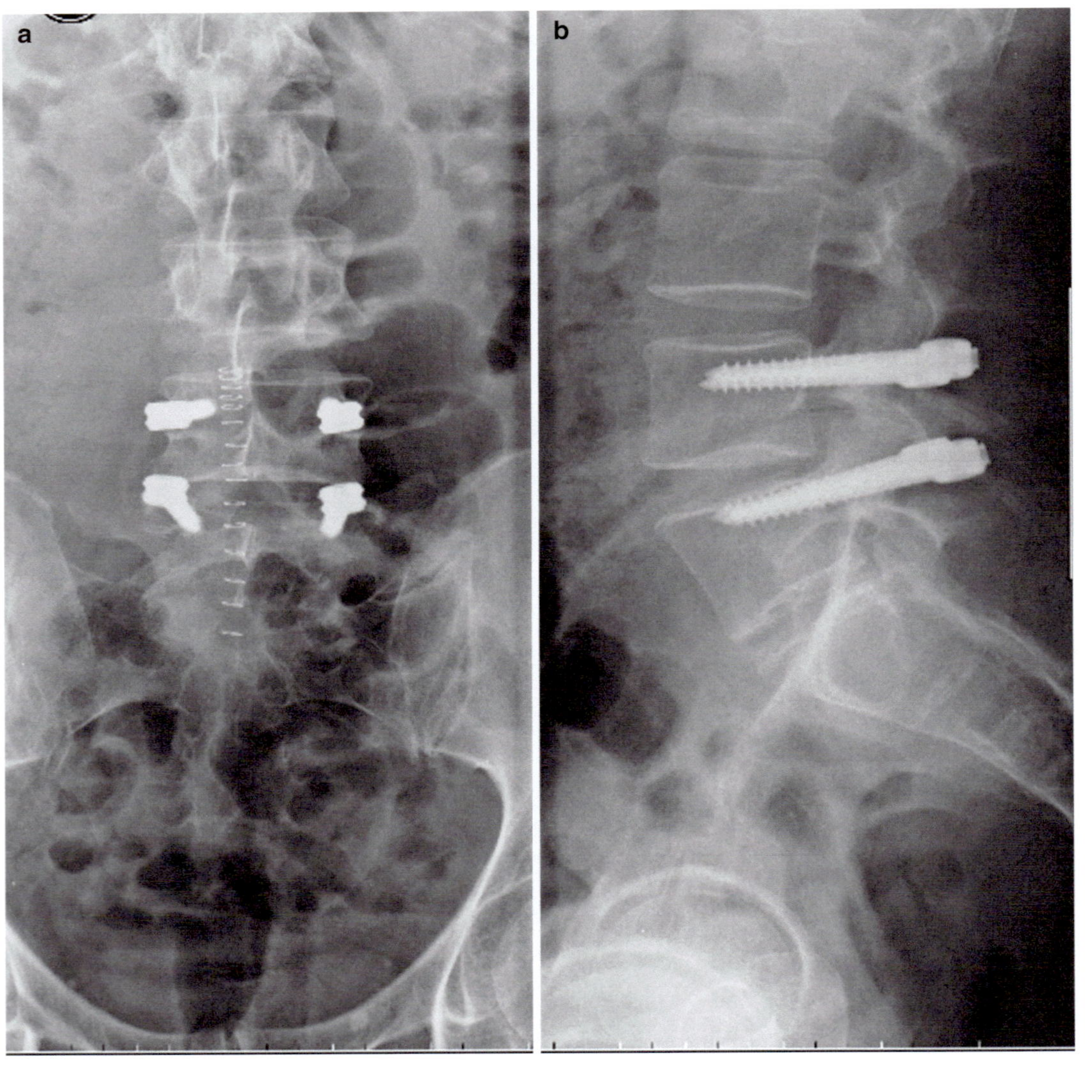

Fig. 46 Coronal (**a**) and sagittal (**b**) X-rays of L4L5 dynamic stabilization

segments frequently end up fused eventually [48]. This technique is claimed to decrease the rate of adjacent segment disease.

4 Pelvic Fixation

Fixations to the pelvis are commonly performed in degenerative and deformity surgery. Thus, it is essential to know the different techniques that can be used. Fixation to the pelvis includes almost systematically pedicle screws in S1. Similarly to the pedicle screws in the lumbar or thoracic spine, these screws are placed on the lateral aspect of the articular process base. However, as sacral bone is often of poor quality, it is recommended that pedicle screws cross the anterior cortex of S1 [49]. Rarely used, mainly in the setting of pelvic fractures, S2 screws can be placed. Their trajectory is divergent to maximize intraosseous length. However, their mechanical grip in the bone is rarely satisfactory.

It is recommended to add a fixation to the ilium whenever the construct spans higher than L3: the three main types are S2AI, iliac, and ilio-sacral screws [50]. S2-alar-iliac (S2AI) screws are inserted on a little ridge between the first and the second dorsal sacral foramen. The trajectory of the screw is orientated ventrally and caudally, crosses the sacro-iliac joint and ends in the iliac bone (Fig. 47). These screws can be placed under navigation control or "tear drop" incidence fluoroscopy.

Iliac screws do not cross the sacro-iliac joint and are implanted only in the iliac bone. It is recommended to avoid any issue related with screws prominence [51]. Due to the lateral entry point of these screws, a connector is usually required to compensate for this offset with S1 screw. Iliac screws trajectory is generally more caudally and ventrally orientated than S2AI screws (Fig. 48).

Ilio-sacral screws require a small lateral incision as the screw is implanted from lateral to medial. Through the median approach, a connector is placed at the usual location of S1 pedicle screw. This connector is composed of a tulip head linked to a ring within the S1 pedicle. The screw is then placed from the iliac bone to the S1 body through the connector, using dedicated instrumentation (Fig. 49). Intraoperative navigation is useful in this case to help position the screw [52].

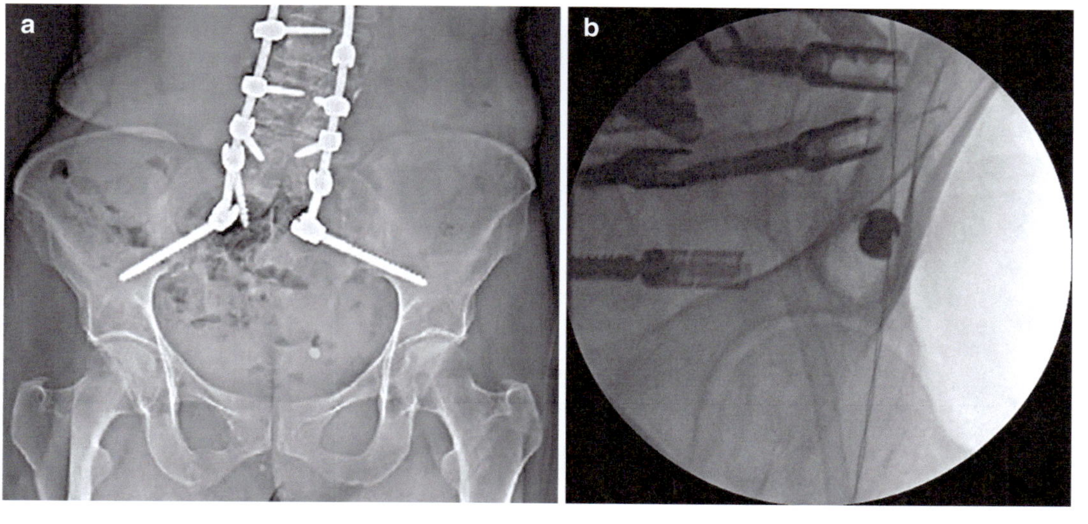

Fig. 47 Coronal X-rays of S2AI screws (**a**) and tear drop incidence (**b**)

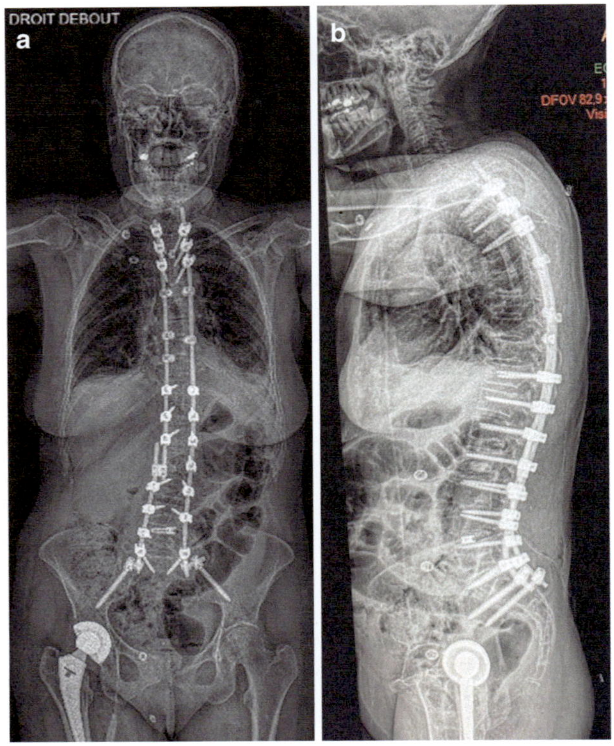

Fig. 48 Coronal (**a**) and sagittal (**b**) X-rays of iliac screws for ASD surgery

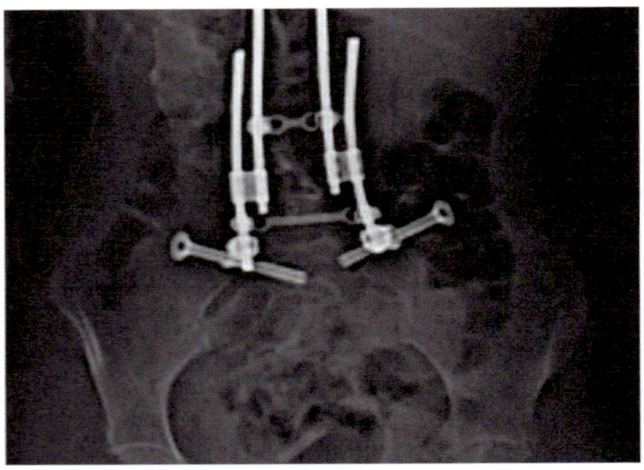

Fig. 49 Coronal X-rays of ilio-sacral screws for neurologic scoliosis

5 Conclusion

Numerous implants are available for spinal instrumentation. While the techniques for implants insertion are well defined, their use is wild.

Before using them, therefore, it is essential to clearly define the surgical objectives in order to choose the right instrumentation technique. It is also necessary to assess spinal anatomy and bone density, as well as whether root canal release or deformity correction is indicated, in order to choose the right implants. Thus, a complete preoperative planning adapted to the patient is important.

Statements and Declarations

E Ferrero: consulting for Implanet and Medtronic

M Khalifé: stock options in Novaspine

L. Chatelain: none

Fundings None.

References

1. Coe JD, Vaccaro AR, Dailey AT, et al. Lateral mass screw fixation in the cervical spine: a systematic literature review. J Bone Joint Surg Am. 2013;95:2136–43. https://doi.org/10.2106/JBJS.L.01522.
2. Abumi K, Kaneda K. Pedicle screw fixation for nontraumatic lesions of the cervi-

cal spine. Spine. 1997;22:1853–63. https://doi.org/10.1097/00007632-199708150-00010.
3. Shin HK, Jeon SR, Roh SW, Park JH. Benefits and pitfalls of O-Arm navigation in cervical pedicle screw. World Neurosurg. 2022;159:e460–5. https://doi.org/10.1016/j.wneu.2021.12.077.
4. Harms J, Melcher RP. Posterior C1-C2 fusion with polyaxial screw and rod fixation. Spine. 2001;26:2467–71. https://doi.org/10.1097/00007632-200111150-00014.
5. Schulz R, Macchiavello N, Fernández E, et al. Harms C1-C2 instrumentation technique: anatomo-surgical guide. Spine. 2011;36:945–50. https://doi.org/10.1097/BRS.0b013e3181e887df.
6. Heywood AW, Learmonth ID, Thomas M. Internal fixation for occipito-cervical fusion. J Bone Joint Surg Br. 1988;70:708–11. https://doi.org/10.1302/0301-620X.70B5.3192565.
7. Fagerström T, Hedlund R. Cotrel Dubousset instrumentation in occipito-cervico-thoracic fusion. Eur Spine J Off Publ Eur Spine Soc Eur Spinal Deform Soc Eur Sect Cerv Spine Res Soc. 2002;11:364–74. https://doi.org/10.1007/s00586-002-0392-z.
8. Dossani RH, Shaughnessy J, Kalakoti P, Nanda A. William Edward Gallie (1882–1959): father of the Gallie wiring technique for atlantoaxial arthrodesis. J Neurosurg. 2018;128:938–41. https://doi.org/10.3171/2016.12.JNS161224.
9. Nikolaidis I, Fouyas IP, Sandercock PA, Statham PF. Surgery for cervical radiculopathy or myelopathy. Cochrane Database Syst Rev. 2010;2010:CD001466. https://doi.org/10.1002/14651858.CD001466.pub3.
10. Castellvi AE, Castellvi A, Clabeaux DH. Corpectomy with titanium cage reconstruction in the cervical spine. J Clin Neurosci Off J Neurosurg Soc Australas. 2012;19:517–21. https://doi.org/10.1016/j.jocn.2011.06.029.
11. Pojskic M, Saβ B, Nimsky C, Carl B. Application of an expandable cage for reconstruction of the cervical spine in a consecutive series of eighty-six patients. Med Kaunas Lith. 2020;56:642. https://doi.org/10.3390/medicina56120642.
12. Perna F, Borghi R, Pilla F, et al. Pedicle screw insertion techniques: an update and review of the literature. Musculoskelet Surg. 2016;100:165–9. https://doi.org/10.1007/s12306-016-0438-8.
13. Roy-Camille R, Saillant G, Mazel C. Internal fixation of the lumbar spine with pedicle screw plating. Clin Orthop. 1986;203:7–17.
14. Roy-Camille R, Petchot P. The treatment of dorsal and lumbar spinal injuries using posterior plates screwed into the pedicle. Acta Orthop Belg. 1991;57(Suppl 1):184–90.
15. Dick W. The "fixateur interne" as a versatile implant for spine surgery. Spine. 1987;12:882–900. https://doi.org/10.1097/00007632-198711000-00009.
16. Kolz JM, Pinter ZW, Bydon M, Sebastian AS. Controversies in spine surgery: is a cortical bone trajectory superior to traditional pedicle screw trajectory? Clin Spine Surg. 2022;35:225–8. https://doi.org/10.1097/BSD.0000000000000965.
17. Dubousset J, Cotrel Y. Application technique of Cotrel-Dubousset instrumentation for scoliosis deformities. Clin Orthop. 1991;264:103–10.
18. Helenius I, Remes V, Yrjönen T, et al. Harrington and Cotrel-Dubousset instrumentation in adolescent idiopathic scoliosis. Long-term functional and radiographic outcomes. J Bone Joint Surg Am. 2003;85-A:2303–9.
19. Cotrel Y, Dubousset J, Guillaumat M. New universal instrumentation in spinal surgery. Clin Orthop. 1988;227:10–23.
20. Lonstein JE. The Galveston technique using Luque or Cotrel-Dubousset rods. Orthop Clin North Am. 1994;25:311–20.
21. McMaster MJ. Luque rod instrumentation in the treatment of adolescent idiopathic scoliosis. A comparative study with Harrington instrumentation. J Bone Joint Surg Br. 1991;73:982–9. https://doi.org/10.1302/0301-620X.73B6.1955449.
22. Ilharreborde B, Sebag G, Skalli W, Mazda K. Adolescent idiopathic scoliosis treated with posteromedial translation: radiologic evaluation with a 3D low-dose system. Eur Spine J Off Publ Eur Spine Soc Eur Spinal Deform Soc Eur Sect Cerv Spine Res Soc. 2013;22:2382–91. https://doi.org/10.1007/s00586-013-2776-7.
23. Gazzeri R, Faiola A, Galarza M, Tamorri M. Universal Clamp system in thoracolumbar spinal fixation: technical note. Acta Neurochir. 2009;151:1673–80. https://doi.org/10.1007/s00701-009-0495-y.
24. Sales de Gauzy J, Jouve J-L, Ilharreborde B, et al. Use of the Universal Clamp in adolescent idiopathic scoliosis. Eur Spine J Off Publ Eur Spine Soc Eur Spinal Deform Soc Eur Sect Cerv Spine Res Soc. 2014;23(Suppl 4):S446–51. https://doi.org/10.1007/s00586-014-3341-8.
25. Doodkorte RJP, Vercoulen TFG, Roth AK, et al. Instrumentation techniques to prevent proximal junctional kyphosis and proximal junctional failure in adult spinal deformity correction-a systematic review of biomechanical studies. Spine J Off J North Am Spine Soc. 2021;21:842–54. https://doi.org/10.1016/j.spinee.2021.01.011.
26. Sursal T, Kim HJ, Sardi JP, et al. Use of tethers for proximal junctional Kyphosis prophylaxis in adult spinal deformity surgery: a review of current clinical evidence. Int J Spine Surg. 2023;17:S26–37. https://doi.org/10.14444/8515.
27. Viswanathan VK, Minnema AJ, Viljoen S, Farhadi HF. Sublaminar banding as an adjunct to pedicle screw-rod constructs: a review and technical note on novel hybrid constructs in spinal deformity surgery. J Neurosurg Spine. 2019:1–7. https://doi.org/10.3171/2018.11.SPINE181154.
28. Safaee MM, Deviren V, Dalle Ore C, et al. Ligament augmentation for prevention of proximal junctional kyphosis and proximal junctional failure in adult spi-

nal deformity. J Neurosurg Spine. 2018;28:512–9. https://doi.org/10.3171/2017.9.SPINE1710.
29. Hall JE. Dwyer Instrumentation in anterior fusion of the spine. J Bone Joint Surg Am. 1981;63:1188–90.
30. Hammerberg KW, Rodts MF, DeWald RL. Zielke instrumentation. Orthopedics. 1988;11:1365–71. https://doi.org/10.3928/0147-7447-19881001-05.
31. Lonner B, Weiner DA, Miyanji F, et al. Vertebral body tethering: rationale, results, and revision. Instr Course Lect. 2022;71:413–25.
32. Mariscal G, Morales J, Pérez S, et al. Meta-analysis on the efficacy and safety of anterior vertebral body tethering in adolescent idiopathic scoliosis. Eur Spine J Off Publ Eur Spine Soc Eur Spinal Deform Soc Eur Sect Cerv Spine Res Soc. 2023;32:140–8. https://doi.org/10.1007/s00586-022-07448-9.
33. Boriani S, Biagini R, De Iure F, et al. Two-level thoracic disc herniation. Spine. 1994;19:2461–6. https://doi.org/10.1097/00007632-199411000-00018.
34. Ha AS, Cerpa M, Lenke LG. State of the art review: Vertebral Osteotomies for the management of Spinal Deformity. Spine Deform. 2020;8:829–43. https://doi.org/10.1007/s43390-020-00144-y.
35. Kumar N, Madhu S, Pandita N, et al. Is there a place for surgical repair in adults with spondylolysis or grade-I spondylolisthesis-a systematic review and treatment algorithm. Spine J Off J North Am Spine Soc. 2021;21:1268–85. https://doi.org/10.1016/j.spinee.2021.03.011.
36. Patil CG, Sarmiento JM, Ugiliweneza B, et al. Interspinous device versus laminectomy for lumbar spinal stenosis: a comparative effectiveness study. Spine J Off J North Am Spine Soc. 2014;14:1484–92. https://doi.org/10.1016/j.spinee.2013.08.053.
37. Schenck CD, Terpstra SES, Moojen WA, et al. Interspinous process device versus conventional decompression for lumbar spinal stenosis: 5-year results of a randomized controlled trial. J Neurosurg Spine. 2022;36:909–17. https://doi.org/10.3171/2021.8.SPINE21419.
38. Sun D, Liang W, Hai Y, et al. OLIF versus ALIF: which is the better surgical approach for degenerative lumbar disease? A systematic review. Eur Spine J Off Publ Eur Spine Soc Eur Spinal Deform Soc Eur Sect Cerv Spine Res Soc. 2023;32:689–99. https://doi.org/10.1007/s00586-022-07516-0.
39. Than KD, Wang AC, Rahman SU, et al. Complication avoidance and management in anterior lumbar interbody fusion. Neurosurg Focus. 2011;31:E6. https://doi.org/10.3171/2011.7.FOCUS11141.
40. Yuan W, Kaliya-Perumal A-K, Chou SM, Oh JY-L. Does Lumbar interbody cage size influence subsidence? A biomechanical study. Spine. 2020;45:88–95. https://doi.org/10.1097/BRS.0000000000003194.
41. Loubeyre J, Ferrero E, Jmal MM, et al. Surgical treatment of degenerative lumbar spondylolisthesis: Effect of TLIF and slip reduction on sagittal alignment. Orthop Traumatol Surg Res OTSR. 2023;109:103541. https://doi.org/10.1016/j.otsr.2022.103541.
42. Guigui P, Ferrero E. Surgical treatment of degenerative spondylolisthesis. Orthop Traumatol Surg Res OTSR. 2017;103:S11–20. https://doi.org/10.1016/j.otsr.2016.06.022.
43. Gurr KR, McAfee PC. Cotrel-Dubousset instrumentation in adults. A preliminary report Spine. 1988;13:510–20. https://doi.org/10.1097/00007632-198805000-00014.
44. Lonner BS, Auerbach JD, Boachie-Adjei O, et al. Treatment of thoracic scoliosis: are monoaxial thoracic pedicle screws the best form of fixation for correction? Spine. 2009;34:845–51. https://doi.org/10.1097/BRS.0b013e31819e2753.
45. Liu P-Y, Lai P-L, Lin C-L. A biomechanical investigation of different screw head designs for vertebral derotation in scoliosis surgery. Spine J Off J North Am Spine Soc. 2017;17:1171–9. https://doi.org/10.1016/j.spinee.2017.04.010.
46. Elder BD, Lo S-FL, Holmes C, et al. The biomechanics of pedicle screw augmentation with cement. Spine J Off J North Am Spine Soc. 2015;15:1432–45. https://doi.org/10.1016/j.spinee.2015.03.016.
47. Shekouhi N, Vosoughi AS, Zavatsky JM, et al. Biomechanical comparison of multi-rod constructs by satellite rod configurations (in-line vs. lateral) and screw types (monoaxial vs. polyaxial) spanning a lumbar pedicle subtraction osteotomy (PSO): is there an optimal configuration? Eur Spine J Off Publ Eur Spine Soc Eur Spinal Deform Soc Eur Sect Cerv Spine Res Soc. 2022;31:3050–9. https://doi.org/10.1007/s00586-022-07331-7.
48. Khalifé M, Devriese F, Ferrero E, et al. Dynesys® dynamic stabilization outcomes in degenerative spine surgery. Acta Orthop Belg. 2021;87:795–803. https://doi.org/10.52628/87.4.28.
49. Coskun E, Wellington IJ, Bellas N, et al. Determination of a neurologic safe zone for bicortical S1 pedicle screw placement. Spine J Off J North Am Spine Soc. 2022;22:1708–15. https://doi.org/10.1016/j.spinee.2022.04.016.
50. Cunningham BW, Sefter JC, Hu N, et al. Biomechanical comparison of iliac screws versus interbody femoral ring allograft on lumbosacral kinematics and sacral screw strain. Spine. 2010;35:E198–205. https://doi.org/10.1097/BRS.0b013e3181c142bf.
51. De la Garza RR, Nakhla J, Sciubba DM, Yassari R. Iliac screw versus S2 alar-iliac screw fixation in adults: a meta-analysis. J Neurosurg Spine. 2018;30:253–8. https://doi.org/10.3171/2018.7.SPINE18710.
52. Dubousset J, Gaume M, Miladi L. Ilio-sacral screw pelvic fixation when correcting spinal deformities with or without pelvic obliquity: our experience over 40 years. Spine Deform. 2021;9:665–70. https://doi.org/10.1007/s43390-020-00263-6.

Biomaterials in Spine Surgery

Jérôme Tonetti and Mehdi Boudissa

1 Introduction

A raw definition of biomaterials could be "materials that could be implanted in biological organism." Since surgeons aim to implant devices, they had to choose solution tolerable, at their time, regarding the service they gave. Surgeons sometimes were not aware of unexpected drawback effects but look at immediate properties as this copper sleeve, which made bone restore [1]. Lane [2] in 1895 used metal plate and screws to fix recent limb fractures with a great immediate effect [2]. Corrosion appearance leads surgeons to change for stainless steel (316 L alloy). Jules Guérin did the first spine surgery attempt in 1839 [3]. No device was implant but tenotomy of para spinous muscles was made. Hadra used the first known device to fix C6–C7 instability in trauma a Pott's disease [4]. It was silver-made wire.

2 Expected Properties

Nowadays, what are the mandatory properties we are looking for?

J. Tonetti (✉) · M. Boudissa
Department of Surgical Orthopedics and Traumatology, CHU Grenoble Alpes, Grenoble, France
e-mail: JTonetti@chu-grenoble.fr; mboudissa@chu-grenoble.fr

2.1 Biocompatibility

Materials for implanted device should be biocompatible. Biostable or bioinert means no reaction of the body against the device or no toxicity of the device against the body. Becker et al. give a definition of biocompatibility: "the capability of a prosthesis implanted in the body to exist in harmony with tissue without causing deleterious changes" [5]. Wear debris or ions released locally or in the general circulation could be involved. High levels of biocompatibility mean they are rejected less often by the patient or cause less likely allergic reactions. The corrosion is the main issue. A classification of the corrosion ability is proposed after in vitro testing of the metals flowed into saline solution under galvanic conditions (Fig. 1) [6]. Out of 118 stainless steel (316 L) retrieved thoracolumbar plates, Majid et al. show 70% of the plates with galvanic corrosion, mainly at the screw–plate interface. They found reductions in nickel content in corroded areas. The design of the device might facilitate this high incidence of corrosion by fretting [7]. Other materials may be able to corrodate. Surgeons fear of galvanic corrosion complications when mix differing metal classes for spinal constructs, especially stainless steel (SS) and titanium. In vitro studies tell us that, despite the mixture of titanium alloy with SS is not advocated, galvanic corrosion is less pronounced in SS–titanium mixed interfaces than in all SS constructs

C. Y. Barrey (ed.), *Spine Surgery*, SFCR Experts Series 1,
https://doi.org/10.1007/978-3-031-85446-0_7

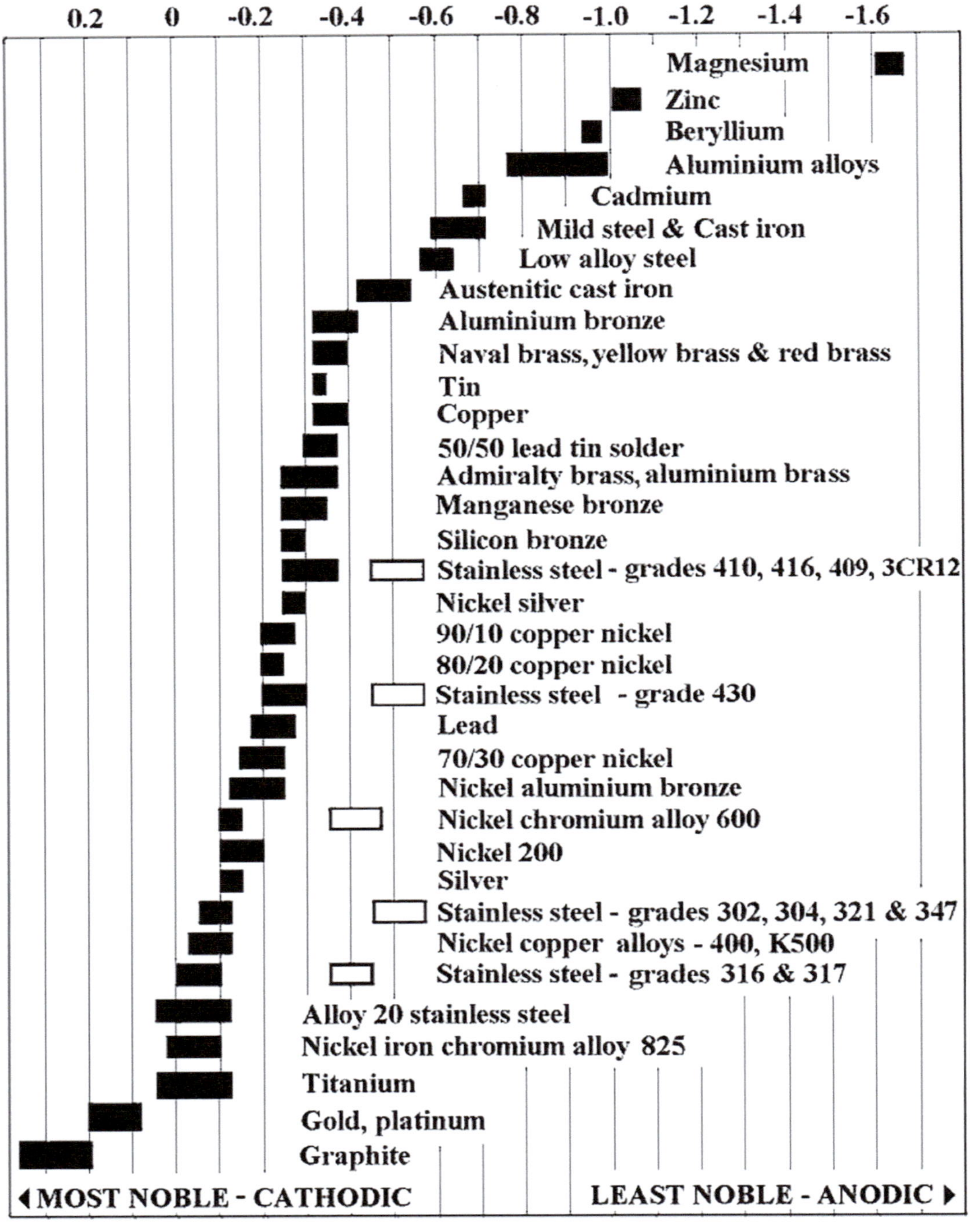

Fig. 1 Galvanic corrosion series for metal flowing into sea water [6]

[8]. Corrosion significantly raised metal levels, including nickel and chromium, in serum and urine [9]. Corrosion exposes the patient to allergenic hypersensibility. The most frequent allergenic metals are cobalt, titanium, chromium, nickel, zirconium [10]. They are contained in stainless steel, Vitallium (cobalt chromium molybdenum), titanium alloy, nitinol, and Oxinium (zirconium niobium). In addition, titanium allergy is described. The cytotoxicity and carcinogenicity role of nickel, chromium, and cobalt are suggested by some studies on the epithelial–mesenchymal transition process [11]. We have no rational to link plasmatic detection of this ions and damage to male reproductive system, anemia, or higher risk of cancers [11]. However, we should avoid or reduce the chance of toxic heavy metals ion delivery by corrosion of spinal implants. The FDA developed the criteria of permitted daily exposure (PDE) in plasma for each heavy metal (μg/cm^2). Efforts are done to found alloy with less ions release. Recent testing on Molybdenum-47.5 Rhenium alloy (MoRe®) are promising with good mechanical properties associated with low rates of ions release after prolonged immersion in physiologic and inflammatory environments [12].

2.2 Mechanical Properties

The mechanical properties of biomaterials should be optimal. They could be quantified as elastic modulus (Young's modulus, which is the stress-to-strain ratio), stiffness (ultimate strength to rupture in tension), fatigue resistance (strength apply on 10^7 loading cycles to rupture), hardness, and ductility (% of elongation to break). These properties are very well studied before sales authorization. Information is precise and studied ex vivo. The quest for mechanically ideal biomaterial is centered on research on elastic modulus (Young's modulus) to be like that of the bone. A classification of metals is done regarding this property (Fig. 2) [13]. Dynamical characteristics in fatigue did not raise great attention. Surgeons are not

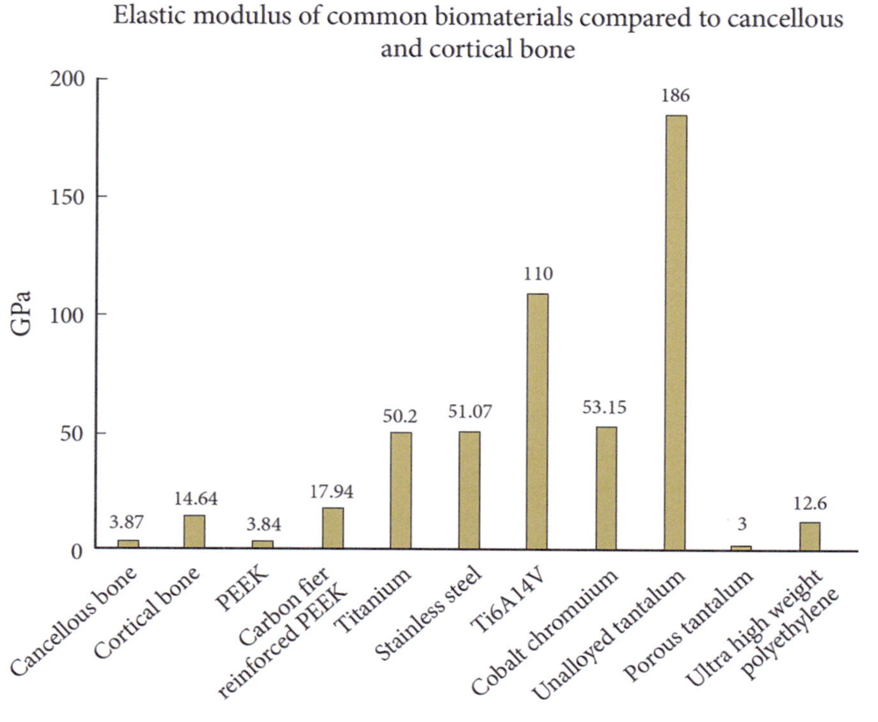

Fig. 2 Young's modulus of principal metals is shown. (Figure from Warburton et al. [13])

confident to use implant for their elastic properties. The repeated solicitations of long construct, which ended up with rods breakage, are more or less a materialization of an evolution toward nonunion during arthrodesis. Attempts at flexible posterior fixation have all ended with failure of the device. Ductility is interesting to bend rods during implantation. It is also linked to appearance of cold welding. That could be an issue, especially in case of device removal. The implant design plays a major role on mechanical properties. The change from original screw–plates devices to screw–rods, in the mid-1990s, makes dropped-down fretting corrosion at the screw–plate interface [14, 16]. Then, the rigid screw–rod connection through monoaxial screw tulip-like head became a problem. Some intraoperative difficulties to connect screws and rods appeared. Adjacent junctional syndrome was generated by the high level of stress at the ends the constructs. Polyaxial screws solved this problem. Nowadays, we are back to fretting issues when the strength of polyaxial screw–rod connection is not strong enough.

2.3 Image Passivity

Imaging compatibility became a mandatory property for spinal device. Surgeons follow the stability of their constructs and intervertebral fusions. Thus, they need for repetitive and objective monitoring by images aside with clinical monitoring. For CT scan images, dense metal is disturbing, since it produces flashing aspects on images. The classification of X-ray beam perturbating materials follows the density scale of implant components. From least to worst, we classify PEEK, UHW polyethylene, ceramics, tricalcium phosphate (TCP), hydroxyapatite (HAp), zirconium (ZrC), titanium alloy, nitinol, stainless steel 316 L, cobalt chrome alloy, and tantalum. This could be a choice when the surgeon is keen to seek the bone bonding around the devices. In spine, MRI is a popular imaging system that shows bone, soft tissues, and disc. The presence of ferric material does not allow good MRI images. The magnetic susceptibility measures the deformation magnetic signal for each biomaterial. A classification of magnetic perturbating materials, from least to worst, might be ceramics materials (TCP, HAp, ZrC, polymeric materials, tantalum, titanium alloy, cobalt chromium alloy, stainless steel 316 L) [17].

Other discriminant properties are examined by surgeons for choosing the best materials: bacterial adhesion and osseointegration.

2.4 Bacterial Adhesion

Biofilms cause 65% of nosocomial infections, about 80% of chronic infections, and 60% of all human bacterial infections, as chronic infection such as periodontitis or acute implant-related device infections [18]. The first stage of reversible bacterial adhesion to biomaterials is favored by different forces: Van der Walls, acid–base phase, electrostatic charge, and hydrophobicity [19, 21] (see Fig. 3). Then proliferation and polysaccharides secretion turn to a slime, which then becomes a biofilm. Materials elemental type influences adhesivity. Ag, Zn, and Cu are known from the age as bactericidal elements. They can be coated on the surface of the implants [22]. Compared adhesivity analysis on alumina ceramic, polyethylene, titanium, and stainless steel show similar adhesivity of titanium versus stainless steel. Ceramic has the lower adhesivity rate compared to polyethylene for *Staphylococcus aureus* and compared to polyethylene, titanium, and stainless steel for *Pseudomonas aeruginosa* [23]. Adhesion forces are linked to surface-finishing treatment of the materials. It modifies hydrophobicity, as well as positive electrostatic charge. The surface roughness of the biomaterials enhance hydrophilicity and affects cell adhesion [19, 20]. A water droplet on a hydrophilic surface will have a low contact angle (<90°). This is the rational to treat the surface of the implant by increasing the roughness to create more hydrophilicity. Bactericidal coating has been developed to decrease bacteria inoculum by releasing positive ions and antibiotics into the immediate environment of the device (silver, zinc, antibiotic).

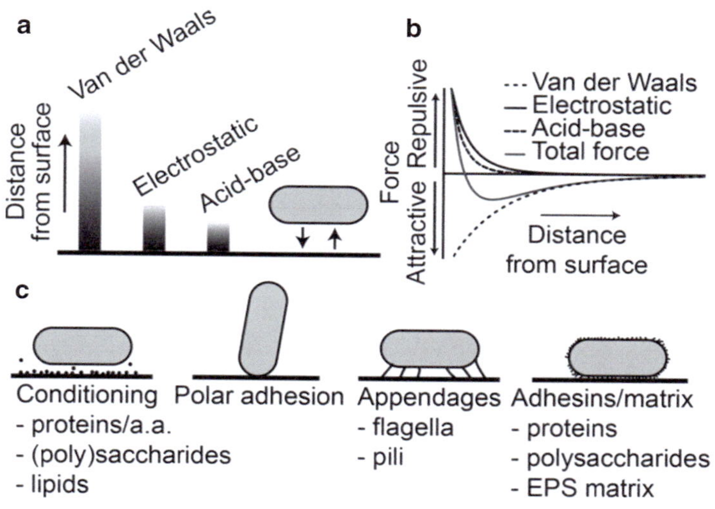

Fig. 3 Forces involve in bacterial adhesion to device. (**a**) Schematic representation of forces. (**b**) Adhesion forces as a function of distance from the surface. (**c**) Strategies employed by bacteria to achieve a smaller separation from the surface. (Sketches from Kimkes T.E.P., Heinemann M. publication [21])

2.5 Osseointegration

Osteoconduction is the ability for a device to facilitate development of growing bone around the device. This phenomenon is regularly seen in the case of bone implants. In spine surgery, it facilitates osseous intervertebral fusion by bone bonding ability. Osseointegration makes implant anchorage stable, by achieving a direct bone-to-implant contact, without fibrous layer. In cranio-facial implantology, this mode of anchorage is the only one for which high success rates have been reported. Osseointegration is mandatory in spinal fixation too (screws). Without osteoconduction there is no osseointegration [26]. Good osseointegration also decreases the appearance of biofilm. Osseointegration process can be viewed as a race between the microorganism that seeks to form the biofilm versus the endogenous tissue that seeks to grow on the implant surface [27]. Osteoinduction is different of osseointegration. Osteoinduction is provoked by protein as dibotermin alfa (rhBMP-2). Osteoinduction implies the recruitment of immature cells and the stimulation of these cells to develop preosteoblasts. In situation, such as a fracture, most of the bone healing depends on osteoinduction. Bone tissue engineering explores innovative strategies using integration of stem cells, dibotermin alfa, and nanomaterial into printed scaffolds. Ongoing research shows success, in vivo, on rat and sheep [28]. Each material might be characterized by osseointegration property, which could be hydrophilicity. To enhance osseointegration at the implant's surface, two methods are used: additive methods (coating) and subtractive methods (acid etching, sandblasting, laser methods, polishing, electromagnetic). Porous-coated implant is proposed to facilitate osteointegration. Physicochemical characteristics of coating includes roughness, porosity, phase, elemental composition, and adhesivity. Ideal design of porous metal implant materials is about pore size, porosity, and pore connectivity. Pores in the range of 200–400 μm in size are thought to promote osteoblast adhesion, migration, and proliferation [30]. Porosity is the ratio of the pore volume to the overall volume of material. The porosity of the trabecular bone is around 80%. Metal loses its mechanical properties when porosity reaches 40% (i.e., tantalum). Powder metallurgy, plasma spray coating, anodic oxidation, micro-arc oxidation, sol–gel technologies lead to small pore porous-coat [31, 32], but elastic modulus and strength of the implant are not modified. Hydroxyapatite (HAp) coatings have been proposed for a while with good results on osseointegration [29]. HAp-based coatings could be doped by various elements as Ag^{+}, Zn^{++}, Cu^{++}, Mg^{++}, Sr^{+}. They combine osseointegration and bactericidal effects. Strontium (Sr^{+}) supports bone growth in osteoporotic bone. Mg^{++} enhance the biodegradability of HAp-based coatings.

3 Biomaterials Review and Clinical Application

We present below the different biomaterials components with their characteristics. The different properties are summarized in Tables 1 and 2.

3.1 Metal Alloys

Metal was the first materials known to be used [1, 33]. Before stainless steel (SS) invention, iron, copper, gold, and silver were used [1, 33]. Patients probably experienced ions toxicity after corrosion, for iron and copper, but we had no record on that. Metal materials are mainly used on rods, plates, hooks, screws, intervertebral cages, and disc arthroplasty. Young's modulus of metal is usually way higher than bone. In Fig. 2, the Young's modulus of principal metal is shown [13]. The surgeons are looking for the ability to be on-site adaptable with great strength. However, we should keep in mind that each bender applied on whatever metal rod is notching it. This mark generates a stress riser that could lead to local fragility of the metal to repetitive solicitations [15]. That is why some brands propose already shaped rods.

3.1.1 Stainless Steel (SS)

Stainless steel 316 L is a low carbon version of steel that gives resistance to intergranular corrosion for heavy section, welding ability, and good machinability. It is an austenitic alloy with 61.9–72% of iron, 16–18% of chromium, 10–14% of nickel, and 2–3% of molybdenum. SS is the most corrodible metal used in spine surgery. Especially fretting corrosion is more frequent with SS than with titanium or cobalt alloys. It generates wear debris [34]. SS contains nickel (Ni) and chromium (Cr), which are the most common metal allergens. The Young's modulus is 193 GPa (versus 14.54 GPa for cortical bone). It is magnetic because of ferric atoms. This high density, around 8000 g/m^3, makes it very visible on X-ray and CT scan. That could be an issue to follow the bone-to-bone bonding progression of intervertebral fusion. Its hydrophilicity is poor, except after surface treatment. It is still very useful because of low cost and its ductility. This allows easy bending of rods on-site to promote the adaptation of long constructs to deformed

Table 1 Summary of major metal materials component properties used in spinal surgery. Mechanical properties are referred to Matweb charts [70]

Property	SS 316 L	Co-28Cr-6Mo	Ti-6Al-4 V	Tantalum	Nitinol 60
Corrosion fretting and galvanic	++++	+++	+	–	++
Wear release	++++	+++	+	–	++
Allergic reaction	++++	++	+	–	+++
Young's modulus (GPa)	193	211	110	186	83
Ultimate tensile stress (MPa)	560	1060	880	900	1240
Hardness	79 (Rockwell B)	30 (Rockwell C)	36 (Rockwell C)	200 (Vickers)	58 (Rockwell C)
Ductility (% elongation at break)	50	25	14	35–70	8
Fatigue strength MPa (10^7 cycles)	145.45	560	240	230	1300
Density (kg/m^3)	8000	8800	4430	16,600	6500
MRI susceptibility (μ emu/g)	2×10^5	8.7	1.8×10^{-4}	9×10^{-7}	3.7×10^{-6}
Hydrophilicity	–	+	++	++++	+++
Cost	–	++	+	++++	+++

Table 2 Summary of principal polymers and ceramic materials properties used in spinal surgery. Mechanical properties are referred to Matweb charts [70]

Property	Cortical bone	PEEK 450G	UHW polyethylene	Ceramic $CaOSiO_2P_2O_5B_2O_3$	Zirconium ZrC	HAp $Ca_{10}(PO_4)_6(OH)_2$	TCP $CA_3(PO_4)_2$
Corrosion	–	0	0	0	0	0	0
Wear release	–	+	+++	++	–	–	–
Allergic reaction	–	–	–	0	+	–	–
Young's modulus (GPa)	11–22	4	0.716	64	345–400	7–13	
Ultimate tensile stress (MPa)	52–133	98	36		83 at 980 °C	38–48	
Hardness		84.5 (shore D)	64.2 (shore D)		2310 (Vickers)		
Ductility (% elongation at break)	0.7–3.1	45	247				
Fatigue strength (MPa) (10^7 cycles)	67	70	16.6	826–2858			120
Density (kg/m^3)	2000	1300	1800	2400	6560	3150	3140
MRI susceptibility (μ emu/g)		0	0	2.6×10^{-5}	2.6×10^{-5}		
Hydrophilicity	+++	Hydrophobic	Hydrophobic	++	+	++++	+++
Cost	–	–	–	+++	++++	++	+

scoliosis spine. However, it stays the worst metal for corrosion.

3.1.2 Cobalt Chromium Alloy (CoCr)

Alternative metal to SS was developed with cobalt-based alloy with 28% of chromium and 5% of molybdenum. Vitallium is another alloy with 65% of cobalt, 30% of chromium, and 5% of molybdenum. CoCr is characterized by its especially high strength as well as good ductility, which is closed to SS. It effectively corrects and stabilizes scoliosis deformation. It is more resistance to notch effect than titanium alloy. It is more resistant at corrosion. It is passive to MRI imaging. The Young's modulus is high. The great difference with the spongious bone modulus makes it non-proper to manufacture pedicular screws. Another drawback of lack of elasticity is stress shielding, which occurs at the end of the posterior thoracolumbar fusion and leads to proximal junctional kyphosis [34]. The biocompatibility of CoCr is among the standard alloys used in medical and dental technologies. However, Co and Cr are involved in cytotoxic activities. Cr is also a common metal allergen. The effort to prevent the release of Co ions is done to coat the implants by calcium phosphate ceramics [35].

3.1.3 Titanium Alloy (Ti-6Al-4 V)

Titanium alloy is made of titanium, aluminum, and vanadium. This second generation of titanium alloy has a Young's modulus closer to cortical bone. It has a great biocompatibility as we know. It has low density and is passive to X-ray imaging. Its strength at rupture and fatigue comportment makes it the preferred materials for posterior constructs. The low Young's modulus is appropriate to screw manufacturing. The drawback of titanium is its ductility with fragility generated by notching when surgeons bend the rods.

A cold welding could also be an issue, especially in case of device removal. It is the most corrosionless metal because a passive oxide film (TiO_2) forms on the surface of titanium when it is exposed to air. Another great property of titanium alloy is magnetic passivity, which is very useful in MRI imaging. Despite its weakest strength, there is no clinical difference between SS, Ti-6Al-4 V, and CoCr for deformation correction ability [24]. Serhan et al. show that, because of titanium elasticity, the corrective force produced by the Ti-6Al-4 V, 30° pre-bend rod was approximately 67% that of a CoCr and SS rods [25]. It has poor osseointegration and hydrophilicity. Titanium allergy is getting more frequent since the skin exposure to titanium is also increasing because it is found in watches, jewelry, body creams, make-ups, deodorants, toothpastes, and food. Surgeon should be aware for titanium allergy. Titanium debris from spinal arthrodesis releases cytokines, which increases osteoclastic activity and cellular apoptosis [36]. This may explain the delayed inflammatory-infectious complications and long-term aseptic osteolysis around screws [37]. New titanium alloys, beta-type titanium–molybdenum and oxygen-modified beta-type titanium–chromium, were designed to enhance mechanical properties (ultimate tensile strength to rupture). Currently, they did not reach out human application because of cytotoxicity concerns [38].

3.1.4 Nitinol (NiTi)

Nitinol presents a unique feature known as superelasticity. This material returns to its original shape after large deformation stops. Its Young's modulus is very close to the bone modulus. It may prevent the adjacent deformation syndrome and the screw loosening. Like titanium, it presents a passive oxide film at its surface. This confers great resistance to galvanic corrosion and its biocompatibility is like titanium alloy. However, some fretting corrosion could appear and may release nickel ions into the blood. The enhancement of rod-head screw connection is a key-point of constructs with nitinol rods. Coating with protecting layers on the rods is also proposed [34].

3.1.5 Tantalum

Surgical use of tantalum is promising. Pure tantalum has great ductility. Adjunction of 2.5% tungsten gives it great resistance. Principal properties of tantalum are hydrophilicity, osseointegration, noncorrodible, magnetic passivity, and high radio opacity [39–41]. It is too strong to be bend onsite. In spine surgery, porous tantalum is used for intervertebral cages. It has a very good porosity, up to 80%, and the Young's modulus is low, closed to spongious bone, at 3 GPa [42]. Roughness gives high coefficient of friction for primary stability in the intervertebral space. A very good osseointegration is observed at bone–cage interface. Altogether, it explains the good clinical outcome of revision surgery for complicated infectious spondylitis [42]. It is also used as positioning landmarks into PEEK cages. It is the more expensive material used in spinal surgery.

3.2 Polymeric Materials

3.2.1 PolyEtherEtherKetone (PEEK)

PEEK is used mainly in intervertebral cages. Its Young's modulus is like cancellous bone (4 GPa versus 3.87 GPa). It seems to be ideal to be placed next to the fragile cortical plateau. The low Young's modulus prevents cage against subsidence inside the underlying vertebral body. That is established by comparative study of cages in PEEK versus titanium [43, 44]. This easy-to-machine and mold material allows numerous and creative designs. Its great advantage is the perfect radiolucency and magnetic passivity to control the growing bone bonding plateau surface inside and around the cage. Other properties such as low cost and perfect biocompatibility drive the industry to develop hardly this option. However, this implant, proposed to achieve intervertebral fusion, has the worst hydrophilicity than osseointegration. Proposal to fulfill the cage with osteoconductive ceramics or spongious autograft is done. Secondary displacement of PEEK cages is observed in the clinical practice. They could go backward into the canal or the foramina. Addressing this problem, treatment of the surface in contact with the plateau could be done. It enhances the porosity to get friction moment and osseointegration for better primary et secondary stability [46]. Composite implant with PEEK dopped by titanium at the interface with vertebral plateau is proposed for the same achievement [45]. The objective to get a fixation that favored intervertebral fusion prompted surgeons to try PEEK rods as posterior lumbar fixation. In literature, the follow-up time of studies is short [47]. We need results on long-term efficacy and on adverse events. What is the fatigue comportment of the implants? Is there an increase of infection rate on this pro-biofilm hydrophobic surfaces? What happens on the adjacent segments of fusion?

We assume that coating, for example, with HAp or antibiotics could help to modify the bactericidal adhesion on PEEK. Other drawback is the impossibility to adapt the posterior rods in PEEK to the shape of the spine. This suggests preoperative design and custom casting of patient-specific implants.

3.2.2 PolyEtherKetoneKetone (PEKK)

Polymer PEKK are a group where the ether of PEEK is switched to a ketone. The ketone link is more rigid and gives to PEKK a better stability in high temperature. This allows production of printed 3D object. This material is stronger in compression and has more friction resistance than PEEK. Its excellent biocompatibility and resistance to temperature made possible application of tantalum coating, HAp coating, and surface treatment [48, 49].

3.2.3 Ultra-High Molecular Weight Polyethylene (UHMWPE)

UHMWPE was first introduced to orthopedics in 1962 by Sir John Charnley through hip replacements and remains the gold standard as orthopedic-bearing material in joint replacements. It is highly hydrophobic. UHMWPE is used clinically because of its significant resistance to abrasion. Then, disc replacement designers choose the bearing couple metal-on-UHMWPE. No other materials currently dethrone UHMWPE from its preeminent position [50]. We know that wear on the prosthesis triggers inflammatory responses resulting in osteolysis, pain, and implant failure on knee and hip arthroplasty [51]. However, nowadays, even in large series at 10 years, no objective macroscopic granuloma was observed [52].

3.2.4 Viscoelastic Elastomer

Total disc arthroplasty imposes cinematic by design of the implant. Adverse effects could appear such as facets pain, pedicular fracture, and adjacent level hyper solicitation. This was the rational to provide implants with six degrees of freedom [53]. Thus, non-articulating prosthesis with viscoelastic core are proposed by different firm. The core is made of silicone, polycarbonate urethane, or polyurethane. The core is fixed on rigid endplates made of titanium, PEEK, or surrounded by an embroidered polyester fiber jacket. The main concern on this technology is the wear debris issue. We do not have long history of using elastomers in the orthopedic field. Long-term studies of viscoelastic total disc replacements are mandatory before large diffusion [54].

3.2.5 PolyMethylMethAcrylate (PMMA)

PMMA is an acrylic polymer used in vertebral augmentation such as vertebroplasty and kyphoplasty. It could fix the reduction obtained by expandable intracorporeal implant [55]. It is very used to enhance primary stability of pedicular screws in osteoporotic spine. An isolated trial was made in the intervertebral space [56]. The polymeric PMMA shows lack of osteoconduction. Biofilm and bacterial adhesion encouraged provider to add antibiotic to PMMA. Antibiotic diffusion is effective for 7 days. After this time laps, the biofilm isolates the PMMA from the surrounding tissues with no further diffusion of the bactericidal effect. Exogenic temperature elevation during polymerization, up to 112 °C, could cause thermal necrosis of osteocytes [57]. The immediate efficiency of vertebroplasty on pain is proved. However, histomorphological observation on rabbits shows the appearance of osteoclasts around the PMMA over the long-term. This phenomenon induces bone resorption, which is eventually greater than bone formation [58]. It results in bone loss around the hard core of PMMA. Thermal necrosis, as well as PMMA low osseointegration characteristic, finally leads to create a pebble into a hole.

3.2.6 Polyester (Polyethylene-Terephthalate—PET)

Some sublaminar bands, made of polyester, do provide a safe alternative to sublaminar Luque-type wires to apply high corrective forces in great scoliosis deformation [59]. Polyester mesh is also used to envelop interspinous spacer in PEEK. Polyester is easy to use and resistant as long as it works in traction. Repetitive shear forces and flexion moments could break the fibers in fatigue.

4 Ceramic Materials

Ceramic has a high biocompatibility rate and low allergic response rate. Spinal implant designers are increasingly investing in ceramics or developing multi-material prosthetics that use a mixture of ceramic and plastic to mimic the human body's spinal discs. Structural ceramics are used to compose intervertebral cages. Clinical studies show good outcome for ceramics cage ($CaO–SiO_2–P_2O_5–B_2O_3$) [60]. Other silicium-based ceramics proposed include Si_3N_4 [13]. Ceramics are too fragile to make big fenestration inside the cages. We attempt primary stability with a high friction ratio at the bone–implant interface and durable stability by osseointegration. Bone substitutes are also ceramics. They are used to fulfill intervertebral space around and into cages. Their osteoconduction is useful to bond the intervertebral space. In this category, we found ceramics made of hydroxyapatite (HAp), calcium phosphate such as tricalcium phosphate (TCP), and glass. Studies on lumbar and cervical fusion compare bone substitute, ceramics, and spongious bone. Associated with the radiolucent cage, no difference between substitute and bone was shown [61].

5 Surface Finishing Issues

5.1 Surface Treatment

The interacting surface of the device could present different aspects. Modification to the surface and bulk characteristics of intervertebral cages (titanium, alloy, tantalum, and PEEK) has been shown to maximize osseointegration and long-term stability (see chapter above) [64]. This effect is recognized when the holes inside the structure are interconnected and larger than 200 μm. Some roughness favors the thickness of the biofilm and bacterial adhesion, whereas others do not. There is no linear relation between size of the irregularity and bacterial adhesion [19]. It suggests that bacteria preferentially adhere to irregularities that conform to their size.

5.2 Coating

5.2.1 Osteoconductive Ceramic Coat (HAp, TCP)

Ceramic coating does not modify material properties. They are chosen to enhance the bone–material interface in order to get a better osseointegration along the device. On pedicular screws, the consequence is a better control of shear forces. HAp ceramic is one of the best osteointegrating coating. It gives mechanical properties at bone–implant interface [62]. Another benefit is lower thickness of the biofilm. No difference is made on titanium between HAp and TCP coating [63]. We understand that the osseointegration does not give immediate primary stiffness. That is why PMMA augmentation is still used in osteoporotic spines as an alternative to coating for screw primary stability. Glass-based bone substitute shows in vitro good osteoconduction properties [65].

Aside from ceramic coating, tantalum coating is also a solution to enhance pedicular screw anchorage [66]. Like ceramics, the osteointegration effect is objective after 12 weeks. There is no biological and mechanical difference with the ceramic coating, for a cost way much higher.

Pedicle screws coated with collagen/chondroitin sulfate shows amazing bone growth on implant surface. That was compared, with success, to HAp coating and coating-less titanium alloy [69]. However, no superior mechanical properties, such as pull-out strength, appear with collagen/chondroitin sulfate coating.

5.2.2 Bactericidal Coating

The antic Mediterranean sailors use silver coating inside the amphora to prevent bacterial contamination of drinkable water during long oversea cruise. The electrostatic effect of positive ions, Ag^+, acts as repellant for bacteria's membrane. The current clinical proposal combines silver and hydroxyapatite (Ag–HA) [68]. The major drawback could be plasma release of Ag^+ ions. Copper is not used because of the toxicity of Cu^{++} ions. Antibiotic coating is known to have a short-lasting time effect, around 7 days. The basic idea was to add antibiotics to ceramics coating such as in PMMA. Unfortunately, the prevention effect is not much than spreading antibiotic powder into the surgical wound before closing. Some hope raised up with glass-based ceramics mixed to antibiotics in sceptic surgical revision for spondylodiscitis [67].

6 Conclusion

The topic on biomaterials used in spinal surgery could seem boring to surgeons. Because we have the choice between different options, the objective of this chapter is to show that making a choice is also dealing with some drawback effects that could affect the clinical result. Biocompatibility is controlled by certification boards (FDA, CE), but the surgeons should be aware of possible corrosion, allergy, and cytotoxicity. The rise of implanted devices infection and the occurrence of pseudarthrosis lead to seek for the best material regarding biofilm and osseointegration. Loosening after circumferential interbody fusion makes us start a reflexional about our choice on intrinsic mechanical properties of each implant. It also helps to understand further development and ongoing proposal from the industry.

References

1. Hallbäck D-A. A medieval (?) bone with a copper plate support indicating an open surgical treatment. OSSA 1976–1977. 3/4:63–82. Lund ISSN 0345-8865
2. Lane WA. Some remarks on the treatment of fractures. BMJ. 1895;1:861–3.
3. Malpas C. Jules Guérin makes his market: the social economy of Orthopaedic medicine in Paris, c. 1825–1845. In: Blécourt WD, Usborne C, editors. Cultural approaches to the history of medicine. UK: Palgrave Macmillan; 2004. p. 148–70.
4. Hadra BE. The classic: wiring of the vertebrae as a means of immobilization in fracture and Potts' disease. Berthold E Hadra Med Times and Register, 1891. Clin Orthop Relat Res. 1975;22(112):4–8.
5. Becker EL, Landau SI, Manuila A. International dictionary of medicine and biology. New York: Wiley; 1986.
6. John P. Atlas steel technical handbook of stainless steel. Atlas Steels Inc. p. 3–4. Australia Available at [www.atlassteels.com.au] Revised: 27/03/2023
7. Majid K, Crowder T, Baker E, Baker K, Koueiter D, Shields E, Herkowitz HN. Analysis of in vivo corrosion of 316L stainless steel posterior thoracolumbar plate systems: a retrieval study. J Spinal Disord Tech. 2011;24(8):500–5. https://doi.org/10.1097/BSD.0b013e3182064497. PMID: 21336173
8. Serhan H, Slivka M, Albert T, Kwak SD. Is galvanic corrosion between titanium alloy and stainless steel spinal implants a clinical concern? Spine J. 2004;4(4):379–87. https://doi.org/10.1016/j.spinee.2003.12.004. PMID: 15246296
9. del Rio J, Beguiristain J, Duart J. Metal levels in corrosion of spinal implants. Eur Spine J. 2007;16(7):1055–61. https://doi.org/10.1007/s00586-007-0311-4. Epub 2007 Jan 26. PMID: 17256156; PMCID: PMC2219664
10. Schalock PC, Menné T, Johansen JD, Taylor JS, Maibach HI, Lidén C, Bruze M, Thyssen JP. Hypersensitivity reactions to metallic implants – diagnostic algorithm and suggested patch test series for clinical use. Contact Derm. 2012;66(1):4–19. https://doi.org/10.1111/j.1600-0536.2011.01971.x. Epub 2011 Sep 29. PMID: 21957996
11. Chen XL, Xu YM, Lau ATY. Toxic metals in the regulation of epithelial-mesenchymal plasticity: demons or angels? Cancer Cell Int. 2022;22(1):237. https://doi.org/10.1186/s12935-022-02638-3. PMID: 35897065; PMCID: PMC9327425
12. Mok JM, Poelstra K, Ammar K, McGirt M, Cormier J, Hart R, Bauman J, Cowart P, Sheth I, Singh P, Yadav J. Characterization of ion release from a novel bio-

material, Molybdenum-47.5Rhenium, in physiologic environments. Spine J. 2023;23(6):900–11. https://doi.org/10.1016/j.spinee.2023.01.007. Epub 2023 Jan 25. PMID: 36706920

13. Warburton A, Girdler SJ, Mikhail CM, Ahn A, Cho SK. Biomaterials in spinal implants: a review. Neurospine. 2020;17(1):101–10. https://doi.org/10.14245/ns.1938296.148. Epub 2019 Nov 4. PMID: 31694360; PMCID: PMC7136103
14. Roy-Camille R, Saillant G, Mazel C. Internal fixation of the lumbar spine with pedicle screw plating. Clin Orthop Relat Res. 1986;203:7–17. PMID: 3955999
15. Lindsey C, Deviren V, Xu Z, Yeh RF, Puttlitz CM. The effects of rod contouring on spinal construct fatigue strength. Spine (Phila Pa 1976). 2006;31(15):1680–7. https://doi.org/10.1097/01.brs.0000224177.97846.00. PMID: 16816763
16. Dubousset J, Cotrel Y. Application technique of Cotrel-Dubousset instrumentation for scoliosis deformities. Clin Orthop Relat Res. 1991;264:103–10. PMID: 1997225
17. Matsuura H, Inoue T, Ogasawara K, Sasaki M, Konno H, Kuzu Y, Nishimoto H, Ogawa A. Quantitative analysis of magnetic resonance imaging susceptibility artifacts caused by neurosurgical biomaterials: comparison of 0.5, 1.5, and 3.0 tesla magnetic fields. Neurol Med Chir (Tokyo). 2005;45(8):395–8; discussion 398–9. https://doi.org/10.2176/nmc.45.395. PMID: 16127256
18. Assefa M, Amare A. Biofilm-associated multi-drug resistance in hospital-acquired infections: a review. Infect Drug Resist. 2022;15:5061–8.
19. Katsikogianni M, Missirlis YF. Concise review of mechanisms of bacterial adhesion to biomaterials and of techniques used in estimating bacteria-material interactions. Eur Cell Mater. 2004;7(8):37–57. https://doi.org/10.22203/ecm.v008a05. PMID: 15593018
20. De-la-Pinta I, Cobos M, Ibarretxe J, Montoya E, Eraso E, Guraya T, Quindós G. Effect of biomaterials hydrophobicity and roughness on biofilm development. J Mater Sci Mater Med. 2019;30(7):77. https://doi.org/10.1007/s10856-019-6281-3. PMID: 31218489
21. Kimkes TEP, Heinemann M. How bacteria recognise and respond to surface contact. FEMS Microbiol Rev. 2020;44(1):106–22. https://doi.org/10.1093/femsre/fuz029. PMID: 31769807; PMCID: PMC7053574
22. Fosca M, Streza A, Antoniac IV, Vadalà G, Rau JV. Ion-doped calcium phosphate-based coatings with antibacterial properties. J Funct Biomater. 2023;14(5):250. https://doi.org/10.3390/jfb14050250. PMID: 37233360; PMCID: PMC10219342
23. Poli E, Ouk TS, Barrière G, Lévèque G, Sol V, Denes E. Does low hydroxyl group surface density explain less bacterial adhesion on porous alumina? Orthop Traumatol Surg Res. 2019;105(3):473–7. https://doi.org/10.1016/j.otsr.2018.11.018. Epub 2019 Jan 3. PMID: 30612953
24. Bowden D, Michielli A, Merrill M, Will S. Systematic review and meta-analysis for the impact of rod materials and sizes in the surgical treatment of adult spine deformity. Spine Deform. 2022;10(6):1265–78. https://doi.org/10.1007/s43390-022-00556-y. Epub 2022 Jul 29. PMID: 35904725; PMCID: PMC9579115
25. Serhan H, Mhatre D, Newton P, Giorgio P, Sturm P. Would CoCr rods provide better correctional forces than stainless steel or titanium for rigid scoliosis curves? J Spinal Disord Tech. 2013;26(2):E70–4. https://doi.org/10.1097/BSD.0b013e31826a0f19. PMID: 22832558
26. Albrektsson T, Johansson C. Osteoinduction, osteoconduction and osseointegration. Eur Spine J. 2001;10(Suppl 2):S96–101. https://doi.org/10.1007/s005860100282. PMID: 11716023; PMCID: PMC3611551
27. Vranceanu DM, Ungureanu E, Ionescu IC, Parau AC, Pruna V, Titorencu I, Badea M, Gălbău CȘ, Idomir M, Dinu M, Dragomir AV, Cotrut CM. In vitro characterization of hydroxyapatite-based coatings doped with mg or Zn electrochemically deposited on nanostructured titanium. Biomimetics (Basel). 2024;9(4):244. https://doi.org/10.3390/biomimetics9040244. PMID: 38667255; PMCID: PMC11047857
28. Garot C, Schoffit S, Monfoulet C, Machillot P, Deroy C, Roques S, Vial J, Vollaire J, Renard M, Ghanem H, El-Hafci H, Decambron A, Josserand V, Bordenave L, Bettega G, Durand M, Manassero M, Viateau V, Logeart-Avramoglou D, Picart C. 3D-printed Osteoinductive polymeric scaffolds with optimized architecture to repair a sheep metatarsal critical-size bone defect. Adv Healthc Mater. 2023;12(30):e2301692. https://doi.org/10.1002/adhm.202301692. Epub 2023 Sep 17. PMID: 37655491.
29. Lemons JE. Hydroxyapatite coatings. Clin Orthop Relat Res. 1988;235:220–3. PMID: 3416527
30. Ran Q, Yang W, Hu Y, Shen X, Yu Y, Xiang Y, Cai K. Osteogenesis of 3D printed porous Ti6Al4V implants with different pore sizes. J Mech Behav Biomed Mater. 2018;84:1–11. https://doi.org/10.1016/j.jmbbm.2018.04.010. Epub 2018 Apr 18. PMID: 29709846
31. Wang R, Ni S, Ma L, Li M. Porous construction and surface modification of titanium-based materials for osteogenesis: a review. Front Bioeng Biotechnol. 2022;25(10):973297. https://doi.org/10.3389/fbioe.2022.973297. PMID: 36091459; PMCID: PMC9452912
32. Clement S, Mehdi A. Sol-gel chemistry: from molecule to functional materials. Molecules. 2020;25(11):2538. https://doi.org/10.3390/molecules25112538. PMID: 32486041; PMCID: PMC7321306
33. Colton C. Orthopedic challenges in ancient Egypt. Bone & Joint 360. 2013;2(2):2–7.
34. Litak J, Szymoniuk M, Czyżewski W, Hoffman Z, Litak J, Sakwa L, Kamieniak P. Metallic implants used in lumbar Interbody fusion. Materials (Basel). 2022;15(10):3650. https://doi.org/10.3390/ma15103650. PMID: 35629676; PMCID: PMC9146470

35. Bandyopadhyay A, Shivaram A, Isik M, Avila JD, Dernell WS, Bose S. Additively manufactured calcium phosphate reinforced CoCrMo alloy: Bio-tribological and biocompatibility evaluation for load-bearing implants. Addit Manuf. 2019;28:312–24. https://doi.org/10.1016/j.addma.2019.04.020. Epub 2019 May 2. PMID: 31341790; PMCID: PMC6656377
36. Cunningham BW, Orbegoso CM, Dmitriev AE, Hallab NJ, Sefter JC, McAfee PC. The effect of titanium particulate on development and maintenance of a posterolateral spinal arthrodesis: an in vivo rabbit model. Spine (Phila Pa 1976). 2002;27(18):1971–81. https://doi.org/10.1097/00007632-200209150-00004. PMID: 12634556
37. Płusa T, Baranowska A, Baranowski P, Dudek J, Baranowska-Kijewska J. Metal hypersensitivity in hip, knee and spine surgery. Postepy Dermatol Alergol. 2023;40(2):215–9. https://doi.org/10.5114/ada.2023.127640. Epub 2023 May 31. PMID: 37312923; PMCID: PMC10258695
38. Liu H, Niinomi M, Nakai M, Cho K, Narita K, Şen M, Shiku H, Matsue T. Mechanical properties and cytocompatibility of oxygen-modified β-type Ti-Cr alloys for spinal fixation devices. Acta Biomater. 2015;12:352–61. https://doi.org/10.1016/j.actbio.2014.10.014. Epub 2014 Oct 23. PMID: 25449914
39. Lebhar J, Kriegel P, Guillin R, Chatellier P, Ropars M, Huten D. Role of MRI in the assessment of interbody fusion with tantalum intervertebral implant. Orthop Traumatol Surg Res. 2020;106(2):285–9. https://doi.org/10.1016/j.otsr.2019.11.018. Epub 2020 Mar 10. PMID: 32169395
40. Patel MS, McCormick JR, Ghasem A, Huntley SR, Gjolaj JP. Tantalum: the next biomaterial in spine surgery? J Spine Surg. 2020;6(1):72–86. https://doi.org/10.21037/jss.2020.01.01. PMID: 32309647; PMCID: PMC7154344
41. Mani G, Porter D, Grove K, Collins S, Ornberg A, Shulfer R. A comprehensive review of biological and materials properties of tantalum and its alloys. J Biomed Mater Res A. 2022;110(6):1291–306. https://doi.org/10.1002/jbm.a.37373. Epub 2022 Feb 13. PMID: 35156305
42. Yang SC, Chen HS, Kao YH, Tu YK. Single-stage anterior debridement and reconstruction with tantalum mesh cage for complicated infectious spondylitis. World J Orthop. 2017;8(9):710–8. https://doi.org/10.5312/wjo.v8.i9.710. PMID: 28979855; PMCID: PMC5605357
43. Seaman S, Kerezoudis P, Bydon M, Torner JC, Hitchon PW. Titanium vs. polyetheretherketone (PEEK) interbody fusion: meta-analysis and review of the literature. J Clin Neurosci. 2017t;44:23–9. https://doi.org/10.1016/j.jocn.2017.06.062. Epub 2017 Jul 21. PMID: 28736113
44. Chen Y, Wang X, Lu X, Yang L, Yang H, Yuan W, Chen D. Comparison of titanium and polyetheretherketone (PEEK) cages in the surgical treatment of multilevel cervical spondylotic myelopathy: a prospective, randomized, control study with over 7-year follow-up. Eur Spine J. 2013;22(7):1539–46. https://doi.org/10.1007/s00586-013-2772-y. Epub 2013 Apr 9. PMID: 23568254; PMCID: PMC3698331
45. Chahlavi A. Reduced subsidence with PEEK-titanium composite versus 3D titanium cages in a retrospective, self-controlled study in Transforaminal lumbar Interbody fusion. Global Spine J. 2024;23:21925682241253168. https://doi.org/10.1177/21925682241253168. Epub ahead of print. PMID: 38780086
46. Torstrick FB, Safranski DL, Burkus JK, Chappuis JL, Lee CSD, Guldberg RE, Gall K, Smith KE. Getting PEEK to stick to bone: the development of Porous PEEK for interbody fusion devices. Tech Orthop. 2017;32(3):158–66. https://doi.org/10.1097/BTO.0000000000000242. Epub 2017 Sep 1. PMID: 29225416; PMCID: PMC5720158
47. Li W, Zhao H, Li C, Liu T, Guan J, Yang Y, Yu X. Polyetheretherketone (PEEK) rods versus titanium rods for posterior lumbar fusion surgery: a systematic review and meta-analysis. J Orthop Surg Res. 2023;18(1):348. https://doi.org/10.1186/s13018-023-03817-2. PMID: 37170362; PMCID: PMC10173510
48. Hu X, Mei S, Wang F, Qian J, Xie D, Zhao J, Yang L, Wu Z, Wei J. Implantable PEKK/tantalum microparticles composite with improved surface performances for regulating cell behaviors, promoting bone formation and osseointegration. Bioact Mater. 2020;6(4):928–40. https://doi.org/10.1016/j.bioactmat.2020.09.021. PMID: 33102936; PMCID: PMC7560583
49. Yuan B, Chen Y, Lin H, Song Y, Yang X, Tang H, Xie E, Hsu T, Yang X, Zhu X, Zhang K, Zhang X. Processing and properties of bioactive surface-porous PEKK. ACS Biomater Sci Eng. 2016;2(6):977–86. https://doi.org/10.1021/acsbiomaterials.6b00103. Epub 2016 May 17. PMID: 33429506
50. Taksali S, Grauer JN, Vaccaro AR. Material considerations for intervertebral disc replacement implants. Spine J. 2004;4(6 Suppl):231S–8S. https://doi.org/10.1016/j.spinee.2004.07.012. PMID: 15541671
51. Werner JH, Rosenberg JH, Keeley KL, Agrawal DK. Immunobiology of periprosthetic inflammation and pain following ultra-high-molecular-weight-polyethylene wear debris in the lumbar spine. Expert Rev Clin Immunol. 2018;14(8):695–706. https://doi.org/10.1080/1744666X.2018.1511428. Epub 2018 Aug 21. PMID: 30099915; PMCID: PMC6287907
52. Kontakis M, Marques C, Löfgren H, Mosavi F, Skeppholm M, Olerud C, MacDowall A. Artificial disc replacement and adjacent-segment pathology: 10-year outcomes of a randomized trial. J Neurosurg Spine. 2021;36(6):945–53. https://doi.org/10.3171/2021.9.SPINE21904. PMID: 34920425
53. Lazennec JY. Lumbar and cervical viscoelastic disc replacement: concepts and current experience. World J Orthop. 2020;11(8):345–56. https://doi.org/10.5312/wjo.v11.i8.345. PMID: 32904082; PMCID: PMC7448204

54. Jacobs CAM, Siepe CJ, Ito K. Viscoelastic cervical total disc replacement devices: Design concepts. Spine J. 2020;20(12):1911–24. https://doi.org/10.1016/j.spinee.2020.08.007. Epub 2020 Aug 15. PMID: 32810609
55. Renaud C. Treatment of vertebral compression fractures with the cranio-caudal expandable implant SpineJack®: technical note and outcomes in 77 consecutive patients. Orthop Traumatol Surg Res. 2015;101(7):857–9. https://doi.org/10.1016/j.otsr.2015.08.009. Epub 2015 Oct 29. PMID: 26521157
56. Varga PP, Jakab G, Bors IB, Lazary A, Szövérfi Z. Experiences with PMMA cement as a stand-alone intervertebral spacer: percutaneous cement discoplasty in the case of vacuum phenomenon within lumbar intervertebral discs. Orthopade. 2015;44(Suppl 1):S1–7. https://doi.org/10.1007/s00132-014-3060-1. PMID: 25875227
57. Belkoff SM, Molloy S. Temperature measurement during polymerization of polymethylmethacrylate cement used for vertebroplasty. Spine (Phila Pa 1976). 2003;28(14):1555–9. PMID: 12865844
58. Quan R, Ni Y, Zhang L, Xu J, Zheng X, Yang D. Short- and long-term effects of vertebroplastic bone cement on cancellous bone. J Mech Behav Biomed Mater. 2014;35:102–10. https://doi.org/10.1016/j.jmbbm.2014.03.007. Epub 2014 Apr 12. PMID: 24762857
59. Canavese F, Samba A. Sublaminar polyester bands for the correction of idiopathic and neuromuscular scoliosis. Ann Transl Med. 2020;8(2):32. https://doi.org/10.21037/atm.2019.08.109. PMID: 32055623; PMCID: PMC6995906
60. Kwon JW, Lee YH, Lee BH, Kim JH, Suk KS. Clinical and radiological outcomes of non-window-type bioactive glass-ceramic cage in single-level ACDF versus PEEK cage filled with autologous bone. Sci Rep. 2024;14(1):4035. https://doi.org/10.1038/s41598-024-54786-3. PMID: 38369553; PMCID: PMC10874951
61. Zadegan SA, Abedi A, Jazayeri SB, Bonaki HN, Vaccaro AR, Rahimi-Movaghar V. Clinical application of ceramics in anterior cervical discectomy and fusion: a review and update. Global. Spine J. 2017;7(4):343–9. https://doi.org/10.1177/2192568217699201. Epub 2017 Apr 20. PMID: 28815162; PMCID: PMC5546682
62. Hasegawa T, Inufusa A, Imai Y, Mikawa Y, Lim TH, An HS. Hydroxyapatite-coating of pedicle screws improves resistance against pull-out force in the osteoporotic canine lumbar spine model: a pilot study. Spine J. 2005;5(3):239–43. https://doi.org/10.1016/j.spinee.2004.11.010. PMID: 15863077
63. Tandon V, Franke J, Kalidindi KKV. Advancements in osteoporotic spine fixation. J Clin Orthop Trauma. 2020;11(5):778–85. https://doi.org/10.1016/j.jcot.2020.06.028. Epub 2020 Jul 6. PMID: 32904223; PMCID: PMC7452352
64. Levy HA, Karamian BA, Yalla GR, Canseco JA, Vaccaro AR, Kepler CK. Impact of surface roughness and bulk porosity on spinal interbody implants. J Biomed Mater Res B Appl Biomater. 2023;111(2):478–89. https://doi.org/10.1002/jbm.b.35161. Epub 2022 Sep 8. PMID: 36075112
65. Fred EJ, Minardi S, Goodwin AM, Nandurkar TS, Plantz MA, Lyons JG, Paul JT, Foley JP, Wintring AJ, Furman AA, Jeong S, Yun C, Stock SR, Hsu WK, Hsu EL. A mechanistic and preclinical assessment of BioRestore bioactive glass as a synthetic bone graft extender and substitute for Osteoinduction and spine fusion. Clin Spine Surg. 2024; https://doi.org/10.1097/BSD.0000000000001597. Epub ahead of print. PMID: 38531819
66. Shi LY, Wang A, Zang FZ, Wang JX, Pan XW, Chen HJ. Tantalum-coated pedicle screws enhance implant integration. Colloids Surf B Biointerfaces. 2017;160:22–32. https://doi.org/10.1016/j.colsurfb.2017.08.059. Epub 2017 Sep 7. PMID: 28915498
67. Borde MD, Menon VK, Kanade UP, Rajale SS, Mane AV, Varma H. Drug eluting bioactive glass ceramics for fusion in spondylodiscitis: a pilot study. Neurosurg Rev. 2024;47(1):80. https://doi.org/10.1007/s10143-024-02317-z. PMID: 38355838
68. Morimoto T, Hirata H, Eto S, Hashimoto A, Kii S, Kobayashi T, Tsukamoto M, Yoshihara T, Toda Y, Mawatari M. Development of silver-containing hydroxyapatite-coated antimicrobial implants for Orthopaedic and spinal surgery. Medicina (Kaunas). 2022;58(4):519. https://doi.org/10.3390/medicina58040519. PMID: 35454358; PMCID: PMC9029955
69. Liu GM, Kong N, Zhang XY, Bai HT, Yao Y, Han HZ, Luo YG. Extracellular matrix-coating pedicle screws conduct and induce osteogenesis. Eur J Orthop Surg Traumatol. 2014;24(Suppl 1):S173–82. https://doi.org/10.1007/s00590-013-1270-6. Epub 2013 Jul 11. PMID: 23842658
70. MatWeb: Online Materials Information Resource. Available on www.matweb.com (2024-06-21).

Bone Substitutes

Théo Broussolle and Cédric Y. Barrey

1 Introduction

In spinal arthrodesis, fusion is sometimes not achieved. This phenomenon, known as pseudarthrodesis, is quite common: 15–17% of lumbar arthrodesis surgeries and up to 24–39% in spinal deformity surgery [1–5]. It is rarer in cervical surgery and about 2.6% (1.2–21.2%) [6–9]. Pseudarthrodesis is responsible for spinal pain and treatment failure, as well as recurrence of anterior sagittal imbalance [1–3]. But 30% of peudarthrodeses are asymptomatic (particularly in elderly patients) [9]. It involves biological mechanisms similar to pseudarthrosis and may be due to inadequate instrumentation, postoperative mechanical stress, or other biological or infectious factors [10]. However, when the instrumentation is solid and the patient's mobility is limited, the remaining therapeutic options (to prevent or cure pseudarthrosis) are biological processes that stimulate osteogenesis and bone remodeling, which brings us to consider bone substitutes to help achieve fusion, in addition to autologous bone graft.

In order to obtain the bone remodeling that leads to fusion, it is necessary to obtain a contact between the cancellous bone surfaces and therefore to provide a bone graft. The spine surgeon can either use a bone graft harvested from the patient (autograft) or a bone graft harvested from other individuals (allograft), animals (allograft), or a synthetic bone graft (bone substitute). Autologous bone graft is currently considered to be the gold standard [11].

As a reminder, cortical (or compact) bone is made up of osteons, formed by cylinders of dense bone surrounding the Haversian canal (linked by the Volkmann's canals) [12]. It provides a real framework for the autograft [13]. However, cortical bone loses some of its mechanical strength when it is harvested for grafting [14]. Cancellous (or trabecular) bone is made up of bone trabeculae surrounding red (hematopoietic) and yellow (adipocytic) bone marrow. It is more vascularized and renews itself more rapidly than cortical bone. Revascularization during a graft starts within a few hours and is complete in a couple of weeks (compared with 2 months for cortical bone) [14]. Cancellous bone can be harvested from the iliac crest, tibia, radius, femur, mandible, rib, or calvaria [13, 15]. It has better osteoconductive, osteoinductive, osteogenic, and angiogenic

T. Broussolle
Department of Spine and Spinal Cord Surgery, Hôpital Neurologique, GHE, Hospices Civils de Lyon, University Claude Bernard of Lyon 1, Lyon, France

C. Y. Barrey (✉)
Department of Spine and Spinal Cord Surgery, Hôpital P. Wertheimer, GHE, Hospices Civils de Lyon (HCL), and University Claude Bernard of Lyon 1, Lyon, France

C. Y. Barrey (ed.), *Spine Surgery*, SFCR Experts Series 1,
https://doi.org/10.1007/978-3-031-85446-0_8

properties than cortical bone, thanks in particular to its concentrations of mesenchymal and hematopoietic stem cells and growth factors [15]. Decortication is essential for fusion, and is even more important than the use of cancellous rather than cortical bone grafts [16, 17]. Decortication involves exposing the bone and partially removing the cortical bone to uncover the cancellous bone in the area where the bone graft (of whatever type) will be placed.

Local bone autografting is sometimes contraindicated (in the case of spinal tumors or infections, for instance) or unavailable (in the case of a revision surgery or an anterior interbody fusion, for example). Autologous bone harvesting, especially remotely, is fraught with comorbidities: infection, pain, hematoma, nerve, vascular, or ureteral injury, sacroiliac joint damage, Tredelenburg gait, or even fracture [15, 18, 19]. The reported rates of minor complications following this procedure range from 7.1% to 39%, and major complications from 1.8% to 10% [15]. Autografting also increases operating duration [20].

When autograft cannot be used, we also consider the alternative use of bone substitutes. These are biomaterials, i.e., materials that are biocompatible (compatible with the human body) and bioactive (not inert). These materials can be osteoconductive (serving as a support for cellular and vascular bone growth) and/or osteoinductive (stimulating osteogenesis by means of cellular growth and differentiation factors, inducing differentiation of mesenchymal stem cells into bone-forming osteoblasts). "Osteostimulating" materials have properties somewhere between osteoconductive and osteoinductive materials. "Osteopromotive" materials enhance bone healing that is already taking place [20]. A good biomaterial must also be biodegradable. A good biomaterial should also have a certain stiffness (like bone) and porosity (to allow cell adhesion). Finally, "osteointegration" describes the surface bonding between the host bone and the grafting material [21]. Bone substitutes are used in around 35,000 patients a year in France [22]. There are a multitude of forms and compositions.

2 Allograft

Allograft is the most frequently chosen bone substitute [23]. It can be fresh, frozen, or freeze-dried, with cortical or cancellous bone. Cortical allograft has the advantage of a better structural strength [24]. Fresh allografts might ignite an immune response or transmit diseases [25]. Indeed, fresh frozen allograft has better osteoinductive and mechanical properties compared to freeze-dried allograft, but induce stronger immune responses and has already transmitted human immune-deficiency virus [24].

Comparative studies of allograft in humans sometimes show similar results but also often inferior results to autograft [26–30] (Fig. 1).

Fig. 1 Example of a viro-inactivated allograft: Osteopure® (Laboratoires O.S.T., Saint-Beauzire, France) (With the kind permission of the respective company to quote their product and use their picture)

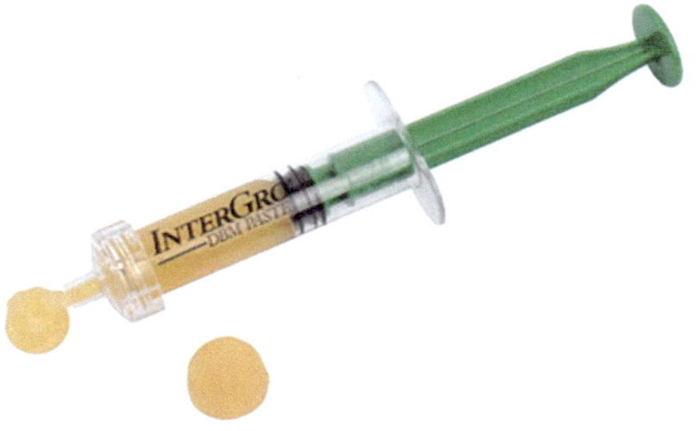

Fig. 2 Example of a demineralized bone matrix: InterGro® (Zimmer Biomet Spine, Inc., Westminster)

3 Demineralized Bone Matrix

Demineralized bone matrix (DBM) is produced through decalcification of corticocancellous bone via acid extraction, retaining the collagenous and non-collagenous proteins of the original tissue and making the growth factors bioavailable and giving this material an osteoinductive character [20, 24]. Because DBM is derived from human tissue, its disease transmission rates are similar to those of allograft bone [20]. However, these rates are variable and depend (as do the BMPs rates) on the mineralization process [20].

The results are thus not uniform, but animal and clinical studies seem to find rates of spinal fusion higher than those of allograft and similar to those of iliac crest bone graft [20, 24, 31]. In the end, DBM is most often used as a bone graft extender [20, 24, 31]. It is available in multiple forms, including gel, malleable putty, flexible strips, bone-chips, or injectable bone paste [24, 31] (Fig. 2).

4 Bioceramics

Bioceramics are synthetic bone substitutes, biocompatible (without risk of infection or toxicity), with the ability for osteointegration, osteoconduction, and maybe even osteostimulation but not for osteoinduction or osteogenicity and demonstrate minimal immediate structural support [24, 31]. Attached to the bone, ceramics induce production and mineralization of osteoid tissue, leading to intramembranous ossification and bone remodeling [24, 31]. Their pore size is critical for cell migration and vascularization [24, 31].

The two main ceramics are hydroxyapatite (HA) and tricalcium phosphate (TCP). HA constitutes the majority of the mineral extracellular matrix of bone. HA is moderately soluble and slowly absorbable, thus more stable than TPC, which releases calcium more quickly as it resorbs (faster, over several months) [20, 24]. However, there is also bicalcium phosphate (BCP), which is a combination of both. The results in terms of spinal fusion are good, but these ceramics are unable to outperform autograft [20, 31].

Finally, there is bioactive glass, another bioceramic made from silicon dioxide (SiO_2), sodium oxide (Na_2O), calcium oxide (CaO), and even phosphorus oxide (P_2O_5) [22]. By varying the proportions of these ions, all range of forms can be produced, from soluble to non-resorbable, and from putty to granules [22, 24]. The minerals it contains have the ability to bind bone proteins and trigger the production of hydroxyapatite [32]. There are few comparative studies on the use of bioactive glass in the spine. A recent systematic review of the literature analyzed 12 preclinical and 12 clinical studies of its use in the spine [33]. The meta-analysis found no significant difference in fusion rates (either preclinically or clinically) between the use of autograft alone or in combination with bioactive glass, but fusion rates with bioactive glass alone were significantly lower than with autograft alone [33]. However, its use, in association with local autograft, is easily achievable for spinal fusion and appears to give promising results [34] (Fig. 3).

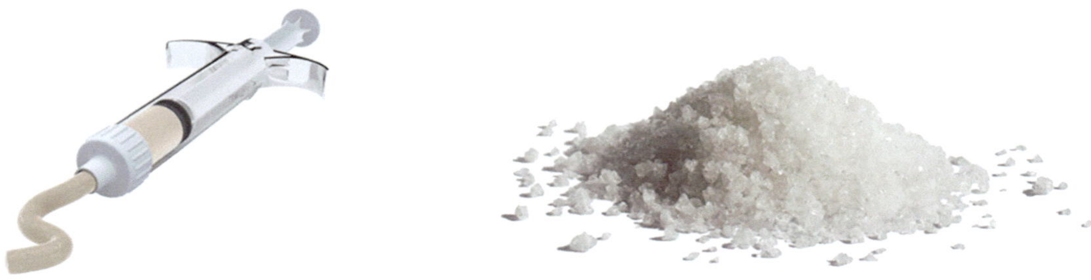

Fig. 3 Example of a bioceramic (bioactive glass): GlassBone® (Laboratoire Noraker, Lyon, France) in putty (left) or granules (right) form (With the kind permission of the respective company to quote their product and use their picture)

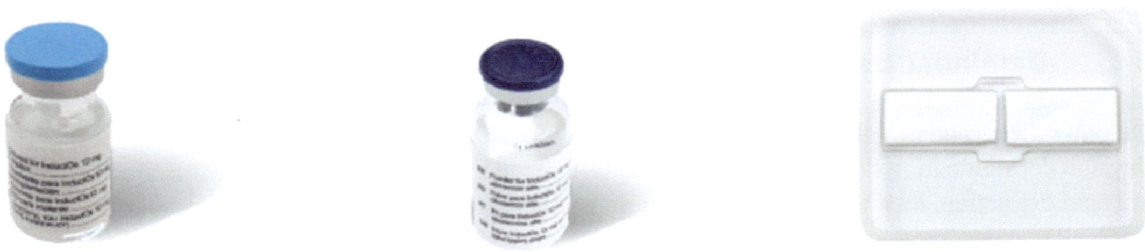

Fig. 4 Example of a BMP: InductOs™—rhBMP-2 (Medtronic): solvent (left), powder (middle), and matrix (right) (With the kind permission of the respective company to quote their product and use their picture)

5 Growth Factors—BMPs

The most commonly used growth factors are BMPs, members of the TGF-β family. The binding of these proteins to their receptors induces a cascade of intracellular events leading to enchondral ossification [31].

The use of BMP-2 and -7 in animals, as well as recombinant BMP-2 (rhBMP-2) and recombinant BMP-7 (OP-1) in humans, has been shown to be effective in spinal fusion [1, 35–37]. However, BMP-7 was withdrawn from the global market in 2014. Numerous studies have found very good results in terms of fusion, close to or equal to 100%, often as good as or better than autograft [20, 31, 38].

However, BMP is no longer reimbursed in France because its Medical Return Service was considered low. In fact, rhBMP-2 seems to be associated with more postoperative complications, in particular mechanical complications, pseudoarthrodesis, and more repeat surgeries [39]. Complications such as anterior neck swelling (after cervicotomy), osteolysis, retrograde ejaculation and urinary retention (after anterior lumbar approach), bony overgrowths, seromas, and radiculitis (after posterior approach) have also been reported [20]. A review of the literature estimated a rate of 10–50% of adverse events associated with rhBMP-2 [40]. Nevertheless, BMP-2 remains on the list of pharmaceutical specialties approved, in authorized indications (for instance, not for cervical surgery). In comparison, BMP-7 has been much less studied and there is less data on its safety (but it is now off the market anyway) [20].

All in all, BMP can be considered an effective tool for patients at risk of pseudoarthrodesis, particularly in the case of posterolateral revision surgery [20]. Other growth factors are less commonly used. Autologous growth factor (AGF) concentrate, for instance, is prepared from the ultra-concentration of platelets but has mixed results [31] (Fig. 4).

6 Other Bone Substitutes

We have not covered all the bone substitutes available in this chapter, but only the main ones.

Collagen is sometimes used, but in combination with other substitutes, as it has had mixed results [24].

Coralline hydroxyapatite (a porous structure made by calcium phosphate and derived from the sea coral) can be harvested from the nature or manufactured and used as a bone substitute [24]. It is similar to human cancellous bone and offers good mechanical qualities but is less osteogenic and is therefore used as a scaffold for osteoinductive bone substitutes [24].

Gene therapy and mesenchymal stem cells-based therapy shows promising osteoinductive results on in vivo animal and ex vivo studies, but they have not yet been developed for use in humans [31]. Xenografts are not used either, for infectious and immunogenic reasons.

7 Conclusion

The gold standard remains local autografting, as it is generally easily accessible, well-tolerated, and has good fusion rates. However, the surgeon can use various bone substitutes as a supplement or alternative. We classify these substitutes into two types: osteoconductive materials and osteoinductive materials [20, 24, 41].

Osteoconductive materials act like as a scaffold on which fusion can be built through osteoblasts migration, or as a mineral repository for cartilaginous calcification following their own resorption [20]. This includes deproteinized allografts or xenografts and bioceramics. However, it seems that if an osteoconductive scaffold is seeded with bone marrow aspirate, it would make it osteoinductive [24].

Osteoinductive materials act by recruiting or differentiating cells (into chondroblastic or osteoblastic lines) to the fusion site to facilitate fusion. Theoretically, they can induce bone production even in the absence of bone [20]. This includes growth factors (like BMPs), demineralized bone matrix, and products based on stem cells.

There is a vast literature on their in vitro effects, but few clinical studies comparing them to each other. This is mainly a question of habit and local availability. The reported fusion rates for each material seem to suggest that osteoinductive materials are superior to osteoconductive materials (Table 1) [42]. However, there is no clear evidence of an advantage in using the former over the latter [41]. One of the most promising emerging surgical options may be the use of a "composite

Table 1 Summary table of the main bone graft materials used for spinal fusion, classified as osteoinductive or osteoconductive

Bone graft material	Advantage	Disadvantage	Fusion rate (%)[a]	Range (%)[a]
Osteoinductive				
Autologous ICBG	Available and inexpensive	Responsible to comorbidities	79	40–100
Local autograft alone	Current gold standard	Sometimes unavailable or contraindicated	89	65–95
BMP-2	Highly effective	Various side effects described	94	90–100
DBM	Available in many forms	Variable results	89	63–97
Osteoconductive				
Bioceramics	Resorbable, in multiple forms	Poor biomechanical properties	87[b]	5–100[b]
Allograft	Structural strength if cortical	Immune and infectious risk if fresh	52	0–92

[a]Data from Hsu et al. [42]
[b]Only as an extender

graft" that contains osteogenic cells and osteoinductive growth factors along with a synthetic osteoconductive matrix, through tissue engineering, for instance [24].

References

1. Galimberti F, Lubelski D, Healy AT, Wang T, Abdullah KG, Nowacki AS, et al. A systematic review of lumbar fusion rates with and without the use of rhBMP-2. Spine. 2015;40(14):1132–9.
2. Campbell RC, Mobbs RJ, Lu VM, Xu J, Rao PJ, Phan K. Posterolateral fusion versus Interbody fusion for degenerative spondylolisthesis: systematic review and meta-analysis. Global Spine J. 2017;7(5):482–90.
3. Levin JM, Tanenbaum JE, Steinmetz MP, Mroz TE, Overley SC. Posterolateral fusion (PLF) versus transforaminal lumbar interbody fusion (TLIF) for spondylolisthesis: a systematic review and meta-analysis. Spine J. 2018;18(6):1088–98.
4. Kim YJ, Bridwell KH, Lenke LG, Rhim S, Cheh G. Pseudarthrosis in long adult spinal deformity instrumentation and fusion to the sacrum: prevalence and risk factor analysis of 144 cases. Spine. 2006;31(20):2329–36.
5. Lee KY, Lee JH, Kang KC, Shin SJ, Shin WJ, Im SK, et al. Strategy for obtaining solid fusion at L5-S1 in adult spinal deformity: risk factor analysis for nonunion at L5-S1. J Neurosurg Spine. 2020:1–9.
6. Badiee RK, Mayer R, Pennicooke B, Chou D, Mummaneni PV, Tan LA. Complications following posterior cervical decompression and fusion: a review of incidence, risk factors, and prevention strategies. J Spine Surg. 2020;6(1):323–33.
7. Shriver MF, Lewis DJ, Kshettry VR, Rosenbaum BP, Benzel EC, Mroz TE. Pseudoarthrosis rates in anterior cervical discectomy and fusion: a meta-analysis. Spine J. 2015;15(9):2016–27.
8. Hofler RC, Swong K, Martin B, Wemhoff M, Jones GA. Risk of Pseudoarthrosis after spinal fusion: analysis from the healthcare cost and utilization project. World Neurosurg déc. 2018;120:e194–202.
9. Leven D, Cho SK. Pseudarthrosis of the cervical spine: risk factors, diagnosis and management. Asian Spine J. 2016;10(4):776–86.
10. Steinmann JC, Herkowitz HN. Pseudarthrosis of the spine. Clin Orthop Relat Res. 1992;284:80–90.
11. Fischer CR, Cassilly R, Cantor W, Edusei E, Hammouri Q, Errico T. A systematic review of comparative studies on bone graft alternatives for common spine fusion procedures. Eur Spine J. 2013;22(6):1423–35.
12. Rho JY, Kuhn-Spearing L, Zioupos P. Mechanical properties and the hierarchical structure of bone. Med Eng Phys. 1998;20(2):92–102.
13. Dissaux C, Wagner D, George D, Spingarn C, Rémond Y. Mechanical impairment on alveolar bone graft: a literature review. J Craniomaxillofac Surg. 2018;7
14. Yaszemski MJ, Payne RG, Hayes WC, Langer R, Mikos AG. Evolution of bone transplantation: molecular, cellular and tissue strategies to engineer human bone. Biomaterials. 1996;17(2):175–85.
15. Myeroff C, Archdeacon M. Autogenous bone graft: donor sites and techniques. J Bone Joint Surg Am. 2011;93(23):2227–36.
16. Canto FRT, Garcia SB, Issa JPM, Marin A, Del Bel EA, Defino HLA. Influence of decortication of the recipient graft bed on graft integration and tissue neoformation in the graft-recipient bed interface. Eur Spine J. 2008;17(5):706–14.
17. Boden SD, Schimandle JH, Hutton WC. An experimental lumbar intertransverse process spinal fusion model. Radiographic, histologic, and biomechanical healing characteristics. Spine. 1995;20(4):412–20.
18. Fernyhough JC, Schimandle JJ, Weigel MC, Edwards CC, Levine AM. Chronic donor site pain complicating bone graft harvesting from the posterior iliac crest for spinal fusion. Spine. 1992;17(12):1474–80.
19. Silber JS, Anderson DG, Daffner SD, Brislin BT, Leland JM, Hilibrand AS, et al. Donor site morbidity after anterior iliac crest bone harvest for single-level anterior cervical discectomy and fusion. Spine. 2003;28(2):134–9.
20. Grabowski G, Cornett CA. Bone graft and bone graft substitutes in spine surgery: current concepts and controversies. J Am Acad Orthop Surg. 2013;21(1):51–60.
21. Costantino PD, Friedman CD. Synthetic bone graft substitutes. Otolaryngol Clin N Am. 1994;27(5):1037–74.
22. HAS. Commission nationale d'evaluation des dispositifs medicaux Et Des Technologies De Sante : glassbone, substitut osseux synthétique. 2018. p. 10.
23. Carter G. Harvesting and implanting allograft bone. AORN J. 1999;70(4):660–70. quiz 672–6
24. Giannoudis PV, Dinopoulos H, Tsiridis E. Bone substitutes: an update. Injury. 2005;36(Suppl 3):S20–7.
25. Friedlaender GE, Strong DM, Tomford WW, Mankin HJ. Long-term follow-up of patients with osteochondral allografts. A correlation between immunologic responses and clinical outcome. Orthop Clin North Am. 1999;30(4):583–8.
26. Gibson S, McLeod I, Wardlaw D, Urbaniak S. Allograft versus autograft in instrumented posterolateral lumbar spinal fusion: a randomized control trial. Spine (Phila Pa 1976). 2002;27(15):1599–603.
27. Samartzis D, Shen FH, Matthews DK, Yoon ST, Goldberg EJ, An HS. Comparison of allograft to autograft in multilevel anterior cervical discectomy and fusion with rigid plate fixation. Spine J. 2003;3(6):451–9.
28. Follmar KE, Prichard HL, DeCroos FC, Wang HT, Levin LS, Klitzman B, et al. Combined bone allograft and adipose-derived stem cell autograft in a rabbit model. Ann Plast Surg. 2007;58(5):561–5.
29. Jorgenson SS, Lowe TG, France J, Sabin J. A prospective analysis of autograft versus allograft in posterolateral lumbar fusion in the same patient. A

minimum of 1-year follow-up in 144 patients. Spine. 1994;19(18):2048–53.
30. An HS, Lynch K, Toth J. Prospective comparison of autograft vs. allograft for adult posterolateral lumbar spine fusion: differences among freeze-dried, frozen, and mixed grafts. J Spinal Disord. 1995;8(2):131–5.
31. Gupta A, Kukkar N, Sharif K, Main BJ, Albers CE, El-Amin SF III. Bone graft substitutes for spine fusion: a brief review. World J Orthop. 2015;6(6):449–56.
32. Lefebvre L. Développement de bioverre poreux ostéoinducteur pour application à l'orthopédie et à l'ingénierie tissulaire.
33. Cottrill E, Pennington Z, Lankipalle N, Ehresman J, Valencia C, Schilling A, et al. The effect of bioactive glasses on spinal fusion: a cross-disciplinary systematic review and meta-analysis of the preclinical and clinical data. J Clin Neurosci. 2020;78:34.
34. Barrey C, Broussolle T. Clinical and radiographic evaluation of bioactive glass in posterior cervical and lumbar spinal fusion. Eur J Orthop Surg Traumatol. 2019;29:1623.
35. Lane JM. Bone morphogenic protein science and studies. J Orthop Trauma. 2005;19(10 Suppl):S17–22.
36. Vaccaro AR, Patel T, Fischgrund J, Anderson DG, Truumees E, Herkowitz H, et al. A pilot safety and efficacy study of OP-1 putty (rhBMP-7) as an adjunct to iliac crest autograft in posterolateral lumbar fusions. Eur Spine J. 2003;12(5):495–500.
37. Burkus JK, Gornet MF, Dickman CA, Zdeblick TA. Anterior lumbar interbody fusion using rhBMP-2 with tapered interbody cages. J Spinal Disord Tech. 2002;15(5):337–49.
38. Boden SD, Kang J, Sandhu H, Heller JG. Use of recombinant human bone morphogenetic protein-2 to achieve posterolateral lumbar spine fusion in humans: a prospective, randomized clinical pilot trial: 2002 Volvo Award in clinical studies. Spine (Phila Pa 1976). 2002;27(23):2662–73.
39. James AW, LaChaud G, Shen J, Asatrian G, Nguyen V, Zhang X, et al. A review of the clinical side effects of bone morphogenetic Protein-2. Tissue Eng Part B Rev. 2016;22(4):284–97.
40. Carragee EJ, Hurwitz EL, Weiner BK. A critical review of recombinant human bone morphogenetic protein-2 trials in spinal surgery: emerging safety concerns and lessons learned. Spine J. 2011;11(6):471–91.
41. Kurd M, Cohick S, Park A, Ahmadinia K, Lee J, An H. Fusion in degenerative spondylolisthesis: comparison of osteoconductive and osteoinductive bone graft substitutes. Eur Spine J. 2015;24(5):1066–73.
42. Hsu WK, Nickoli MS, Wang JC, Lieberman JR, An HS, Yoon ST, et al. Improving the clinical evidence of bone graft substitute technology in lumbar spine surgery. Global Spine J. 2012;2(4):239–48.

Spinal Cord Injury and Regeneration

Florence E. Perrin, William Haynes,
Yannick N. Gerber, and Nicolas Lonjon

1 Epidemiology

Overall, the symptoms of spinal cord lesion positively correlate with the extent of the damage and the location along the rostrocaudal segment of the spinal cord. They can include loss of sensorimotor and autonomic functions (including blood pressure, bladder and bowel control, breathing and heart rate).

The number of people living with spinal cord injury is unclear; however, in the most recent WHO report, albeit published some time ago, the estimated worldwide number of people who suffer a traumatic spinal cord injury every year is between 250,000 and 500,000 [1]. Due to availability of the data, methodological approaches, composition in the population (children and adults) and exposure to risk, the incidence rates of traumatic spinal cord injury (TSCI) strongly vary across the world from 13 to 53 cases per million (cpm) population. The national spinal cord injury statistical center recently reported an incidence rates of 54 cpm people in the United States [2]. In a recent literature review including data from 49 countries, the incidence of TSCI ranged from 3.3 to 195.4 cpm [3]. However, there are some unavoidable limitations such as the availability of data (49 out of 200 countries) and country-specific methodologies to collect data.

Studies indicate that among adults, there are consistently higher incidence rates of TSCI among males, with a minimum male-to-female ratio of 2:1, whereas in the pediatric population, the sex ratio is more balanced. TSCI displays two common age-associated peaks: young adults (females: 15–19 years and males: 20–29 years) and older people (females >60 and males >70) [1].

Based on data across WHO regions, the foremost common causes of TSCI are transport (road traffic crashes in particular), falls, violence, and sports (see Fig. 1). However, strong fluctuations are observed depending on the region. For instance, transport accounts for 40% in the Americas and up to 70% in Africa, falls range from 15% in Africa to 40% in Asia, violence varies from 2% in Canada to 60% in Afghanistan,

F. E. Perrin (✉)
MMDN, Univ. Montpellier, EPHE, INSERM, Montpellier, France

Institut Universitaire de France (IUF), Paris, France
e-mail: florence.perrin@umontpellier.fr

W. Haynes
Department of Neurosurgery, CHU, Montpellier, France
e-mail: w-haynes@chu-montpellier.fr

Y. N. Gerber
MMDN, Univ. Montpellier, EPHE, INSERM, Montpellier, France
e-mail: Yannick.gerber@umontpellier.fr

N. Lonjon
MMDN, Univ. Montpellier, EPHE, INSERM, Montpellier, France

Department of Neurosurgery, CHU, Montpellier, France
e-mail: n-lonjon@chu-montpellier.fr

C. Y. Barrey (ed.), *Spine Surgery*, SFCR Experts Series 1,
https://doi.org/10.1007/978-3-031-85446-0_9

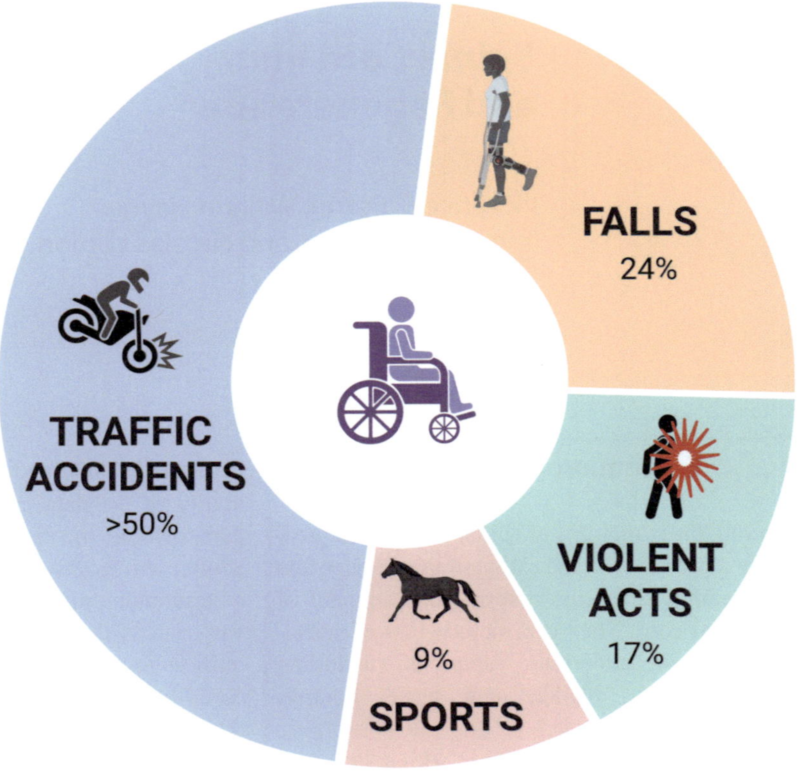

Fig. 1 Causes of spinal cord injury. Traffic accidents are the most recent leading cause of SCI, followed by falls. Violent acts and sports/recreation activities are also relatively common causes. (Data from the WHO [1] and NSCISC [2] reports. Source: Author)

and sports range from less than 5% in Africa/Asia to 10% in the Americas. The etiology of TSCI also varies depending on age and gender. Among children and young adults, transport represents the most common cause of TSCI, while falls become the predominant cause after the age of 60 [1]. Violence and sports are more common among males after the age of 5 and 13 years, respectively.

In high-income countries, the average age at the injury has increased. In the United States, it changed from 29 years during the 1970s to 43 since 2015 [2].

Overall, people with SCI are 2 to 5 times more likely to die prematurely, either directly from the injury or from secondary conditions, than people without SCI, with significant variation depending on the location worldwide and the level and severity of the lesion. Mortality is higher for tetraplegics than for paraplegics, and people with complete lesions die earlier than people with incomplete injuries.

The highest risk of death occurs during the first year after TSCI, and in low-income countries, many patients die from preventable secondary conditions such as urologic complications and pressure ulcers. In high-income countries, improvements in medical management have resulted in longer life expectancy since 1950s, particularly through a decreased risk of mortality from secondary conditions such as urosepsis and respiratory problems; however, these risks remain higher compared to the general population [1]. Though, in the United States, the average remaining years of life for persons with SCI have not improved since the 1980s [2].

2 Pathophysiology

The pathophysiological progression of SCI involves an initial mechanical trauma (see Fig. 2b), inducing the primary injury (see Fig. 2c), followed by subsequent secondary inju-

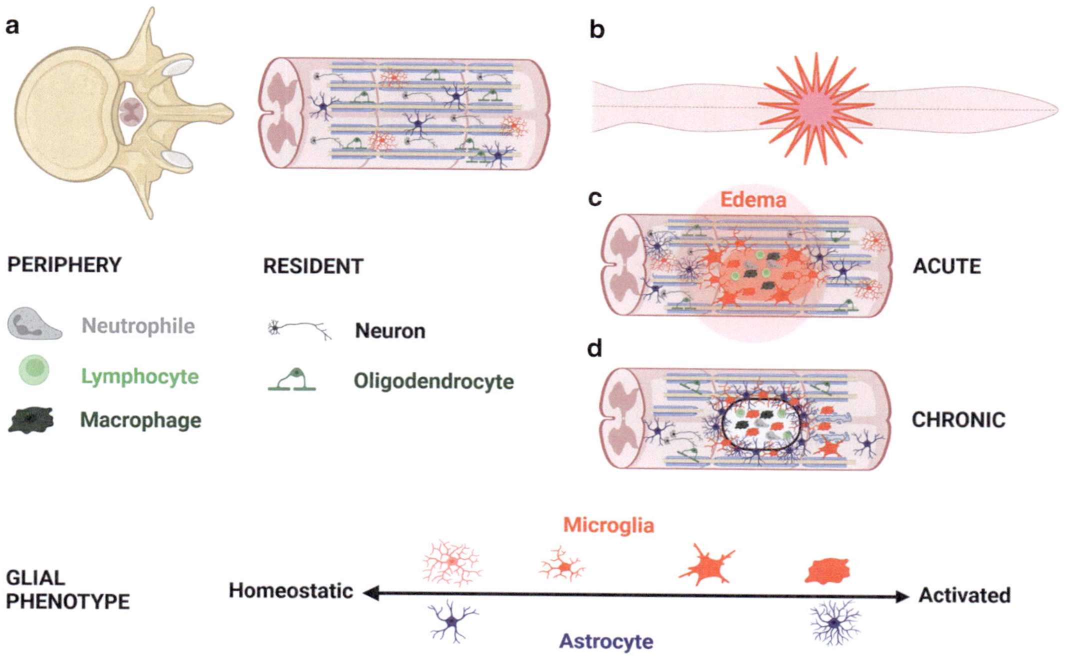

Fig. 2 Pathophysiology. (**a**) Schematic view of the uninjured spinal cord. (**b**) Spinal cord trauma. (**c**) Cellular responses and tissue reorganization at the acute stage following SCI. (**d**) Cellular responses and tissue reorganization at the chronic stage following SCI. (Source: Author)

ries that can persist for several weeks, months, and even years (see Fig. 2d) after the initial trauma.

The acute phase begins just within minutes after the primary injury, initiating a cascade of cellular and biochemical events that may extend over several weeks or months. Importantly, these events can play both protective and reparative roles, as well as exacerbate damage. While a general pattern of secondary mechanisms has been identified, the nature of the primary injury influences the dynamics of these mechanisms. Therefore, we can broadly categorize that the acute phase typically occurs within seconds to hours, the intermediate phase spans hours to weeks, and the long-lasting or chronic phase extends from months to years.

First, bleeding leads to hypotension and vasospasm, which, on cellular level, result in hypoxia, disruption in molecular homeostasis, and excitotoxicity. At the lesion site, these events induce cell death. In the subacute phase, the evolution of edema (represented in Fig. 2c) plays a critical role after SCI. This phase is also characterized by the activation of resident immune cells (microglia) and the infiltration of peripheral immune cell (macrophage, neutrophils, lymphocytes). Importantly, this inflammatory response is not only detrimental but also exhibits beneficial effects, including the clearance of cellular and myelin debris containing inhibitors that prevent axonal regrowth (see Fig. 2c).

In the latter stages of this phase, a glial scar forms and surrounds the lesion epicenter. The glial scar, primarily composed of microglia, NG2 glia (also known as oligodendrocyte progenitor cells), and astrocytes plays dual roles. It acts as both a barrier to spontaneous axonal regeneration, hindering functional recovery, and as a limit to lesion extension. Glial cells activation involves intricate cellular and molecular interactions, including crosstalk with immune cells. After injury, glial cells proliferate and migrate toward the injury site. During the acute and subacute stages, early microglia activation and infiltration of monocyte derived macrophages (MDM) from the periphery precede immune-cell infiltration and astrocyte activation. At later stage, astrocytes, together with microglia and NG2 cells, contribute to the formation of a dense astroglial border surrounding the lesion. The lesion core, or fibrotic scar, is composed of infiltrating immune cells, and a few activated microglia along with dense extracellular components such as fibronectin, laminin, and collagen (see Fig. 2d) [4].

Importantly, there is a persistent microglia proliferation in the chronic stage after SCI, reflecting the long-lasting dynamics of the scar [5]. Adult rodents and primates exhibit overall similar dynamics of the glial response; however, astrocytic activation in primates is delayed compared to rodents (for review see [6]). Therefore, understanding species-specific glial dynamics after SCI is crucial to identify the correct time windows for potential targets for therapeutic interventions. Furthermore, immune cell responses display sexual dimorphism. Thus, investigations of sex-dependent responses following SCI are also of utmost importance.

All these events occur concomitantly with mechanisms including excitotoxicity and free radical assaults and extend to secondary retrograde and Wallerian degeneration. In the long-lasting or chronic phase, there is overall stabilization of the lesion volume; however, it may expand to secondary scar-encapsulated cavities.

3 Standard of Care

As stated above, complex pathophysiological processes occur immediately after the injury and continue to evolve during the chronic phase. In the acute stage after injury, patients not only develop neurological deficits directly related to the injury but also undergo spinal shock, characterized by respiratory/circulatory disruption, as well as urinary incontinence. During this phase, the primary focus is to ensure adequate respiratory function and provide hemodynamic support.

Within days following the injury, the patient enters the subacute stage or secondary phase, during which they typically recover from spinal shock. However, despite this recovery, neurological deficits and accompanying complications persist from the original trauma. The patient then progresses to the chronic phase of SCI, which is dependent upon the overall condition of the patient and the severity of the lesion. In this phase, patients might undergo partial neurological improvement, development of adaptive mechanisms, or the emergence of delayed neurological symptoms such as urinary bladder dysfunction, neuropathic pain, dysautonomia, lipodystrophy, musculoskeletal atrophy, and abnormal skeletal postures (for review see [7]). Only about 1% of patients with SCI achieve full recovery. Nearly 45% of cases involve severe neurological impairment, which may manifest as complete or incomplete tetraplegia, with or without accompanying respiratory compromise.

One of the major challenges in effectively managing SCI lies in the identification of noninvasive, precise, practical, and sensitive predictive measures for diagnosing the severity of the injury and guiding treatment decisions. Given the availability of reliable diagnostic and predictive tests, treatments, including surgical interventions, can be personalized for each patient. This personalized approach ensures the implementation of better evidence-based practices. However, tools available to evaluate the severity of spinal cord tissue damage and predict recovery are still limited, especially in developing countries. This limitation arises from substantial resources required to perform various imaging tests necessary to determine the best neurosurgical intervention for each case.

To establish reasonable therapy goals and plan for post discharge care, it is essential for patients, families, and health care providers to have accurate information about prognosis of recovery. Discussing prognosis and expected outcomes with patients and families requires a thorough understanding of the neurologic impact and a fair assessment of the severity of the SCI. Therefore, we provide a concise overview of prognosis and outcomes after SCI.

4 Biomarkers

Potential SCI biomarkers used to follow the neurological recovery state could significantly enhance diagnostic and treatment strategies. Of course, the selection of appropriate biomarkers should be based on the stage of the injury. Recent updates in SCI biomarkers have highlighted two methods for identifying possible biomarkers.

During the first few weeks after the injury, the disruption of the blood–spinal cord barrier (BSCB) permits the release of various neurological structural components from the damaged tissue. These components enter the systemic circulation and the cerebrospinal fluid (CSF). As the injury advances, various components resulting from pathological processes such as neuroinflammation, excitotoxicity, reactive oxygen species, and apoptosis become expressed or released. Hence, there is an increasing interest in investigating correlations between these components and the severity or outcomes of the injury. The initial source of biomarkers originates from the breach of the BSCB, allowing cellular components such as proteins, phospholipids, neurotransmitters, and metabolites to leak from the lesion site into the CSF and bloodstream. These components are often derived from both glial cells and neurons.

The second significant origin of biomarkers comprises products generated from neuroinflammatory processes or regenerative attempts occurring in the subacute or chronic phase. Efforts are currently being made to analyze the components of blood and CSF at various timepoints post-injury, although it is important to note the lack of human studies for many suggested potential biomarkers (for review see [8]).

Potential biomarkers in SCI are directly associated with the injury and the loss of cells, including neurons and glial cells. Biomarkers of neuronal death include, but are not restricted to neurofilaments (NF), cleaved Tau, and neuron-specific enolase (NSE). NF that are cytoskeletal proteins expressed in the cytoplasm of axonal fibers, comprise NF-light (NF-L), -medium (NF-M), and -heavy (NF-H) chains and are released from the cytoplasm of injured neurons after SCI. During the evolution of secondary injury, characterized by neuroinflammation and apoptosis, NFs may leak into the extracellular space together with other cytoplasmic components. Therefore, NFs are speculated to potentially reflect the severity of neuronal loss as well as the extent of secondary damage. Several studies support the notion that elevated NF-L and NF-H levels are associated with more severe SCI and poorer neurological prognosis. Tau, a microtubule associated protein, helps to stabilize axons and contributes to axonal transport after an injury. In particular, cleaved Tau is abundant within disrupted axons and is detectable in the sera/CSF upon BSCB disruption. Some studies suggest that higher Tau levels correlate with increased injury severities and predict neurological outcome. However, further research efforts are required to clearly identify Tau potential role as a SCI biomarker.

NSE, an enzyme in neuronal cytoplasm, is an established biomarker for ischemic brain injury. In experimental SCI models, NSE is expressed in both neurons and glial cells at the injury site, therefore suggesting a link between NSE, neuroinflammation, and astrogliosis. Moreover, the severity of the injury models correlates with neurological deficits and protein levels in CSF and serum. However, clinical studies are still lacking and essential to validate these correlations.

Matrix metalloproteinases (MMPs) are crucial for the degradation of extracellular matrix proteins in both neurons and glial cells. MMPs expressed during the subacute phase of SCI may therefore serve as potential biomarkers for predicting neurological outcomes.

Biomarkers of glial cell death and responses include, but are not restricted to, glial fibrillary acidic protein (GFAP), S100-β, and various inflammatory markers. GFAP, an intermediate filament protein, plays a crucial role in the proper assembly and development of astrocyte cytoskeleton. It is upregulated after injury and serves as an established biomarker for traumatic brain injury. Serum concentration of GFAP differs between patients with improved recovery and those without improvement, as defined by a change in American Impairment Scale (AIS) grade and motor score over a 6-month period. After 24 h, the level of GFAP in the serum of patients had been reported as significantly higher than control levels. Additionally, significant variation in GFAP levels were observed between AIS grade A, B, and grades C+ D cases. S100-β, a calcium binding protein in glial cells, is also an established marker for brain injury. However, insufficient studies in SCI have explored S100-β levels in tissue, serum, or CSF. Furthermore, a large number of nonspecific inflammatory factors are reported in the literature, with varying degrees of interest in SCI. Nonetheless, there is a need for large sample size human studies to examine the fluctuation of their serum levels and achieve the best predictive correlations with neurological recovery.

Besides, proteomics is becoming an important approach for biomarker discovery in SCI. This approach uncovers targets that reflect the activity of diverse molecular pathways, whether activated or suppressed following injury. It also offers a chronological overview of physiological responses to injury that can help to predict outcomes and recovery.

5 Modern Clinical Management

Despite significant investment in preclinical research to enhance comprehension of SCI pathophysiology and create efficient targeted therapies, few, if any, have reached clinical practice. Present clinical strategies for SCI treatment encompass aggressive intensive care interventions, early surgical decompression, and stabilization, coupled with blood pressure elevation to mitigate secondary injury. Significant advances have been made in the clinical management of SCI over the past two decades, resulting in rapid changes in guidelines. Particularly notable progress has been achieved in the diagnosis and treatment of blunt cerebrovascular injury, along with advancements in the utilization of imaging techniques and timing of decompression. While these guidelines may offer varying conclusions, they remain precious resources for healthcare practitioners.

5.1 Surgical Decompression (Fig. 4a)

Recent studies provide evidence of neurological benefits from early surgical decompression for SCI (Fig. 3). This has led to the recognition that urgent decompression of the injured spinal cord is crucial. A recent meta-analysis that evaluated the timing of surgery from 1996 to 2012 across 18 studies, revealed significant heterogeneity among these studies. Nonetheless, early surgery consistently demonstrated superior total motor score, greater neurological improvement, and shorter hospital stays compared to late surgery.

The Surgical Timing in Acute Spinal Cord Injury Study (STASCIS) was a prospective multicenter study comparing 6-month surgical outcome after early ($<$24 h) or late ($\geq$24 h) treatment for cervical spinal cord injury. A total of 313 patients were enrolled and patients who underwent early surgery showed a greater likelihood of $\geq$2 improvement in AIS grades at 6-month follow-up. Although criticisms were made regarding the methodology used, these results have increased the important of early SCI treatment.

Further study of outcome data and the timing of surgery is expected in the near future. Given the demonstrated benefits of early surgical treatment for patients with cervical SCI, recent research efforts have evaluated early decompression following thoracolumbar SCI, evaluated methods for earlier transfer of patients for surgical care, earlier rehabilitation after surgery, and the development of imaging methods to stratify patients and predict prognosis before surgical intervention.

The concept of optimal surgical care is becoming increasingly legitimate as soon as possible, and efforts must be made at all levels to transport patients as quickly as possible to a multidisciplinary care platform. Surgical decompression after SCI is nowadays mainly accepted as a neuroprotective measure. Through the modification of both extrinsic and intrinsic pressure on the spinal cord, combined with anatomical realignment and fusion techniques, it is possible to achieve an equalization of intraspinal pressure with cerebrospinal fluid (CSF) pressure. This can enhance

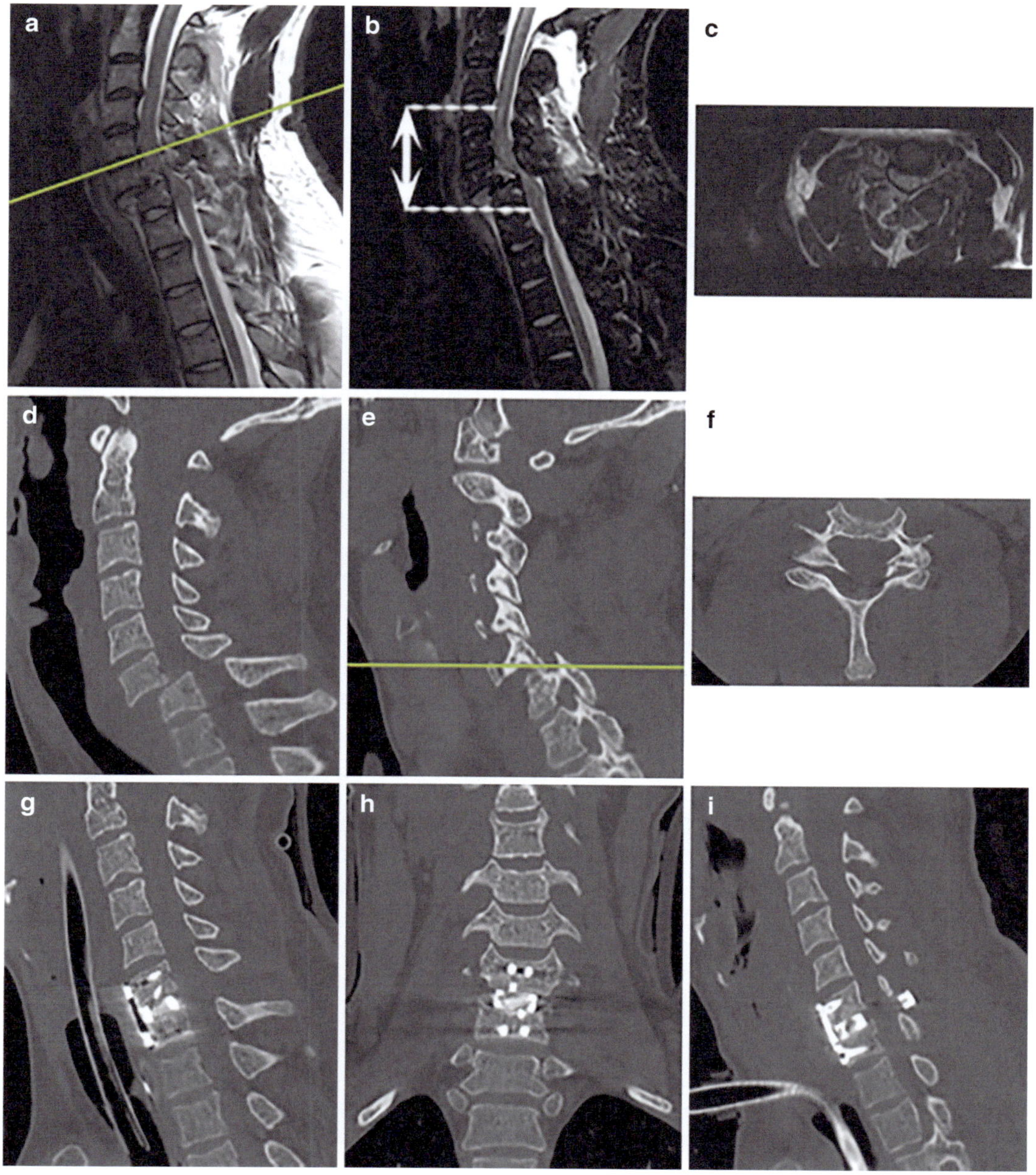

Fig. 3 Neuroimaging. (**a**) Sagittal T2 MRI view of cervical spine after motor vehicle accident. At the level of cervical luxation (C6–C7), we can see a complete reduction in the size of the spinal canal with partial transection of the cord. (**b**) Sagittal T2 STIR MRI view: the spinal cord lesion extension is indicated by the two-way arrows. We can see also an extensive hyperintensity of the interspinous soft tissues between C2–C7 level, indicating a posterior ligamentous injury. (**c**) Axial T2 MRI section, one level above the lesion, taken at the level indicated in yellow in (**a**), showing a diffuse hyperintensity in the cord with focal points of hypointensity indicating a significant edema with points of hemorrhage. (**d**, **e**) Sagittal cervical spine tomodensitometry views before surgery, showing a complete cervical C6–C7 luxation. (**f**) Axial cervical spine tomodensitometry section taken at the level indicated in yellow in (**e**), indicating a complete bilateral C6–C7 facets luxation. (**g**, **h**) Sagittal and coronal cervical spine tomodensitometry views after the first anterior cervical discectomy and fusion surgery with titanium cage and plate. (**i**) Sagittal cervical spine tomodensitometry views after the second posterior fixation surgery with locking band and graft

spinal cord perfusion pressure (SCPP) and facilitate autoregulation.

Furthermore, recent research indicates that expansion duraplasty could potentially mitigate the extent of secondary injury and facilitate neurological recovery by reducing edema and the resulting obstruction of microcirculation. This approach may also help alleviate ischemia and minimize damage to neural tissue at the site of injury [9]. Indeed, some authors argue that bony decompression alone is insufficient for achieving full decompression of the spinal cord. Consequently, expansion duraplasty is essential to reestablish a patent subarachnoid space and to improve SCPP. Some authors also propose an algorithm to predict the need for expansion duraplasty for AIS grades A–C patients. They suggest that complete decompression is most likely achieved with multilevel laminectomy, which reestablished CSF interface posteriorly, anteriorly, or in anterior/posterior aspects of the swollen spinal cord. However, in a small percentage of patients, when the swollen spinal cord continues to be compressed against the dura and is not relieved with the projected laminectomy (as observed through real-time intraoperative ultrasonography), additional duraplasty may still be necessary. Important limitations exist in this retrospective work, and a future randomized controlled trial may help resolve some of these uncertainties.

5.2 Hemodynamic Regulation (Fig. 4a)

Independently of hypovolemic shock, the "spinal shock" resulting from the loss and deregulation of sympathetic centers can sometimes lead to severe arterial hypotension. A vasoplegic circulatory attack of neurogenic origin, characterized by hypotension and an inadequate cardiac response, is sometimes observed with bradycardia. The incidence of the spinal shock varies between 19 and 29% in cases of cervical spinal cord injury. For example, a large retrospective English study analyzing the incidence of spinal shock in patients with isolated spinal cord injuries (without any other significant injury) highlighted that upon arrival at the emergency room, 14.2% of the patients presented clinical signs of spinal shock [10]. Physiopathologically termed "neurogenic shock," this condition can result in spinal cord hypoperfusion and therefore worsened damages to the spinal cord. Several reports have suggested that preventing hypotension after SCI and even augmenting mean arterial pressure (MAP) may be beneficial to neurological recovery. While target parameters remain subject to debate, all studies recommend a mean blood pressure > 85 mmHg. More precisely, hemodynamic support with vasopressor medications has been suggested in recent American Association of Neurosurgical Surgeon and Congress of Neurological Surgeons (AANS/CNS) guidelines to prevent hypotension (defined as a systolic blood pressure < 90 mmHg) and to increase MAPs to >85–90 mmHg [11].

A recent meta-analysis of 11 studies (9 retrospective, 2 prospective) evaluating MAP measurements in SCI suggested that MAP augmentation was achieved in most patients, with lower MAPs correlating with worse outcomes. Commonly used agents included dopamine, norepinephrine, and phenylephrine, although dopamine was associated with more complications than other vasopressors. However, these data remain controversial [12]. Ultimately, no recommendation of a specific type of pressor has been seen from the AANS/CNS Joint Section guidelines and the Consortium for Spinal Cord Medicine recommends dopamine or norepinephrine because of the incorporation of both alpha and beta adrenergic agents [13].

Future studies will further refine how MAP augmentation is achieved and applied after SCI and probably direct intrathecal monitors of cord perfusion, combined by meticulous clinical studies, will further optimize the control of perfusion of preserved and injured spinal cord tissue.

5.3 Invasive Spinal Cord Pressure Monitoring (Fig. 4a)

As mentioned above, current clinical guidelines recommend maintaining the MAP between 85 and 90 mmHg for the first 7 days postinjury. One potential limitation with this approach is the exclusive focus on MAP and not spinal cord perfusion pressure (SCPP). SCPP signifies the net pressure gradient responsible for delivering oxygen to the injured spinal cord. It is determined by subtracting the pressure within the intrathecal space from the MAP. Pressure within the intrathecal space can be measured either by surgically inserting a pressure probe at the site of the injury during spinal decompression/fusion or by percutaneous insertion of a catheter into the lumbar cistern distal to the injury site. Therefore, optimal hemodynamic management should include monitoring of intraspinal pressure to calculate and act upon spinal perfusion pressure.

Furthermore, guidelines for managing hemodynamics in traumatic brain injury offer Level IIB recommendations concerning cerebral perfusion pressure thresholds and Level III recommendations regarding blood pressure thresholds [14]. Likewise, SCPP undergoes regular monitoring during thoracoabdominal aortic aneurysm repair due to the inherent vulnerability of the spinal cord's blood supply. In this scenario, a catheter is percutaneously inserted into the lumbar cistern to perform dual functions: monitoring intrathecal pressure (ITP) and draining CSF to lower ITP, consequently elevating SCPP. Recommendations for CSF drainage following traumatic brain injury advocate for continuous drainage over intermittent drainage to reduce ITP and improve recovery outcomes [15]. Combination of MAP increase and CSF drainage induced a better enhancement of spinal cord perfusion than drainage alone after SCI in a porcine model. Two clinical studies have examined the impact of CSF drainage on pressure within the intrathecal space so far, but neither has shown a definitive correlation between CSF drainage and intrathecal pressure. Recent studies propose that expansion duraplasty, when employed during surgical decompression, shows promises in decreasing ISP and improving SCPP. This approach may diminish secondary injury and promote neurological recovery by reducing edema and preventing subsequent microcirculation obstruction, ischemia, and neural tissue damage at the injury site [16]. Recent studies have expanded the role of epidural and intrathecal pressure monitoring to directly evaluate perfusion in order to improve understanding of spinal cord perfusion and explore potential local therapeutic solutions. Recent work has shown that pressure catheters placed subdurally at the site of injury can predict neurological outcome 9–12 months after injury. Studies in animals indicate that AQP4 channels are pivotal in both the formation and resolution of edema after SCI, underscoring the potential therapeutic value of modulating AQP4 for resolving edema and facilitating functional recovery. Promising novel research regarding interventions aimed at decreasing pressure within the intrathecal space emphasizes potential pharmacological targets. These targets include substances such as substance P, which can help in reducing neurogenic inflammation, as well as methods for decreasing CSF secretion and/or accumulation.

Therefore, new and promising clinical research includes interventions to lower pressure along with approaches aimed at reducing CSF secretion and/or buildup. However, several parameters, including but not restricted to anesthesia, posture, sleep disturbances, and pharmacological intervention, may interfere with CSF physiology and pressure, therefore a better understanding of CSF physiology following SCI may accelerate interventions to reduce pressure around the injured cord.

5.4 Corticosteroids (Fig. 4a)

Corticosteroids are a controversial neuroprotective treatment for acute SCI. The main randomized controlled trials, namely the National Acute Spinal Cord Injury Studies (NASCIS), have evaluated the role of methylprednisolone sodium succinate (MPSS) at different times of injury [17]. Although primary endpoints were not improved with the use of steroids, secondary analysis suggested that treatment within 8 h led to an improvement in Functional Independence Measure scores at 1 year. However, this improvement was accompanied by a significative increase in risks directly linked to corticosteroid such as infections, gastrointestinal hemorrhages, and deaths. Since these studies, controversy has persisted over the interest of this protocol, the AANS/CNS, and many other similar European Surgical and Anesthesiologist associations did not recommend steroid use after SCI citing a lack of supportive evidence. A more recent systematic review from AO Spine (New guidelines from AO Spine on the management of SCI), based on the modest improvements in mean motor scores at 6 and 12 months in the corticosteroid group compared with the control group, suggested making a 24-h infusion of high-dose MPSS available to adult patients within 8 h after SCI [11].

Future clinical studies evaluating possible novel anti-inflammatory or other neuroprotective agents will have to ensure that treatments are provided early, SCI groups are well defined with an adequate control group available, an objective measure of functional outcome is used, and a realistic follow-up time for recovery is provided.

5.5 Modern Neuroimaging (Fig. 4a)

Magnetic resonance imaging (MRI) of intramedullary signal characteristics early (within hours to days) after SCI provides important clinical information for predicting SCI recovery. T2-weighted sagittal images are considered the most useful for prognostic purposes. Conventional MRI techniques, such as T2-weighted or T1-weighted imaging, clarify macrostructural information about the cause, level, presence, and degree of compression, and extent of SCI. MRI techniques also identify disc and ligamentous injuries. The described patterns mostly include hemorrhage, edema, and the absence of abnormal findings [18].

As a result, conventional MRI offers fundamental guidance during the diagnostic of traumatic SCI (Fig. 4). Most patients with SCI develop a posttraumatic cyst within the first month after injury. Tissue bridges located dorsally and/or ventrally adjacent to the cyst become discernible on the midsagittal slice of T2-weighted scans approximately 3 weeks after trauma. During the first year after trauma, the extent of the focal injury site remains stable and tissue bridges persist.

From a prognostic point of view, lack of MRI signal abnormality is associated with less severe grades of injury and the greatest amount of recovery. Patients with no abnormal signals almost always have incomplete injuries. Hemorrhage is seen more consistently with a neurologic complete injury based on physical examination, especially if exceeding a single level and associated with a poor neurologic recovery. Hemorrhage size/length has been associated with a more severe injury and poorer prognosis for neurologic recovery. The upper boundary of the anatomic location of the hemorrhage seems to best correspond to the neurologic level of injury.

Some authors have studied various radiological findings and concluded that the BASIC score, recently described by the Brain And Spinal Injury Center (BASIC), is the best predictor of both neurological severity and AIS conversion. They developed a 5-point scoring system based on MRI, which assesses the extent of signal abnormality and its extension on axial T2-weighted images, as well as the presence or absence of T2 hypointense point in the spinal cord [19]. In addition, axial T2-weighted images enable measurement of the cross-sectional area and shape of the gray and white matters, thus providing quantitative metrics of tissue inflammation or atrophy according to the time from injury. A variety of increasingly advanced quantitative MRI (qMRI) techniques have been utilized in examining the spinal cord, offering the potential to furnish sensitive and specific markers of spinal cord pathology. These qMRI methods are in various stages of development, but diffusion tensor imaging (DTI) is the method most frequently used in routine clinical care. DTI belongs to a family of diffusion MRI techniques that exploit the self-diffusion of water. Microstructural information provided by DTI is expected to complement current approaches to patient assessment and has the potential to monitor disease progression and evaluate the efficacy of therapies. Over the last 20 years, some preclinical studies have also validated DTI metrics as accurate measures of the histopathological changes occurring following SCI. Investigations into the pattern of neurodegeneration in animal models of SCI have estab-

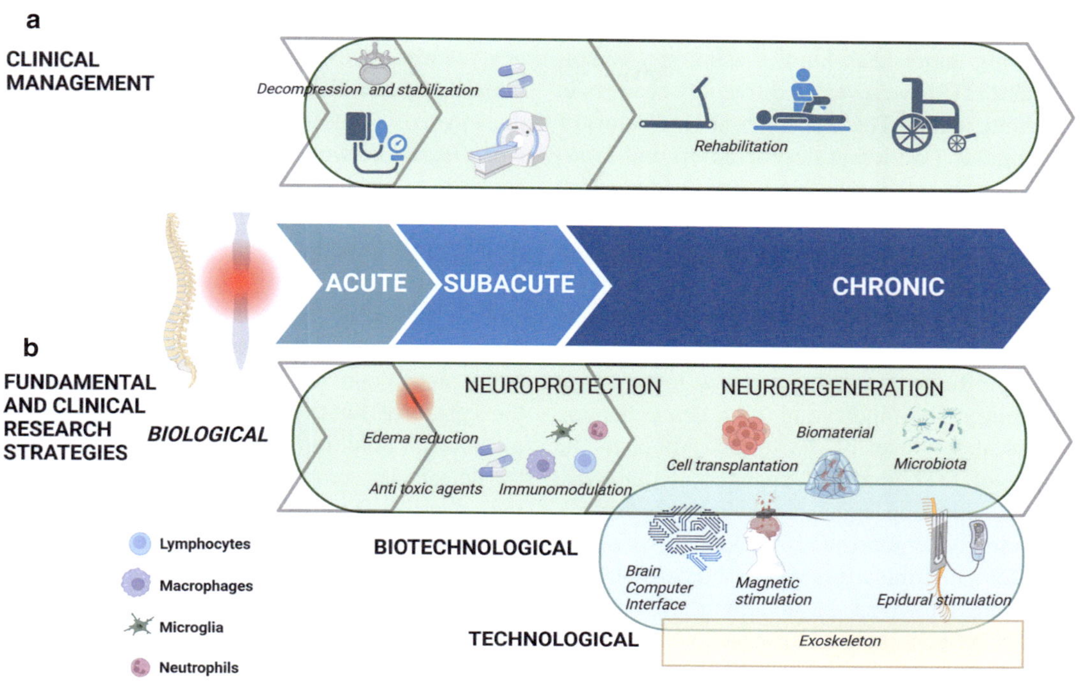

Fig. 4 Pathophysiology. (**a**) Actual clinical management after SCI at different time after traumatism. (**b**) Fundamental and clinical research strategies at different time post injury. (Source: Author)

lished decreased axial diffusivity as a marker for axonal degeneration and increased radial diffusivity as a marker for demyelination [20]. In these studies, histological observation of axon and myelin degeneration was spatially and temporally consistent with changes in diffusivity. However, despite this correlation, DTI metrics are only indirect measures of pathological processes and can also be affected by other physiological factors; for example, inflammation has been found to decrease radial diffusivity values, potentially masking concurrent demyelination.

In clinical studies, accessibility to the injury site with DTI is restricted due to the early surgical treatment undergone by most patients with SCI, involving the insertion of metallic pedicular implants. These implants subsequently create major MRI artifacts, including image distortion, signal loss, and imperfect fat suppression. Although strategies exist for reducing these artifacts, such as view-angle tilting, slice-encoding for metal artifact correction (SEMAC), and compressed sensing multispectral imaging techniques, these strategies have not yet been applied to diffusion MRI. Therefore, most DTI investigations have focused on the acute phase of SCI, with imaging being performed before patients undergo surgery. In patients with acute SCI, baseline measurements (taken <24 h after trauma) of fractional anisotropy, mean diffusivity, and axial diffusivity at the site of injury correlated with the International Standards for Neurological Classification of Spinal Cord Injury (ISNCSCI) motor scores at 1 year after injury [21]. A study, which used presurgical DTI to investigate cervical SCI, showed that patients with lower mean fractional anisotropy of the spinal cord and the corticospinal tract at the C1–C2 level had a lower level of impairment, as measured by the ISNCSCI upper-limb motor score and the ISNCSCI impairment scale.

Regarding the utilization of DTI for outcome prediction, the correlation between DTI metrics and clinical scores acquired during the chronic post-injury phase is particularly intriguing. This is because the majority of SCI patients typically experience improvements within the initial year following injury [22]. Studies using in vivo spinal cord DTI have revealed diffusivity changes in the white matter. These changes are indicators of anterograde (Wallerian degeneration) and retrograde degeneration involving both disintegration of axonal structure and demyelination. A reduction in fractional anisotropy was consistently observed both above and below the level of injury, albeit with changes of lesser magnitude compared to those observed at the injury site. Radial diffusivity was found to be increased at the injury site, indicating that demyelination occurs at the level of the lesion. Although the ability of DTI to detect changes in otherwise normal-appearing spinal cord white matter has been clearly demonstrated, the adoption of spinal cord DTI in clinical practice is hindered by the difficulties involved in obtaining high-quality images, reliable data, and the lack of robust and automated data processing software. Moreover, the correct interpretation of DTI metrics and its correlation to clinical and functional scores is challenging. Nevertheless, DTI has been employed to detect alterations in microstructure both above and below the lesion or stenosis, which remain undetectable with conventional MRI. Furthermore, spinal cord DTI metrics exhibit correlations with neurological and electrophysiological outcomes following traumatic SCI.

Several improvements to existing MRI methods have been introduced over the past decade with the aim of maximizing signal-to-noise ratios and resolution, but the implementation of these methods in a clinical setting remains a challenge. Further advances in data acquisition, processing and modeling are needed to improve the reliability and specificity of quantitative MRI metrics as predictors of patient outcome.

5.6 Rehabilitation (Fig. 4a)

Rehabilitation is an integral part of care as soon as the patient has moved beyond the hyperacute stage. It should be started as early as possible, including in intensive care with trophicity, range and, activity-based exercise although teams are not yet always used to this. The earliness and intensity of rehabilitation is prognostic. Most of the effort is focused on the first 6–12 months when neural networks are most plastic and susceptible to be guided by rehabilitation. Later rehabilitation sessions will be geared toward maintaining function that has already been acquired.

It is important for acute-care physicians to keep in mind that rehabilitation's primary objective is not to cure the physical deficiency (make the legs move) but to restore function in a socially meaningful context (go to the cinema, whether by wheelchair, crutches, or independent walking). Consequently, there are always two parallel strategies at work in a rehabilitation program: restorative and palliative. The former is centered on physical therapy, the second is based on occupational therapy but may also involve various technological or surgical intervention (e.g., tibial stimulation for bladder control, nerve transfer in the upper limb for grip improvement). Each program is adapted to a patient and there is no standard intervention [23].

Basic physiotherapy is based on strength and endurance training using load bearing and repeated contractions [24]. It targets postural muscles, essential for any activity, and restoration of meaningful sublesional contraction. Simply adding thousands of contractions does not improve voluntary control and proprioceptive feedback and input to the cord appear essential. Moreover, proprioceptive feedback and input to the cord appear essential. They are targeted through the use of treadmills for the lower limbs with support coming from parallel bars or harnesses offering a variable degree of support. This improves self-ambulation outcomes compared to basic analytical therapy. Muscle action, and composition, can also be improved by the use of electrical stimulation, preferably in a context relevant to the desired pattern of movement. A typical example is electrical stimulation to improve step activity on the treadmill, with the harness [25], or to improve torque on a cycle ergometer (FES cycling). Fear and lack of self-confidence are known to restrain underlying physical possibilities. This is prompting the development of virtual reality during physiotherapy sessions. Immersed in the game, the patient will lean/reach more and further than he believes possible, using only proprioceptive feedback [26]. There are various games targeting different functions. Exoskeletons could play a role in helping to relearn an adequate body representation but when and how to use it is not yet clear. An additional key benefit of physical therapy is global metabolic health and muscle composition.

Occupational therapy is centered on activities rather than muscles or proprioception. There is a component of therapy not far from analytical techniques used in physical therapy; however, the aim of occupational therapy is to work on a specific activity that is relevant to the individual patient and may be context specific. Restricted activity and consequent limited social participation are at the core of handicap as a social concept. Occupational therapy will use physical exercises, palliative strategies, and environment adaptations tailored to the patient. A cornerstone is restoring the ability for self-movement through the use of various aides. The wheelchair is the most obvious example with sometimes complex command systems through head or chin movement, if not eye tracking for the highest lesions. Other aspects of activity-based rehabilitation include the adaptation of the environment to the patient: adequately weighed cutlery, wheelchair-"friendly" bathrooms, learning to drive modified cars, and so on. One could argue that current legislative evolutions are an extension of that logic. Surgical and technological interventions are another axis of "palliative" rehabilitation: electrical stimulation for bladder control can be external (on the posterior tibial nerve) or implanted on the sacral roots [27]. Bladders can also be enlarged to give more autonomy to patients (self-catheterization can take up to an hour when having to manage transfers and dressing/undressing with a spinal lesion). Nerves can be transferred from one muscle group to another, or tendons moved between joints in the upper limb to restore palmar and/or thumb grimp depending on the level of the lesion [28].

Finally, medical care is focused on preventing (and treating) complications of the spinal cord lesion: pressure sores, neurogenic bladder, and subsequent renal failure; managing spasticity of the skeletal and sphincter muscles through medication or botulinic toxin injections; and treating neuropathic pain among others.

5.7 Neurotechnology (Fig. 4b)

While the search for biological treatments of spinal cord injury tends to be focused on the restoration of damaged spinal circuits, rehabilitation and technological research appears to be focused on palliating the circuits, either through a functional short-circuit or even by providing a fully external compensation.

A strategy that has received a lot of media attention is electrical epidural stimulation. Spinal cord neurons, in vertebrates, are organized in units called central pattern generators. These units are capable of generating oscillatory activity that serves as the basis of left–right alternating movement as well as agonist–antagonist oppositions. While functionally present in the human baby (archaic walk reflex), they disappear in the first years with the appearance of suprasegmental control from the brain, thus requiring one to "relearn" how to walk. Nonetheless, these central pattern generators are still present, if latent, throughout the human spinal cord, including beneath eventual spinal cord lesions [29]. One objective of research is to reactivate these generators to palliate the suprasegmental input that has been disrupted by the lesion.

Electrical fields that are applied transdurally to the dorsal (sensory) aspects of the spinal cord can generate the oscillatory activity with the adequate frequency and intensity parameters. The idea is therefore to reactivate these pattern generators through the use of implants. Some residual long-fiber connections could provide the necessary cerebral input to start/stop these circuits (75% of AIS A patients are considered "discomplete" with existing but nonfunctional cerebrospinal connections).

Beyond the electrophysiological laboratory, various teams have published encouraging clinical results with epidural stimulation, but a wide-ranging, robust clinical trial is still awaited. A number of cases have been published by American teams and show that, with the use of commercially available electrodes and devices, AIS A or B patients can be made to stand + − walk with some form of weight support. However, the improvement requires upward of 6 if not 12 months of intensive rehabilitation. The type of stimulation parameters appears to have an impact, but how they are chosen is not described [30].

In a more exploratory fashion, the Lausanne team models the current waves that happen throughout the cord during walking and tries to reproduce it through the currents that are delivered by the implanted electrode. Motion sensors initiate the electrical stimulation pattern, which is tailored to the patient's movements. With this technique, the Lausanne team has shown the resumption of independent walking (with light technical aides). However, the profile of patients is quite different: AIS C and D; and the amount of engineering time required makes it a strategy still far from the commercial market. The next step is to try to bypass the lesion entirely with an artificial brain–spine connection [31].

Other teams are trying to use similar brain interfaces to control targeted functional electrical stimulation. However, those models are not embedded and so potentially further from clinical use. Energy source and the physical ability for the underlying muscle to perform the task remain limiting factors.

6 Therapeutic Strategies in Preclinical Research (Fig. 4b)

Research strategies typically do not address the primary mechanical injury as it is often considered unavoidable. The intricate pathophysiology of secondary mechanisms presents promising approaches for potential therapeutic strategies, which can be classified into neuroprotective and restorative categories (Fig. 4). Neuroprotective strategies aim to prevent or minimize degeneration and damage, thereby protecting cells and functions that may not have been directly affected by the initial mechanical injury. Restorative strategies refer to the recovery of functional abilities by restoring communication between the brain and the body. This could be achieved through the use of implanted bridges or by regeneration of new nervous tissue to replace damaged areas after SCI.

While historically, repairing the spinal cord after SCI focused on precise restoration of the neuronal network, modern regenerative strategies encompass various forms of tissue restoration, including conduction enhancing stimulation of axonal growth, transplantation of different cell types including stem cells, enhancement of remyelination and neuronal implants.

In research strategies, pharmacological approaches have been developed to limit the injury damage and potentially repair the sensorimotor functions. Different molecules have been suggested to act on various pathways, by promoting axonal regrowth, including through targeting serotonin neurotransmission (for review see [32]), by targeting apoptosis, by decreasing excitotoxicity and oxidative stress, and by modulating inflammation.

In particular, nowadays, understanding the mechanisms underlying the dynamics of harmful and beneficial roles of neuroinflammation is crucial for the development of effective therapeutic strategies aimed at mitigating the detrimental effects of neuroinflammation while harnessing its potential for promoting tissue repair and functional recovery. Interestingly, channel blockers aimed at maintaining homeostasis and reducing inflammation have shown promising results in preclinical studies. In addition, pharmacological approaches aimed at targeting glial scar formation and its dynamic evolution over time after SCI have shown promising results. These approaches involve modulating the composition and organization of the extracellular matrix, as well as influencing the immune cell response and astrocyte behavior.

In addition to classical pharmacological approaches, research and development of biomaterials could not only contribute as scaffold material to bridge the cyst and cavities and constitutes a positive environment for axon regeneration but also serve as drug-eluting biomaterials. Implanted biomaterial can indeed be loaded with various bioactive agents, such as neurotrophic factors, anti-inflammatory drugs, and growth factors and therefore deliver drugs at the site of the lesion. Moreover, they can be engineered to release the therapeutic agent over an extended period after implantation Several types of biomaterials have been engineered, including hydrogels microspheres, and scaffolds composed of natural or synthetic polymers. There are still challenges to overcome, such as achieving optimal release kinetics, ensuring biocompatibility, and promoting long-term tissue integration.

Nanomaterials show promise as nanocarriers by addressing challenges such as low drug permeability and ensuring precise, targeted release. A wide array of nanomaterial types, including metal and polymer-based varieties, along with liposomes, are available. Nanovehicles offer numerous advantages, such as preventing cargo degradation, enhancing drug absorption, facilitating specific interactions with cellular compartments, reducing adverse effects, and boosting drug bioavailability (for review see [33]).

Strategies involving the development of cell-based therapies including stem cells, associated or not with the use of biomaterials, as well as extracellular vesicles are also investigated. Broadly, cell therapies can either consist of transplanting exogenous cells or enhancing and directing endogenous progenitor cells (for review see [33]).

Furthermore, modulating gene expression after SCI to regulate the spinal secondary damage is also developed.

In parallel to the biological advances, technological and engineering improvements in brain–computer interface to bypass neural damage after SCI represent an active multidisciplinary research area. Owing to recent decoding and engineering technologies, this field is currently undergoing an intense and rapid progress with new waves aiming to reestablish bidirectional communications between the brain and the periphery.

7 Spinal Cord Injury and the Gut Microbiota (Fig. 4b)

The gut microbiota has been shown to regulate systemic immunity and modulate CNS disease progression. In clinical studies, intestinal dysfunction and gut dysbiosis are often reported in SCI patients. While not all factors affecting gut microbiota such as dietary intake and antibiotic treatment have always been taken into account, it appears that the gut microbiota is affected by SCI, including alterations in the diversity and abundance of bacterial species in the gut (for review see [34]). In preclinical studies, the severity of gut dysbiosis is influenced by the severity of SCI. For instance, in mice, spinal compression injury induces a shift in the overall bacterial population, conversely to spinal contusion injury [35]. The authors hypothesized that the increased dysbiosis observed after compression injury affects the immune system that in turn modulates pain outcomes, given the important role of the gut microbiota in neuropathic and central pain. Moreover, gut dysbiosis is associated with changes in chemokines and cytokines that can promote local and systemic inflammation. Therefore, SCI-induced alteration of the gut–brain axis, which represents the bidirectional communication between the CNS and the gut microbiota, can aggravate several secondary complications such as gastrointestinal dysfunction, infections, and metabolic disorders. Consequently, research on gastrointestinal microbiome (GIM) modulation, including diet adjustment, probiotics, prebiotics, and fecal microbiota transplantation, may offer therapeutic strategies.

References

1. WHO. International perspectives on spinal cord injury. 2013.
2. NSCISC. Facts and figures at a glance. 2021.

3. Jazayeri SB, et al. Incidence of traumatic spinal cord injury worldwide: a systematic review, data integration, and update. World Neurosurg X. 2023;18:100171.
4. Zhu Y, et al. Fibronectin matrix assembly after spinal cord injury. J Neurotrauma. 2015;32(15):1158–67.
5. Perez JC, et al. CSF1R inhibition at chronic stage after spinal cord injury modulates microglia proliferation. Glia. 2023;71:2782–98.
6. Perez JC, Gerber YN, Perrin FE. Dynamic diversity of glial response among species in spinal cord injury. Front Aging Neurosci. 2021;13:769548.
7. Eckert MJ, Martin MJ. Trauma: spinal cord injury. Surg Clin North Am. 2017;97(5):1031–45.
8. Albayar AA, et al. Biomarkers in spinal cord injury: prognostic insights and future potentials. Front Neurol. 2019;10:27.
9. Garg K, Agrawal D, Hurlbert RJ. Expansive Duraplasty – simple technique with promising results in complete cervical spinal cord injury: a preliminary study. Neurol India. 2022;70(1):319–24.
10. Mallek JT, et al. The incidence of neurogenic shock after spinal cord injury in patients admitted to a high-volume level I trauma center. Am Surg. 2012;78(5):623–6.
11. Fehlings MG, et al. A clinical practice guideline for the Management of Acute Spinal Cord Injury: introduction, rationale, and scope. Global Spine J. 2017;7(3 Suppl):84S–94S.
12. Saadeh YS, et al. The impact of blood pressure management after spinal cord injury: a systematic review of the literature. Neurosurg Focus. 2017;43(5):E20.
13. Consortium for Spinal Cord, M. Early acute management in adults with spinal cord injury: a clinical practice guideline for health-care professionals. J Spinal Cord Med. 2008;31(4):403–79.
14. Carney NA, et al. Guidelines for the acute medical management of severe traumatic brain injury in infants, children, and adolescents. Pediatr Crit Care Med. 2003;4(3 Suppl):S1.
15. Carney N, et al. Guidelines for the management of severe traumatic brain injury, fourth edition. Neurosurgery. 2017;80(1):6–15.
16. Camlar M, et al. Does Decompressive Duraplasty have a neuroprotective effect on spinal trauma?: an experimental study. World Neurosurg. 2019;126:e288–94.
17. Bracken, M.B., et al., Administration of methylprednisolone for 24 or 48 hours or tirilazad mesylate for 48 hours in the treatment of acute spinal cord injury. Results of the third national acute spinal cord injury randomized controlled trial. National acute spinal cord injury study. JAMA, 1997. 277(20): p. 1597–1604.
18. Andreoli C, et al. MRI in the acute phase of spinal cord traumatic lesions: relationship between MRI findings and neurological outcome. Radiol Med. 2005;110(5–6):636–45.
19. Farhadi HF, et al. Impact of admission imaging findings on neurological outcomes in acute cervical traumatic spinal cord injury. J Neurotrauma. 2018;35(12):1398–406.
20. Kozlowski P, et al. Characterizing white matter damage in rat spinal cord with quantitative MRI and histology. J Neurotrauma. 2008;25(6):653–76.
21. Shanmuganathan K, et al. Diffusion tensor imaging parameter obtained during acute blunt cervical spinal cord injury in predicting long-term outcome. J Neurotrauma. 2017;34(21):2964–71.
22. Ahuja CS, et al. Traumatic spinal cord injury. Nat Rev Dis Primers. 2017;3:17018.
23. Devillard X, et al. Effects of training programs for spinal cord injury. Ann Readapt Med Phys. 2007;50(6):490–8, 480–9.
24. Gordon T, Mao J. Muscle atrophy and procedures for training after spinal cord injury. Phys Ther. 1994;74(1):50–60.
25. Field-Fote EC. Combined use of body weight support, functional electric stimulation, and treadmill training to improve walking ability in individuals with chronic incomplete spinal cord injury. Arch Phys Med Rehabil. 2001;82(6):818–24.
26. Sengupta M, et al. Role of virtual reality in balance training in patients with spinal cord injury: a prospective comparative pre-post study. Asian Spine J. 2020;14(1):51–8.
27. Steers WD, et al. A review on functional electrical stimulation of bladder and bowel in spinal cord injury. J Long-Term Eff Med Implants. 2017;27(2–4):307–17.
28. Liew SK, Shim BJ, Gong HS. Upper limb reconstruction in tetraplegic patients: a primer for spinal cord injury specialists. Korean J Neurotrauma. 2020;16(2):126–37.
29. Dimitrijevic MR, Gerasimenko Y, Pinter MM. Evidence for a spinal central pattern generator in humans. Ann N Y Acad Sci. 1998;860:360–76.
30. Angeli CA, et al. Recovery of over-ground walking after chronic motor complete spinal cord injury. N Engl J Med. 2018;379(13):1244–50.
31. Lorach H, et al. Walking naturally after spinal cord injury using a brain-spine interface. Nature. 2023;618(7963):126–33.
32. Perrin FE, Noristani HN. Serotonergic mechanisms in spinal cord injury. Exp Neurol. 2019;318:174–91.
33. Costachescu B, et al. Novel strategies for spinal cord regeneration. Int J Mol Sci. 2022;23(9):4552.
34. Cui Y, et al. Dual-directional regulation of spinal cord injury and the gut microbiota. Neural Regen Res. 2024;19(3):548–56.
35. Bannerman CA, et al. Spinal cord injury in mice affects central and peripheral pathology in a severity-dependent manner. Pain. 2022;163(6):1172–85.

Data Management and Artificial Intelligence in Spine Surgery

Yann Philippe Charles

1 Clinical Registers

Clinical data collection has changed our approach to evaluate patient reported outcome measures (PROMs) to assess health-related quality of life (QoL) for different conditions related to spinal disease. Evidence gathered from large datasets is intended to improve quality in spine care. Epidemiologic data collection and research is conducted to enable prevention and rehabilitation programs for low back pain, which represents as common condition associated with disability [1–3]. Normative datasets have improved diagnostics and help clinicians to formulate accurate treatment plans and to evaluate clinical results. Examples are the validation and cross-cultural adaptions QoL questionnaires [4] or the establishment of age-related full spine sagittal alignment parameters [5, 6]. Large clinical registers investigating surgical outcomes are intended to improve knowledge and provide guidance for best practice. Thus, the likelihood of improving low back pain by surgical treatment has been assessed in the treatment including medico-economic aspects [7]. The role of cervical fusion and total disc replacement has been evaluated from large national datasets [8].

Analyses of clinical registers are traditionally based on statistical methods. Modern concepts of prediction include artificial intelligence (AI). Machine learning (ML), as a branch of AI, originates from computer science and uses algorithms established from previous data analysis. Different machine learning methods are used for clinical prediction models. ML represents a new approach to solve problems in the diagnostic, therapeutic, or scientific process. The management of complex spinal pathologies is challenging when multiple parameters must be taken into consideration. Among these disorders, adult spinal deformity represents a subset of conditions that are associated with a high degree of postoperative complications. Large-scale register data is required to line out associations of risk factors that are significant for clinical practice. Merging of the registers from different continents has made it possible to use large-scale clinical data, patient, and spinal deformity characteristics and associated risk factors as training data for creating a ML algorithm [9]. This tool is aimed to calculate risks and predict the clinical outcomes to support the spine surgeon's decision-making, which might be biased by personal experience and risk perception. The role of additional patient-related factors, such as biologic and genetic factors of aging and frailty, might be better understood and predicted by AI algorithms, which could be implemented as an aid in surgical decision-making [10].

Y. P. Charles (✉)
Service de Chirurgie du Rachis, Hôpitaux Universitaires de Strasbourg, Université de Strasbourg, Strasbourg, France
e-mail: YannPhilippe.CHARLES@chru-strasbourg.fr

C. Y. Barrey (ed.), *Spine Surgery*, SFCR Experts Series 1,
https://doi.org/10.1007/978-3-031-85446-0_10

2 Fundamentals of Machine Learning

The fundamentals of AI are based on a detailed analysis of learning methods and various aspects of human intelligence. These techniques enable machine to simulate these human abilities. The informatic development of processes based on human learning experience made it possible to develop ML techniques. The principle of ML uses a computer system that learns from a dataset and then able to predict a result by applying an algorithm. This algorithm can be built by using two different principles defined as supervised or unsupervised learning [11–13].

Supervised learning is based on a training dataset, which is labeled by a human expert. This information is then integrated into the system as a binary outcome (true or false) related to the input data. The supervised ML technique attempts to reproduce human learning. For example, radiologic features on computed tomography (CT) could be used as training data to create a model that analyzes the presence or absence of a vertebral fracture. Independent data, such as pixels and Hounsfield units, within the CT image are used as threshold values or vectors. This data will then predict the outcome variable location and fracture type. CT images that were not used for training of the system represent non-annotated data. This data is then analyzed by the automated system. To ensure the accuracy of the system, it needs to be validated with respect to its ability to differentiate between the presence or absence of a fracture. The final goal of supervised learning is a linear classification for qualitative data or a linear regression for quantitative data.

Unsupervised learning is based on automatic data analysis without prior human labeling of a training dataset. The system learns the structure of non-labeled data by itself to classify them into homogenous groups. This principle of learning is related to neuropsychology and described by the Hebbian theory [14]. It is based on the associative learning of neurons that are jointly stimulated, where an association is achieved by repeated stimuli. This principle represents the basis of human and animal learning, where relationships between different information are built and then memorized. Computer systems that use unsupervised learning techniques can perceive nonlinear relationships between data in a similar manner. Unsupervised ML enables to identify clusters of related variables and to detect abnormalities. Artificial neural networks can be constructed using these automated learning techniques. While unsupervised learning become more and more important, most models currently used for spinal applications are supervised learning models.

3 Machine Learning Techniques

3.1 Classification and Regression Trees

Classification and regression trees (CART), also called random forests, represent a model of decision-making that is commonly used in medicine, such as in diagnostics or treatment algorithms [15]. The graphical representation of this method is assimilated to a tree, with a starting point, the base knot, and various pathways, the branches, connecting subsequent knots, thus leading a set of choices with a final classification (Fig. 1). Very complex CART using multiple knots and branches usually require dividing the tree into smaller clusters for group-specific analyses of a problem. The principle of pruning can be used to simplify the CART and make it more efficient. However, under-learning carries a risk of approximation and overlearning has a risk of showing to detailed relationships that are not relevant for decision-making.

3.2 Support Vector Machines

Support vector machines (SVM) use a two-dimensional or a three-dimensional representation aiming for discrimination of data. A separation plane is typically used in a *x,y* or *x,y,z* coordinate system to classify data [11, 13]. Three-dimensional SVM models use algorithms with a hyperplane, which represents a space

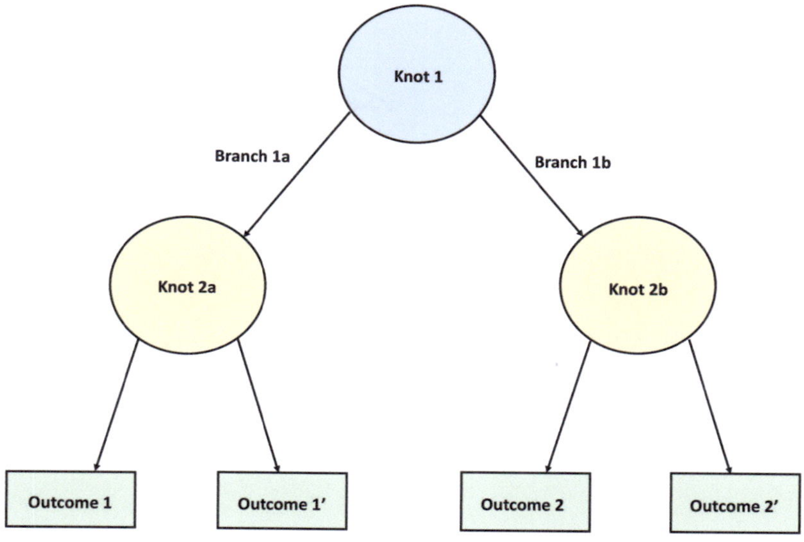

Fig. 1 Classification and regression tree

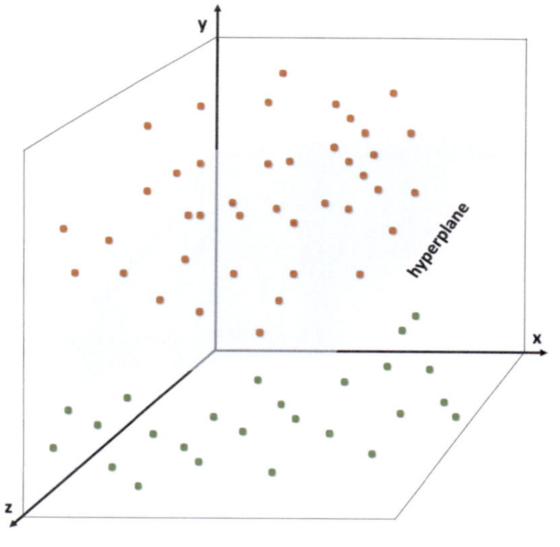

Fig. 2 Support vector machine

dividing data into two classes (Fig. 2). Underfitting and overfitting of models should be avoided in SVM to ensure reliability and without making the model too complex. SVM can be adapted to problems of nonlinear classification to regressions and clustering.

3.3 Artificial Neural Networks

Artificial neural networks (ANN) belong to unsupervised ML techniques, which mimic the human learning model building connections and interactions of neurons in the brain by repeated stimuli according to the Hebbian learning principles [11, 14]. The system of ANN is organized in layers with an input layer at the beginning and an output layer at the end. In between the information passes through different layers of artificial neurons, where combinations of data information are analyzed and refined (Fig. 3). ANN use functions such a linear combinations of input data, multiplied by a weighting factor, which generates a result through a linear or nonlinear activation function. Regularization functions might be used to limit the risk of overlearning. ANN learning consists in finding the optimal values of the weighing factors to ensure that the data processed across different neuronal layers produces an accurate prediction and outcome.

3.4 Convolutional Neural Networks

Convolutional neural networks CNN represent a subtype of ANN where the connection between neurons simulates functions of the human visual cortex [11, 16, 17]. Specific areas of the visual field stimulate specific groups of neurons from the visual cortex. The information from specific areas is processed by multiple layers of sensory neurons that analyze specific morphologic characteristics. The input data is then successively

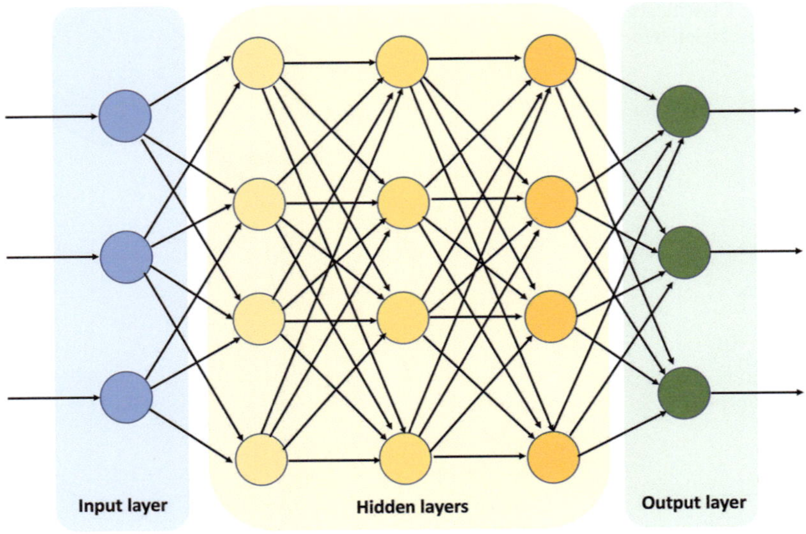

Fig. 3 Artificial neural network

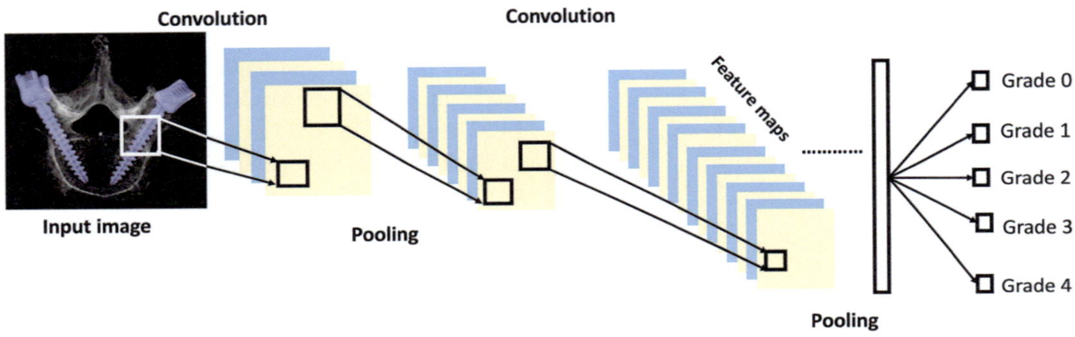

Fig. 4 Convolutional neural network

processed in small portions of information using convolution and pooling steps (Fig. 4). Image or video algorithms use the techniques of CNN, where the visual or audio entry data results in a combination of pieces of information from groups of neurons, which then produces a complete image architecture. Automatic voice recognition is similarly based on the CNN technique, where the outcome can be used for an automatic voice command or result in a written sentence in informatic text processing applications.

3.5 Deep Learning

Deep learning (DL) combines different techniques of ML derived from ANN and CNN [11–13]. Usually, DL techniques are applied when investigating complex relationships with a high degree of abstraction that can be difficult to analyze by humans. Multiple layers of ANN are linked to each other by nonlinear transformations. DL can process data at a very large scale using smart data that feeds the system with multiple parameters. In practice, real-time information and shared data might foster the level of common knowledge by means of automated rapid availability and access.

4 Applications in Spinal Imaging

Diagnostic radiology uses ML algorithms for automatic image interpretation and pathology detection. This principle has been tested for degenerative changes in the lumbar spine on magnetic resonance imaging (MRI). Automatic segmentation of lumbar vertebrae and intervertebral discs can be achieved by CNN, and detailed classification of disc degeneration according to Pfirrmann stages 1–5 is possible [18, 19]. More specific features such as disc herniation or protrusion, spinal canal stenosis, or degenerative spondylolisthesis can be detected as well and accurately predicted by CNN when comparing to human expert radiologist interpretation [20]. DL models were developed to transpose interpretation of disc degeneration from MRI to lateral lumbar X-rays, thus implementing more complex imaging features into standard radiographic imaging [21].

AI algorithms were further investigated for the automatic assessment of posterior–anterior and lateral EOS full-spine radiographs. Normal sagittal spino-pelvic and global alignment such as thoracic kyphosis, lumbar lordosis, pelvic incidence, pelvic tilt, sacral slope, sagittal vertical axis, and spino-sacral angle can be accurately predicted [22, 23]. More complex DL models can assess spinal deformities such as scoliosis. Sagittal alignment and pathologic coronal parameters such as the Cobb angle can be automatically detected and quantified [21].

Intraoperative imaging used for surgical navigation is usually based on cone beam computed tomography (CBCT). This imaging is required for surgical navigation. Vertebral segmentation can be achieved automatically from CBCT two- and three-dimensional reconstructions. A ML algorithm identifies bony vertebral structures and defines their levels and anatomical key points that are necessary for surgical planning a transpedicular approach for vertebroplasty or pedicle screw placement [24, 25]. At the current stage, a verification step by the surgeon is included in most imaging and navigation systems when defining the exact trajectory and targets on the vertebra.

5 Applications in Spine Surgery

ML algorithms have been implemented into standard CBCT imaging to assist the surgeon better with augmented reality surgical navigation. With this technique, images and additional information can be virtually projected in the surgical field [24, 25]. Additional real-time feedback may be given to the operator by filming the position of instruments and implants, thus matching imaging data and surgical maneuvers. The accuracy of this new navigation technique has been evaluated for percutaneous pedicle screw placement and was found to be as accurate as standard navigation techniques [26]. Other systems using augmented reality use an environment of intraoperative CT and microscope, where tumors can be implemented in the surgical field for better visualization and assist the surgeon when dissecting anatomic and pathologic structures [27].

Although the use of robotics has not become the standard in spine surgery yet, there is an increasing interest during the recent years. This technology combines intraoperative imaging and surgical navigation with a robotic arm that enables to drill a transpedicular trajectory and place a pedicle screw safely. The objective of this approach is to optimize pedicle screw placement in an automated and reproducible fashion without subjective perception bias by the surgeon, which could arise in the beginning of a learning curve or due to fatigue during long procedures [28, 29]. Currently, these tools are designed to improve safety, but they remain under the surgeon's control.

6 Applications in Clinical Decision-Making

Clinical decision-making for diagnosis and treatment is usually based on scientific evidence including systematic reviews, clinical practice recommendations by scientific societies or expert groups, and the physician's clinical experience. However, the management of complex spinal pathologies can be challenging when multiple parameters must be taken into consideration. Clinical registers including a very large number of patients from different institutions and countries are valuable because they allow analyses on representative populations, and they limit the risk of a center-based bias. Adult spinal deformity is a typical example of complex situations, which are at high risk for postoperative complications. The interplay between different parameters remains difficult to assess preoperatively when trying to predict clinical outcome and risk for complications accurately. ML algorithms such as SVM can be used to calculate the risk depending on the patient's profile and the proposed surgical technique, and to predict postoperative PROMs [30, 31]. Other techniques trying to implement AI for optimal clinical decision-making are based on cluster analysis using CART models, where cluster hierarchization classifies patients with adult spinal deformity to assist the surgeon in preoperative clinical decision-making when assessing risk versus benefit [9, 32].

7 Ethical and Economic Aspects

The role of AI in spine surgery is rapidly increasing. ML tools are already used to assist surgeons in their practice, especially in the field of image-guided and robotic surgery. Applications that allow to predict quality of life, the intraoperative risks, or the risk–benefit ratio by implementing a health economics dimension have been investigated and might be implemented in routine clinical practice. Today, the course of diagnostics and treatment involve the clinician's responsibility and it remains unclear to what extent this could be taken over by a machine using automated processes. On the other hand, when comparing to human thinking, AI algorithms using large datasets enable more accurate, consistent, and objective benefit versus risk assessment and outcome prediction based on rational analysis. ML might be used as an adjunct to the clinicians' experience, thus facilitating clinical decision-making and analyses of complex problems [33].

Moreover, the medico-economic variable becomes more and more important today. Expenses in a health care system should provide improvement of QoL for the patient at a reasonable price for the society. Quality-Adjusted Life Years (QALYs) consider direct and indirect medical costs to calculate an improvement in QoL for a treatment by multiplying PROMs with a time span. QALYs might therefore be implemented into ML algorithms to align clinical evidence-based and health economics practices on a broader scale.

8 Conclusion

ML represents a branch of AI and groups different techniques that have taken an increasing role in spine surgery. The main applications are automated image analysis providing support to surgical technologies such as navigation, augmented reality, or robotics. In the field of diagnostics and clinical decision-making, ML algorithms have been tested for complex problems. They might be implemented as supportive tool to the clinician's experience, thus improving the analysis of multiple level relationships with indirect links in an objective and reliable manner.

Conflict of Interest None.

References

1. Vos T, Flaxman AD, Naghavi M, et al. Years lived with disability (YLDs) for 1160 sequelae of 289 diseases and injuries 1990–2010: a systematic analysis for the global burden of disease study 2010. Lancet. 2012;380(9859):2163–96. https://doi.org/10.1016/S0140-6736(12)61729-2.
2. Juniper M, Le TK, Mladsi D. The epidemiology, economic burden, and pharmacological treatment of chronic low back pain in France, Germany, Italy, Spain and the UK: a literature-based review. Expert Opin Pharmacother. 2009;10(16):2581–92. https://doi.org/10.1517/14656560903304063. PMID: 19874246
3. Kessler JT, Melloh M, Zweig T, Aghayev E, Röder C. Development of a documentation instrument for the conservative treatment of spinal disorders in the international spine registry, spine tango. Eur Spine J. 2011;20(3):369–79. https://doi.org/10.1007/s00586-010-1474-y. Epub 2010 Jun 9. PMID: 20532924; PMCID: PMC3048233
4. Genevay S, Cedraschi C, Marty M, Rozenberg S, De Goumoëns P, Faundez A, Balagué F, Porchet F, Mannion AF. Reliability and validity of the cross-culturally adapted French version of the Core Outcome Measures Index (COMI) in patients with low back pain. Eur Spine J. 2012;21(1):130–7. https://

doi.org/10.1007/s00586-011-1992-2. Epub 2011 Sep 1. PMID: 21881865; PMCID: PMC3252438
5. Charles YP, Bauduin E, Pesenti S, et al. Variation of global sagittal alignment parameters according to gender, pelvic incidence, and age. Clin Spine Surg. 2022;35(7):E610–20. https://doi.org/10.1097/BSD.0000000000001321. Epub 2022 Apr 5. PMID: 35383599
6. Charles YP, Lamas V, Ilharreborde B, et al. Comparison of spinopelvic configuration and Roussouly alignment types between pediatric and adult populations. Spine (Phila Pa 1976). 2022;47(18):1303–13. https://doi.org/10.1097/BRS.0000000000004411. Epub 2022 Jun 29. PMID: 35797644
7. Peul WC, Bredenoord AL, Jacobs WC. Avoid surgery as first line treatment for non-specific low back pain. BMJ. 2014;16(349):g4214. https://doi.org/10.1136/bmj.g4214. PMID: 25030631
8. MacDowall A, Skeppholm M, Lindhagen L, et al. Artificial disc replacement versus fusion in patients with cervical degenerative disc disease with radiculopathy: 5-year outcomes from the National Swedish Spine Register. J Neurosurg Spine. 2018;30(2):159–67. https://doi.org/10.3171/2018.7.SPINE18657. PMID: 30485205
9. Ames CP, Smith JS, Pellisé F, et al. Artificial intelligence based hierarchical clustering of patient types and intervention categories in adult spinal deformity surgery: towards a new classification scheme that predicts quality and value. Spine (Phila Pa 1976). 2019;44(13):915–26. https://doi.org/10.1097/BRS.0000000000002974. PMID: 31205167
10. Haddad S, Pizones J, Raganato R, et al. Future data points to implement in adult spinal deformity assessment for artificial intelligence modeling prediction: the importance of the biological dimension. Int J Spine Surg. 2023;17(S1):S34–44. https://doi.org/10.14444/8502. Epub 2023 May 10. PMID: 37164480; PMCID: PMC10318909
11. Galbusera F, Casaroli G, Bassani T. Artificial intelligence and machine learning in spine research. JOR Spine. 2019;2(1):e1044. https://doi.org/10.1002/jsp2.1044. PMID: 31463458; PMCID: PMC6686793
12. Mallow GM, Siyaji ZK, Galbusera F, et al. Intelligence-based spine care model: a new era of research and clinical decision-making. Global Spine J. 2021;11(2):135–45. https://doi.org/10.1177/2192568220973984. Epub 2020 Nov 28. PMID: 33251858; PMCID: PMC7882816
13. Chang M, Canseco JA, Nicholson KJ, et al. The role of machine learning in spine surgery: the future is now. Front Surg. 2020;21(7):54. https://doi.org/10.3389/fsurg.2020.00054. PMID: 32974382; PMCID: PMC7472375
14. Topol EJ. High-performance medicine: the convergence of human and artificial intelligence. Nat Med. 2019;25(1):44–56. https://doi.org/10.1038/s41591-018-0300-7. Epub 2019 Jan 7. PMID: 30617339
15. Hayes T, Usami S, Jacobucci R, McArdle JJ. Using classification and regression trees (cart) and random forests to analyze attrition: results from two simulations. Psychol Aging. 2015;30(4):911–29. https://doi.org/10.1037/pag0000046. Epub 2015 Sep 21. PMID: 26389526; PMCID: PMC4743660
16. Saravi B, Hassel F, Ülkümen S, Zink A, et al. Artificial intelligence-driven prediction modeling and decision making in spine surgery using hybrid machine learning models. J Pers Med. 2022;12(4):509. https://doi.org/10.3390/jpm12040509. PMID: 35455625; PMCID: PMC9029065
17. Charles YP, Lamas V, Ntilikina Y. Artificial intelligence and treatment algorithms in spine surgery. Orthop Traumatol Surg Res. 2023;109(1S):103456. https://doi.org/10.1016/j.otsr.2022.103456. Epub 2022 Oct 24. PMID: 36302452
18. Pfirrmann CW, Metzdorf A, Zanetti M, et al. Magnetic resonance classification of lumbar intervertebral disc degeneration. Spine (Phila Pa 1976). 2001;26(17):1873–8. https://doi.org/10.1097/00007632-200109010-00011. PMID: 11568697
19. Harada GK, Siyaji ZK, Younis S, et al. Imaging in spine surgery: current concepts and future directions. Spine Surg Relat Res. 2019;4(2):99–110. https://doi.org/10.22603/ssrr.2020-0011. PMID: 32405554; PMCID: PMC7217684
20. Jamaludin A, Lootus M, Kadir T, et al. ISSLS prize in bioengineering science 2017: automation of reading of radiological features from magnetic resonance images (MRIs) of the lumbar spine without human intervention is comparable with an expert radiologist. Eur Spine J. 2017;26(5):1374–83. https://doi.org/10.1007/s00586-017-4956-3. Epub 2017 Feb 6. PMID: 28168339
21. Galbusera F, Niemeyer F, Wilke HJ, et al. Fully automated radiological analysis of spinal disorders and deformities: a deep learning approach. Eur Spine J. 2019;28(5):951–60. https://doi.org/10.1007/s00586-019-05944-z. Epub 2019 Mar 12. PMID: 30864061
22. Grover P, Siebenwirth J, Caspari C, et al. Can artificial intelligence support or even replace physicians in measuring sagittal balance? A validation study on preoperative and postoperative full spine images of 170 patients. Eur Spine J. 2022;31(8):1943–51. https://doi.org/10.1007/s00586-022-07309-5. Epub 2022 Jul 7. Erratum in: Eur Spine J 2023 Mar;32(3):1095–1097. PMID: 35796837
23. Weng CH, Wang CL, Huang YJ, et al. Artificial intelligence for automatic measurement of sagittal vertical Axis using ResUNet framework. J Clin Med. 2019;8(11):1826. https://doi.org/10.3390/jcm8111826. PMID: 31683913; PMCID: PMC6912675
24. Burström G, Buerger C, Hoppenbrouwers J, et al. Machine learning for automated 3-dimensional segmentation of the spine and suggested placement of pedicle screws based on intraoperative cone-beam computer tomography. J Neurosurg Spine. 2019;31(1):147–54. https://doi.org/10.3171/2018.12.SPINE181397. PMID: 30901757

25. Auloge P, Cazzato RL, Ramamurthy N, et al. Augmented reality and artificial intelligence-based navigation during percutaneous vertebroplasty: a pilot randomised clinical trial. Eur Spine J. 2020;29(7):1580–9. https://doi.org/10.1007/s00586-019-06054-6. Epub 2019 Jul 2. PMID: 31270676
26. Charles YP, Cazzato RL, Nachabe R, et al. Minimally invasive Transforaminal lumbar Interbody fusion using augmented reality surgical navigation for percutaneous pedicle screw placement. Clin Spine Surg. 2021;34(7):E415–24. https://doi.org/10.1097/BSD.0000000000001132. PMID: 33560011
27. Carl B, Bopp M, Saß B, et al. Implementation of augmented reality support in spine surgery. Eur Spine J. 2019;28(7):1697–711. https://doi.org/10.1007/s00586-019-05969-4. Epub 2019 Apr 5. PMID: 30953169
28. Liounakos JI, Chenin L, Theodore N, Wang MY. Robotics in spine surgery and spine surgery training. Oper Neurosurg (Hagerstown). 2021;21(2):35–40. https://doi.org/10.1093/ons/opaa449. PMID: 34017989
29. Lopez IB, Benzakour A, Mavrogenis A, et al. Robotics in spine surgery: systematic review of literature. Int Orthop. 2023;47(2):447–56. https://doi.org/10.1007/s00264-022-05508-9. Epub 2022 Jul 18. PMID: 35849162
30. Joshi RS, Lau D, Scheer JK, et al. State-of-the-art reviews predictive modeling in adult spinal deformity: applications of advanced analytics. Spine Deform. 2021;9(5):1223–39. https://doi.org/10.1007/s43390-021-00360-0. Epub 2021 May 18. PMID: 34003461; PMCID: PMC8363545
31. Pellisé F, Serra-Burriel M, Smith JS, et al. Development and validation of risk stratification models for adult spinal deformity surgery. J Neurosurg Spine. 2019;28:1–13. https://doi.org/10.3171/2019.3.SPINE181452. Epub ahead of print. PMID: 31252385
32. Ames CP, Smith JS, Pellisé F, et al. Development of predictive models for all individual questions of SRS-22R after adult spinal deformity surgery: a step toward individualized medicine. Eur Spine J. 2019;28(9):1998–2011. https://doi.org/10.1007/s00586-019-06079-x. Epub 2019 Jul 19. PMID: 31325052
33. Keskinbora KH. Medical ethics considerations on artificial intelligence. J Clin Neurosci. 2019;64:277–82. https://doi.org/10.1016/j.jocn.2019.03.001. Epub 2019 Mar 14

Emerging Technologies

Stéphane Fuentes, Anis Choucha,
and Kaissar Farah

1 Introduction

The evolution of spinal surgery reflects the relentless march of technological progress, a journey marked by successive industrial revolutions and the convergence of diverse scientific disciplines. Just as the third industrial revolution ushered in an era of electronics and information technology, transforming manufacturing processes with automation, the advent of the fourth industrial revolution heralded the dawn of cyber-physical systems and smart technologies. In this era, the fusion of artificial intelligence, big data, or robots has penetrated various sectors, reshaping paradigms and catalyzing innovation.

Technological advancements in spine surgery have been instrumental in overcoming inherent limitations faced by surgeons, such as touch and sight. Innovations such as advanced imaging systems and robotic assistance aim to revolutionize surgical precision and control, enabling surgeons to navigate complex anatomical structures with unprecedented accuracy. By augmenting human capabilities, these technologies have boasted to significantly improve surgical efficiency, reduced procedural times, and minimized the risk of complications. Furthermore, the integration of real-time feedback mechanisms and enhanced visualization tools has pushed the boundaries of safety and efficacy, fostering greater confidence in surgical outcomes.

This chapter delves into a comprehensive examination of cutting-edge technologies shaping the landscape of spinal surgery. From enhanced surgical environments facilitated by state-of-the-art operating tables to tools designed to minimize intraoperative bleeding, as well as the integration of robotic assistance, the scope of innovation is vast and multifaceted. Are these advancements genuinely beneficial or merely marketing hype? What about economic considerations, learning curves, limitations, and future prospects? Are we truly advancing patient care, or are we merely chasing technological novelty without substantial benefits?

1. Operating Tables

Throughout history, surgical table improvements have paralleled medical breakthrough to ensure a suitable surgical environment. With the advent of aseptic technic popularized by Lister, surgical tables shifted from wood to materials that allow sanitization [1]; with the advent of

S. Fuentes (✉) · K. Farah
Department of Neurosurgery, Aix Marseille Univ, APHM, UH Timone, Marseille, France
e-mail: stephane.fuentes@ap-hm.fr

A. Choucha
Department of Neurosurgery, Aix Marseille Univ, APHM, UH Timone, Marseille, France

Laboratory of Biomechanics and Application, UMRT24, Gustave Eiffel University, Aix Marseille, France

C. Y. Barrey (ed.), *Spine Surgery*, SFCR Experts Series 1,
https://doi.org/10.1007/978-3-031-85446-0_11

C-Arm in 1955, radiolucent frame emerged in the operating room (OR) in the 1960s and so on [2]. In the following sections, we will delve into the latest technological innovations in spinal surgery tables, allowing proper patient positioning while mitigating iatrogenic complications, from ergonomic design to integrated imaging capabilities with low artifact.

2 Spinal Surgical Tables and Patient's Positioning

Surgery starts before the incision, with patient positioning. Also, planning spinal surgery encompasses a wide range of patients' positioning, with approaches spanning from the craniovertebral junction to the pelvic bone; through anterior, posterior, or oblique corridors. The utilization of adjuncts such as the Mayfield head clamp further emphasize the diversity of positionings. Adequate positioning is a key to surgical success.

Indeed, each positioning has its own array of iatrogenic complications [3, 4]. Here are a few examples of complications related to patient positioning that rely on both the surgeon's skill in setup and the surgical table itself. First, rare but devastating, postoperative visual loss can occur in prone position surgery, due to excessive face compression. In a nationwide study over a decade in the United States, Shen et al. found an incidence of postoperative visual loss of 3.09/10,000 (0.03%) in spinal procedures [5]. Second, overstretching of upper brachial plexus or compression of the ulnar nerve have an incidence of 0.03–0.1% as a result of poor arm positioning [6]. In a review of 517, Uribe et al. found that 17 patients experienced postoperative brachial plexopathy in prone position and 44 in supine or lateral position [7]. Lastly, Nicol et al. suggested that intraoperative positioning plays a crucial role in the occurrence of deep vein thrombosis (DVT) and pulmonary embolism (PE) [8].

3 Single-Based Traditional OR Tables

Recent advances have been made in traditional operating tables to enhance surgical results. A wide array of attachments such as side rail allow for the use of mini-invasive surgeries, or the use of robotic arm such as Cirq arm® [9]. Surgical cushion, added to an improved flexibility, enables a variety of position including supine, lateral decubitus, or in varying degrees of Trendelenburg or reverse Trendelenburg. Radiolucent frames facilitate intraoperative fluoroscopy. The base can be mobile or fixed. Main operating room (OR) tables available on the current market are Trumpf TruSystem 7000, Getinge Maquet Meera, Stryker Operon D860, and STERIS AMSCO. The Trumpf TruSystem 7000 boast a table motion and a design well suited to integrate the Da Vinci Xi Robot from Intuitive Surgical (discussed below). The STERIS AMSCO OR table displays a warming system available during the surgery to assist anesthesiologists. Although versatile, the base of these tables can represent an obstacle when using a C-arm. Fig. 1 displays these tables.

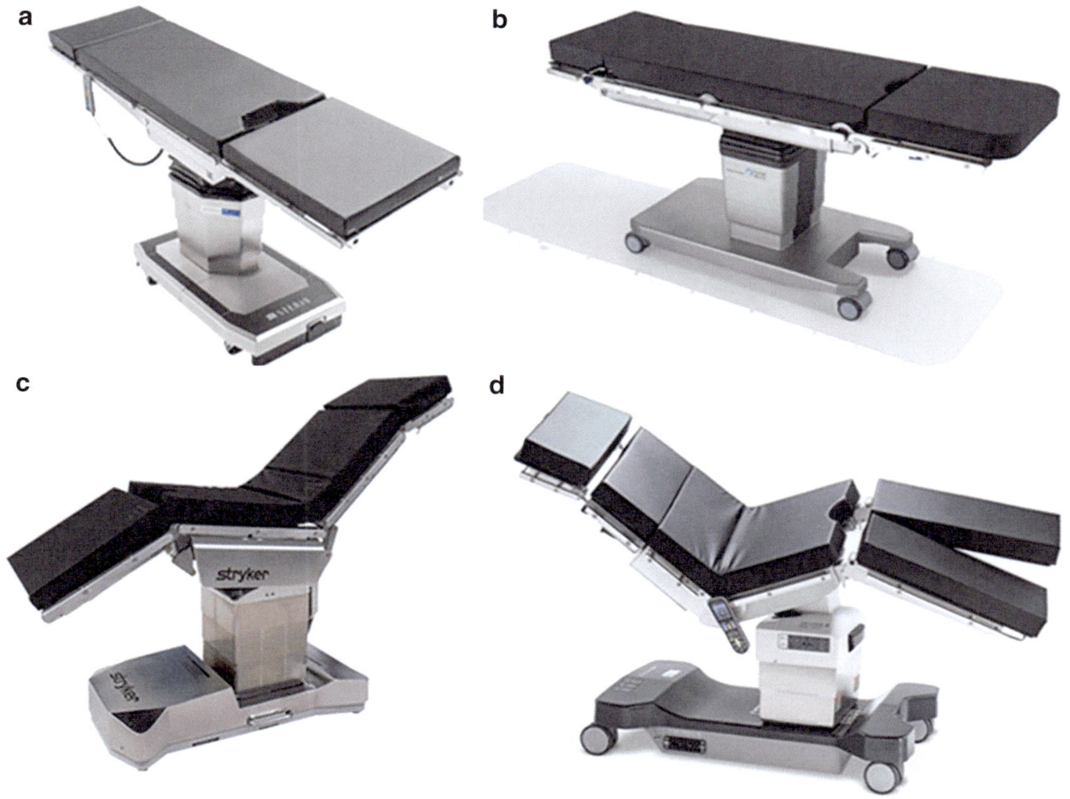

Fig. 1 Single based recent mobile OR tables: (**a**): STERIS AMSCO 5095; (**b**) Trumpf TruSystem 7000; (**c**) Stryker Operon D860; (**d**) Getinge Maquet Meera

4 The Hillrom Allen Positioning System

The Allen Positioning System (Fig. 2) serves as an extension for operating tables. Adding to a radiotransparent frame, it offers suitable access to surgical areas and imaging technologies such as O-arm®. The system enables intraoperative flexion and patient repositioning, ensuring precise alignment of the head and cervical spine through the C-Flex® head positioning system (Fig. 2d). Pressure distribution is well spread with chest, hip, and head supports and accommodates various surgical positions, including prone, lateral, and supine. With lateral tilting up to 20° and its ability to readjust supports intraoperatively with an extensive range of motion make it useful for kyphotic patients, anterior arthroplasty, and lateral procedures. The Allen Bow Frame®, attaching to standard operating tables, creates the reverse lordosis necessary for opening intervertebral spaces, while allowing the patient's abdomen to hang freely during procedures lowering abdominal pressure. The modular system is suitable for all spine surgery types, with a quick-connect coupler for easy attachment to a skull clamp (Fig. 2b).

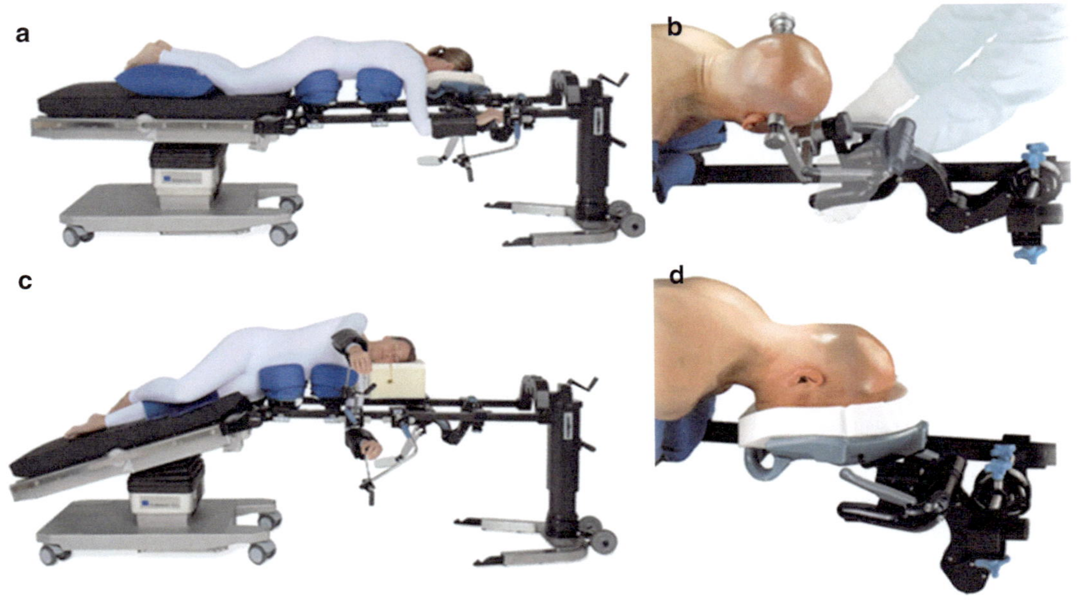

Fig. 2 Hillrom Allen Positioning System: (**a** and **c**) supine and lateral positioning, respectively; (**b**) adjunct of a head clamp; (**d**) adjunct of a C flex

5 The Mitzuho OSI "Jackson Table"

In 1992, Orthopaedic Systems Inc. (OSI) released the modular table system (MTS), the first operating table entirely made of radiolucent carbon fiber composite material. OSI merged with The Mizuho Group in 2002 and the MTS soon became known as the "Jackson table." One unique feature of the MTS is its ability to interchange in three different setups: the "spinal surgery," the "radiolucent imaging," and the "orthopedic trauma" (Fig. 3). Rather than having a single central support as the STERIS AMSCO or the Trumpf TruSystem 7000, the MTS is supported by two posts at each end of the table, which also allow for tilting and height adjustment. This enables more versatility for the C-arm to navigate central parts of the body during an operation. However, this system is limited by its ability to adjust patient positioning during the operation, hence high care must be taken prior to draping, with appropriate use of cushion or bumps and bone foam.

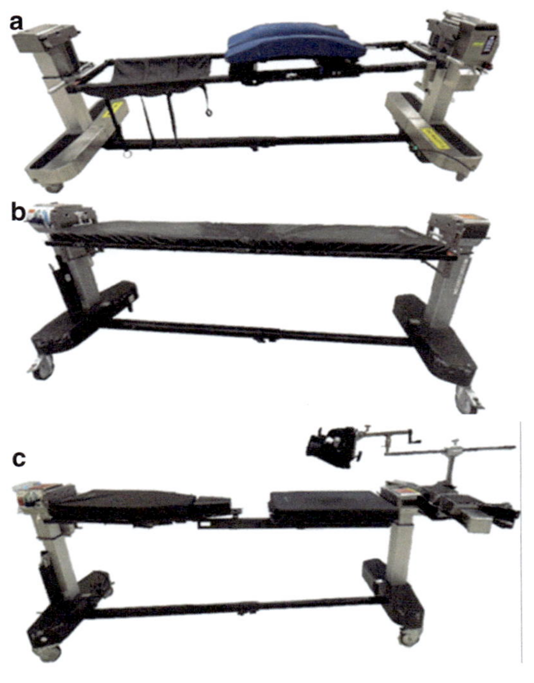

Fig. 3 The OSI Mitzuho "Jackson table": (**a**) spinal surgery top; (**b**) radiolucent top; (**c**) orthopedic trauma top. (Figure from Habibi et al. article 2)

2. Blood Loss Control

Blood loss is a primary concern in spine surgery and a significant source of morbidity. Intraoperative blood loss can trigger blood pressure instability, compromising organ perfusion and leading to organ failure; blood loss can also induce lethal coagulation disorder. Moreover, excessive blood loss influences postoperative recovery and complication such as higher rates of transfusions, infections [10, 11], and longer hospitalization length of stay [12].

With a total number of spinal procedures multiplied by 3 in the last three decades [13, 14], effective intraoperative blood management has emerged as a critical area of research and clinical focus. In this section, we will discuss innovative products and tools aimed at reducing blood loss. *Minimal invasive surgery and endoscopic spinal procedure will be addressed later in a specific section.*

6 Piezosurgery

Piezosurgery uses high-intensity focused ultrasound, leveraging the principles of cavitation, thermal effects, and mechanical forces to cut through the bone (Fig. 4). At its core lies a transducer within a knife, converting electrical energy into mechanical energy [15, 16]. This results in precise high-frequency vibrations, causing water within tissue cells to evaporate, disrupting protein hydrogen bonds, thus facilitating efficient bone tissue cutting [17]. The ultrasonic cutter head operates at a temperature below 38 °C and within a propagation distance of less than 200 microns [18]. Ultimately, its focused ultrasound targets only bone tissue of specific hardness, leaving surrounding blood vessels and nerve tissue unharmed while effectively controlling bleeding at the surgical site. This innovative approach signifies a significant advancement in surgical techniques, ensuring both efficacy and safety in complex procedures adding to traditional high-speed drills and Kerisson rongeurs.

Hidaka pioneered the use of ultrasound bone scalpel (UBS) in a cervical double-door laminoplasty for the first time in 1998 [18]. Subsequently, UBS garnered increasing attention from the spine surgeons community and the range of usages widened with facetectomy [19], foraminotomy [20], hemilaminoplasty [21], thoracolumbar decompression [22], cervical decompression [23], chiari 1 malformation [24], and so on. Many studies outline better outcome with less blood loss [18–23]. Chen et al. conducted a retrospective study on 293 patients and concluded that the combined use of ultrasonic bone scalpel and hemostatic matrix (cf below) is recommended for primary thoracolumbar surgery [25]. Recently in October 2023, Rittipoldech conducted a prospective randomized study on 31 patients and showed significant less blood loss and shorter laminectomy time [26].

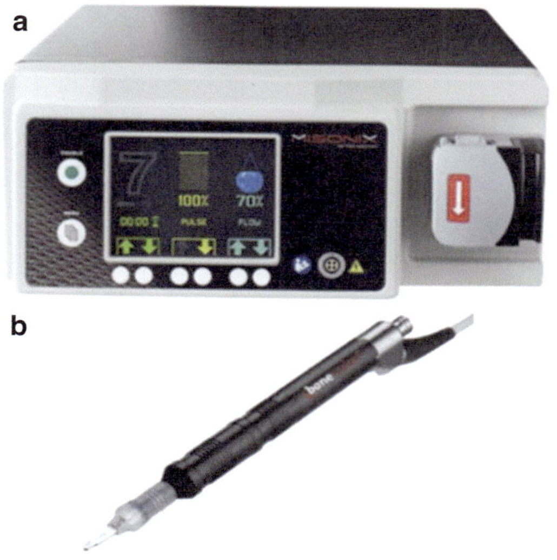

Fig. 4 Example of ultrasonic bone scalpel: (**a**) generator; (**b**) surgical tool

7 Hemostatic Matrix

Intraoperative management of venous bleeding from the spinal epidural space may warrant the application of various products directly at the surgical site. Surgicel®, fibrillar collagen, and Gelfoam® are commonly utilized to staunch bleeding, packed strategically within the operative area. While bipolar coagulation presents

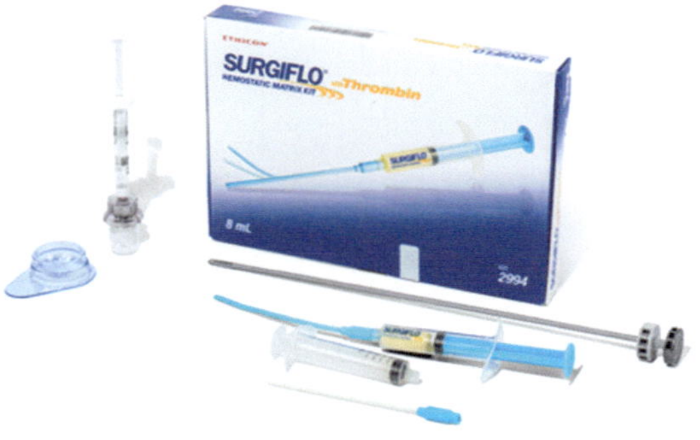

Fig. 5 Example of hemostatic matrix available: Surgiflo (Ethicon)

another option for controlling hemorrhage from the spinal venous plexus, it carries the inherent risk of injuring healthy nervous tissue.

Innovations in hemostatic technology have introduced hemostatic matrices, notably emerging in the late 2000s, with the first retrospective cohort study pertaining to spine surgery published in 2014 [27]. Among these advancements are products such as FloSeal [28] (Baxter Healthcare, Deerfield, Illinois, United States) and Surgiflo [29] (Ethicon, Somerville, New Jersey, United States) (Fig. 5). Derived from blood sources, these local hemostatics operate through chemical and/or mechanical means, fostering platelet aggregation on the surface and providing a substrate for the coagulation cascade [27]. Importantly, they do not stimulate blood cell proliferation but instead facilitate the natural coagulation process.

FloSeal comprises a matrix of bovine gelatin and human thrombin, boasting a preparation time of 168 s and subsequent reabsorption by the organism within 6–8 weeks [28]. Surgiflo, originating from pigs/swine, offers a quicker preparation time of 81 seconds and a reabsorption period of 4–6 weeks, slightly shorter than that of FloSeal [29]. the Floseal Hemostatic Matrix comes in 5 and 10 mL kits, while the Surgiflo Hemostatic Matrix comes in 8 mL kits. Each of these types of various configurations has an independent product description and codes for identification and tracking by hospital facilities and the US Food and Drug Administration (FDA) [30].

One of the main concerns highlighted in various studies regarding these products revolves around their cost. For instance, 8 mL Surgiflo is priced at US$ 295 and 5 mL Floseal costs US$ 199. Nevertheless, numerous prospective randomized clinical trials (RCTs) [31] have demonstrated the clinical efficacy of these products, leading to notable reductions in time to achieve hemostasis and improved control over bleeding, thereby mitigating patient blood loss. Consequently, the seemingly high cost of these hemostatic matrices is offset by several factors such as shorter hospital stays, reduced surgical duration, and less need for blood transfusions. Unfortunately, to date there are no cost-effectiveness study addressing that issue specifically in relation to spine surgery.

3. Minimally Invasive Spine Surgery

Minimally invasive surgery (MIS) has its roots in the nineteenth century, with the advent of the cystoscope for bladder stone management. From then, the ethos of surgery went from "small incision equal small operation" to "doing more with less." The term "MIS" encompass multiple concepts: surgical approaches, systems or products, and a philosophy. Its core principles are to minimize collateral damage, preserve normal anatomy, and reduce the overall stress to the patient, while achieving the same surgical goals as open surgery. Despite the long and winding path marked by fatal side effects and a lack of evidence at an early stage, MIS has now reached the position of scientific, well-established, and genuinely patient-friendly treatment. This philosophy heralded the era of modern surgery.

Technological advancements in cranial surgery, notably the introduction of the operating microscope as early as the 1960s by pioneers such as Yazargyl, have greatly influenced spinal surgery (Fig. 6). Over the past half-century, the field of spinal surgery has made significant strides. The invention of various surgical techniques and the refinement of surgical instruments have enabled surgeons to address a broader range of spinal issues with smaller incisions and minimal structural damage. Minimally invasive spinal surgery (MISS) has expanded its scope, transitioning from basic percutaneous procedures that were not feasible with conventional surgical methods to treating conditions traditionally man-

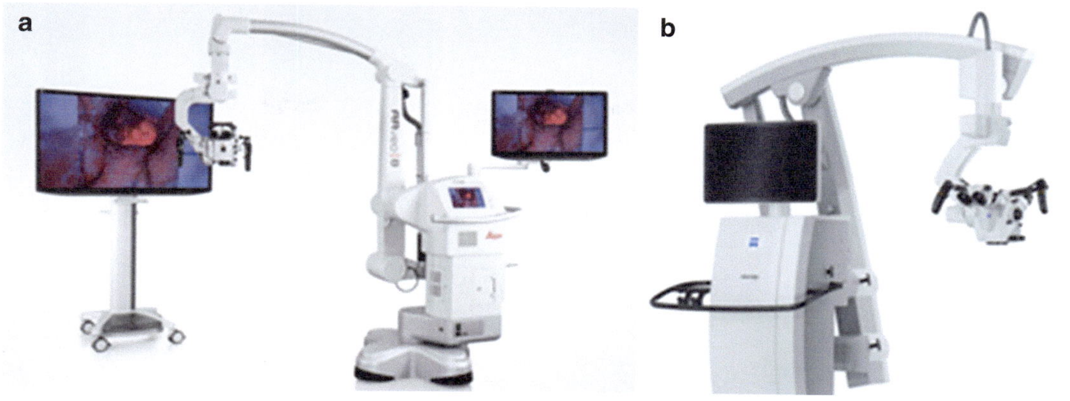

Fig. 6 Examples of surgical microscope: (**a**) Leica Evolved ARveo 8; (**b**) Zeiss Kinevo 900 Microscope

aged through open surgery. These advancements have revolutionized spinal treatment, offering patients less invasive options with potentially shorter recovery times and improved outcomes.

In this section, we will discuss the latest advancements in minimally invasive spine surgery, with a focus on tubular surgery and the more recent rise in popularity of spinal endoscopy.

8 Percutaneous Posterior Spinal Fusion

The emergence of intraoperative imaging with the C-arm in the 1960s (cf below) and its worldwide adoption paved the way for the development of minimally invasive techniques. It served as a catalyst for the ingenuity of spine surgeons, defining new approaches. In 1982, Magerl reported the first percutaneous screw placement for posterior spinal fusion [32] (Fig. 7), utilizing C-arm imaging to enable a comprehensive visualization of the longitudinal axis of the pedicle. Since then, the technique has undergone substantial refinement, with today more than 30 types of systems being made available on the market [33] (when including product revisions), and a proportion of percutaneous screws going from 13% of all screws in 2006 to 52% in 2016 (according to the North American Spine Society) [33]—and the market is expected to keep expanding in the future.

In 1982, Magerl's initial technique differed significantly from contemporary practices adopted worldwide [32] (Figs. 7 and 8). The screws inserted were linked with temporary external spinal skeletal fixation until adequate fusion occurred. Later, in 1995, Mathews and Long reported on a fully percutaneous pedicle screw (PPS) system through subcutaneous rod connection [34]; however, its widespread adoption was hindered by the frequent occurrence of nonunion resulting from its inadequate fixation strength. Subsequently, in 1999, Wiesner et al. introduced a method that remains widely utilized today: the insertion of a K-wire up to the junction of the pedicle and vertebral body with the assistance of C-arm imaging [35]. Finally, Foley et al. in 2001 developed and employed a rod-fixing device based on the sextant principle [36], wherein rods were connected without direct visualization under the guidance of a C-arm, a technique that is currently prevalent. The introduction of the SEXTANT system (Medtronic, Memphis, TN, USA) in 2001 marked the first commercially available percutaneous pedicle screw (PPS) system, with widespread availability in 2005 [33]. This innovative system has since become standard instrumentation utilized globally and has served as a cornerstone for subsequent PPS systems and the minimally invasive spine stabilization procedure.

From 2007 to 2011 a series of second-generation systems emerged such as PathFinder (Abbott Spine, Austin, TX, USA) in 2007; VIPER (DePuy Synthes Spine, Raynham, MA, USA) and MANTIS (Stryker, Kalamazoo, MI, USA) in 2009; or ILLICO SE (Alphatec Spine, Carlsbad, CA, USA)

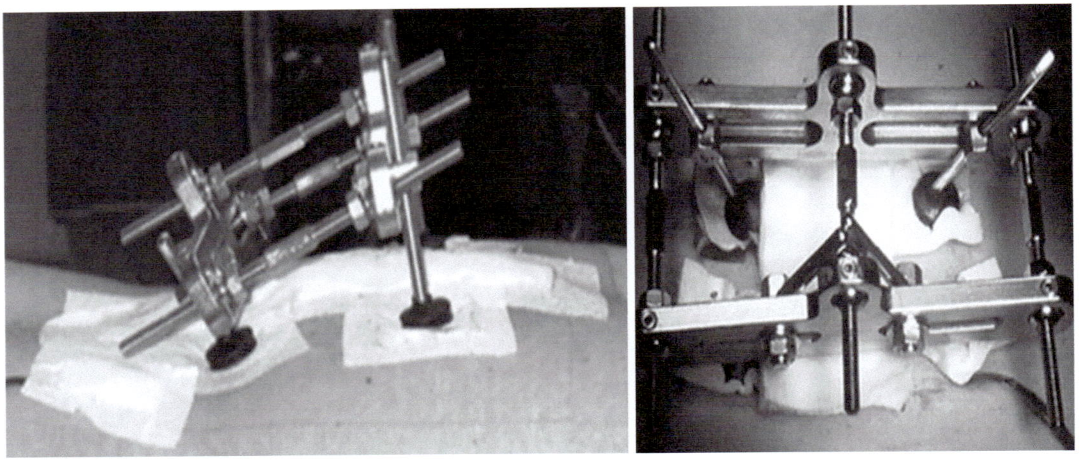

Fig. 7 Magerl's external fixation

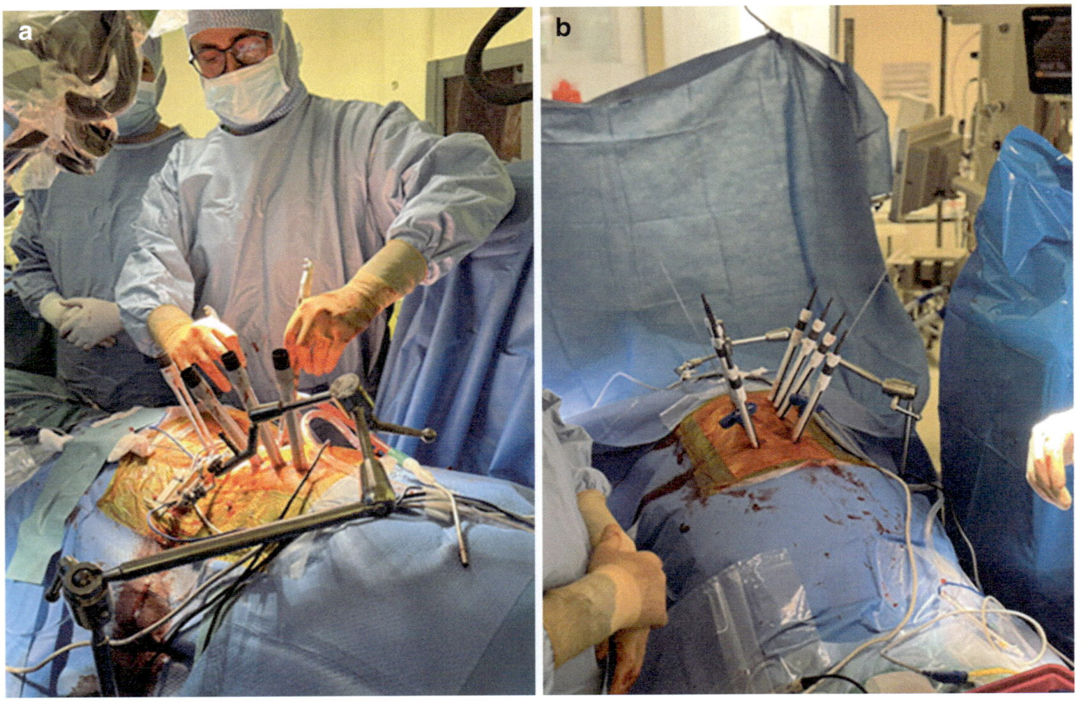

Fig. 8 Minimally invasive posterior spinal screw placement

in 2011. The third generation followed from 2011 to 2020 (Fig. 8), with a new design, integrating an extended tab to easily facilitate slippage correction. These systems are in wide use today and represent most of the currently available systems available on the market. Typical third-generation systems include ES2 (Stryker), VIPER2 X-tab (DePuy Synthes Spine), Voyager (Medtronic), PRECEPT (NuVasive, San Diego, CA, USA), or Saccura (Japan Medical Dynamic Marketing, Tokyo, Japan). More recently, fourth-generation systems that do not require the use of conventional guidewires were introduced from 2019 onwards, including VIPER PRIME (DePuy Synthes Spine) and Voyager ATMAS (Medtronic) [33].

9 Percutaneous Vertebral Augmentation

In 1984, at the University Hospital of Amiens in France, neurosurgeon Galibert and neuroradiologist Deramond introduced percutaneous vertebroplasty (PVP), injecting bone cement to treat large vertebral cavities [37]. The inaugural patient to undergo this novel procedure, presented with severe cervical pain and a vertebral hemangioma spanning the entirety of the C2 vertebral body. Initially aimed at aggressive hemangiomas only, Dusquenel expanded its use to alleviate pain from compression fractures due to osteoporosis and malignancy [38]. Limited awareness of this innovant procedure in North America changed in 1993 when French researcher Depriester-Debussche presented PVP at an American conference, inspiring Jensen and Dion to introduce it in the United States [39]. In 1997, Jensen reported the first US series using polymethyl methacrylate (PMMA) for osteoporotic vertebral fractures, with the University of Virginia Medical Center becoming a teaching center [38, 39]. Concurrent biomechanical studies by Belkoff at Johns Hopkins laid the foundation for clinical application, addressing aspects such as PMMA's temperature effects and injection techniques (unilateral or bilateral) [40]. These studies informed subsequent widespread adoption of PVP. In 2003, the first controlled trial comparing PVP with conservative therapy emphasized its immediate efficacy in pain relief, function enhancement, and reduced analgesia use, highlighting its policy significance [38].

10 Intravertebral Reduction Devices

Despite the growing popularity of vertebroplasty, concerns about cement leakage and damage to the spinal cord and nerves represented significant drawbacks. In 1994, orthopedic surgeon Reiley, engineer Scholten, and biochemist Talmadge collaborated to address these issues. They developed a technique involving the insertion of an inflatable balloon into compressed vertebral bodies before injecting PMMA cement [38]. This approach aimed to reduce cement extrusion, improve localization, and make vertebroplasty safer while restoring vertebral height and reducing kyphotic deformity. After FDA approval in 1998, Reiley performed the first successful kyphoplasty for osteoporotic vertebral compression fractures [41]. Kyphon, holding the patent for the height-restoration device, began selling its balloon device in 1999, reaching US$ 261,000 in sales by the year-end. By 2006, Kyphon reported global sales of approximately US$ 408 million, driven by positive clinical results and effective educational efforts. In 2007, Medtronic acquired Kyphon for US$ 3.9 billion, marking one of the largest medical technology acquisitions in history [42].

More recently, in the early 2010s, the SpineJack (SJ; Vexim, Balma, France) emerged (Fig. 9). This device is inserted inside the vertebral body through the pedicles, guided by C-arm (same way as kyphoplasty balloon). After a template is deployed, it is replaced by the implants. The implant is finally opened, and Cohesion (Vexim) bone cement is injected inside the implant and spread into the adjacent trabecular bone.

A proficient combination of percutaneous spinal fixation, vertebroplasty, and intravertebral reduction devices represent an effective approach, offering a viable minimally invasive treatment option for a broad spectrum of conditions, including traumatic fractures [43], complications of osteoporosis [44], and spinal metastases [45]. This approach facilitates the restoration of spinal stability, anatomical alignment, and alleviate pain. However, there are no consensus regarding the optimal surgical planning tailored to each individual case and the "art of medicine" prevail upon the "evidence-based medicine" at an individual scale. One hope lies in leveraging artificial intelligence to pave the way for personalized medicine, enabling the

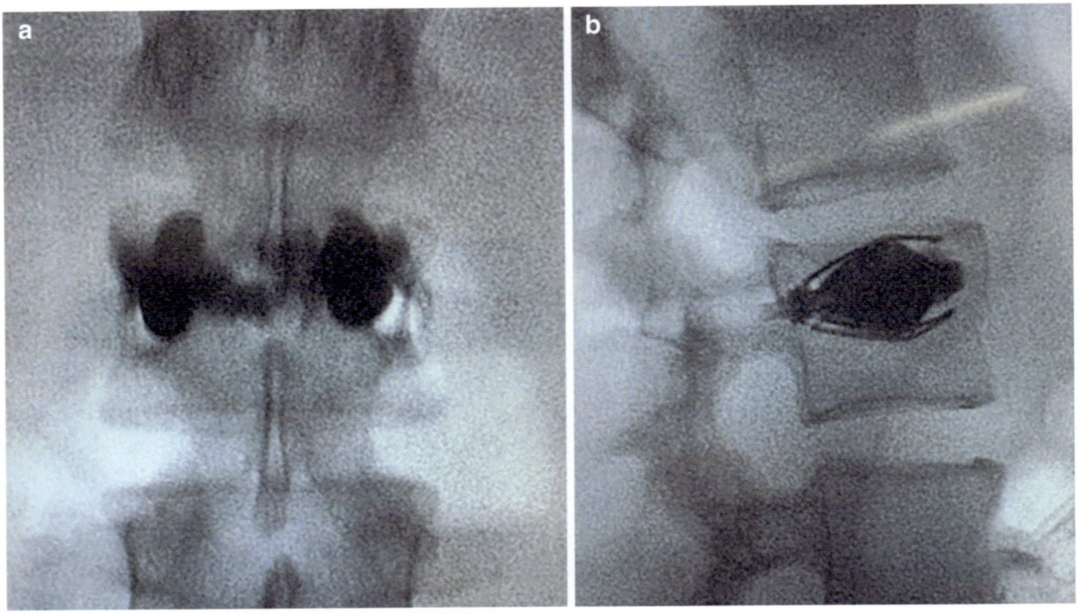

Fig. 9 Intraoperative anteroposterior (**a**) and lateral (**b**) radiographs of a lumbar vertebral augmentation through a SpineJack® for a compression fracture

identification of the most suitable surgical plan for each patient in the future.

11 Tubular Surgery: Overview

One of the main collateral damages of traditional open spinal surgery for decompression or disc herniation surgery is excessive injury to the posterior paraspinal muscles, as well as muscle fascia, that physiologically maintain the integrity of discs, joints, and ligaments. Hence, open posterior spinal surgery bears significant risks of long-term muscle atrophy and subsequent disruption of spinal posture in neutral position. Through a tubular paramedian muscle dilation, tubular microsurgery stands as a robust solution to address this issue. Indeed, it maintains multifidus tendon attachment to the spinous process and integrity of the median dorsolumbar fascia.

Second, traditional "self-retaining" retractors used in open surgery have been proven to cause more retraction pressure, harming neurovascular supply during surgery. By using tubular retractors that are attached to the surgical table, the pressure exerted upon surrounding structures is lowered by up to 50% [46], and the shape of the tubular retractor also spread the pressure optimally by increasing the surface contact area.

The tubular retractor system was introduced by Foley and Smith in 1997 [47]. This innovative system consists of a series of concentric dilators and thin-walled (0.9 mm) tubular retractors of variable length (Fig. 10). An accurate depth of retractors enables a straightforward view to the operating field, keeping muscles aside. METRx system (Medtronic Sofamor Danek, Memphis, TN) was the first commercially available product and has become one of the most extensively used tubular retractor system worldwide. It provides various sizes of dilators, tubular retractors, and flexible arms. The length of tubular retractors ranges from 3 to 9 cm, with diameters varying between 14 and 22 mm (Fig. 11). Beveled MetriX also enables over the top contralateral decompression.

This technology rapidly gained attention from the spine surgeon community, which gradually implemented evidence of safety and efficacy if not superiority compared to traditional tech-

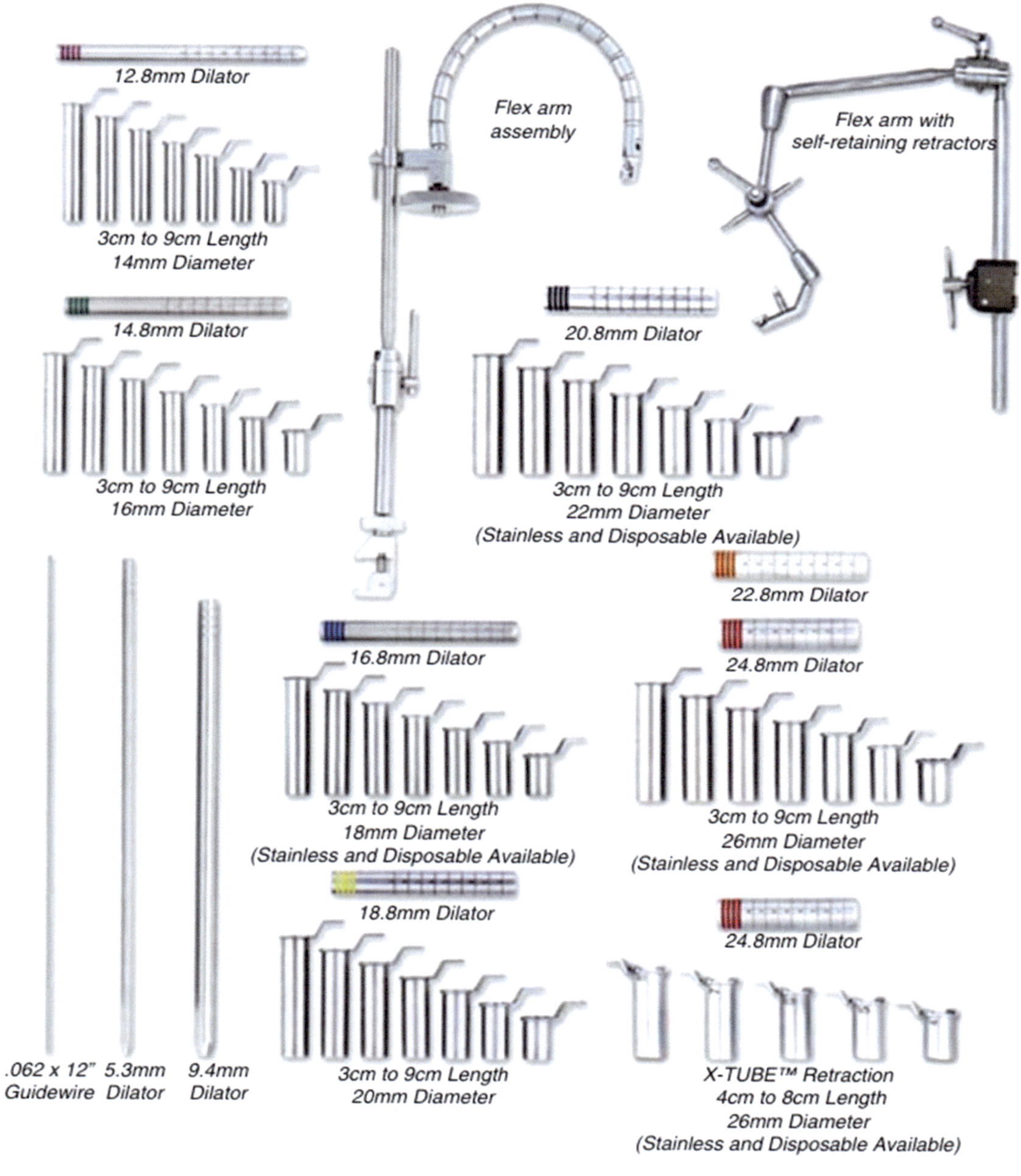

Fig. 10 METRx system part 1

niques. It is now well established as a viable approach for a wide range of indications including decompression, microdiscectomy, and interbody fusion: *noteworthy, the latter benefitted from concomitant emergence of percutaneous posterior spine fusion.* Furthermore, advanced reconstruction including posterior corpectomies and strut fusion for burst fractures, tumors [48], and infections are also described in the current literature.

In microdiscectomy, with the use of a 20 mm diameter and 50–60 mm length tube, large cohort prospective study and meta-analysis showed safety and efficacy [49, 50]. In lumbar decom-

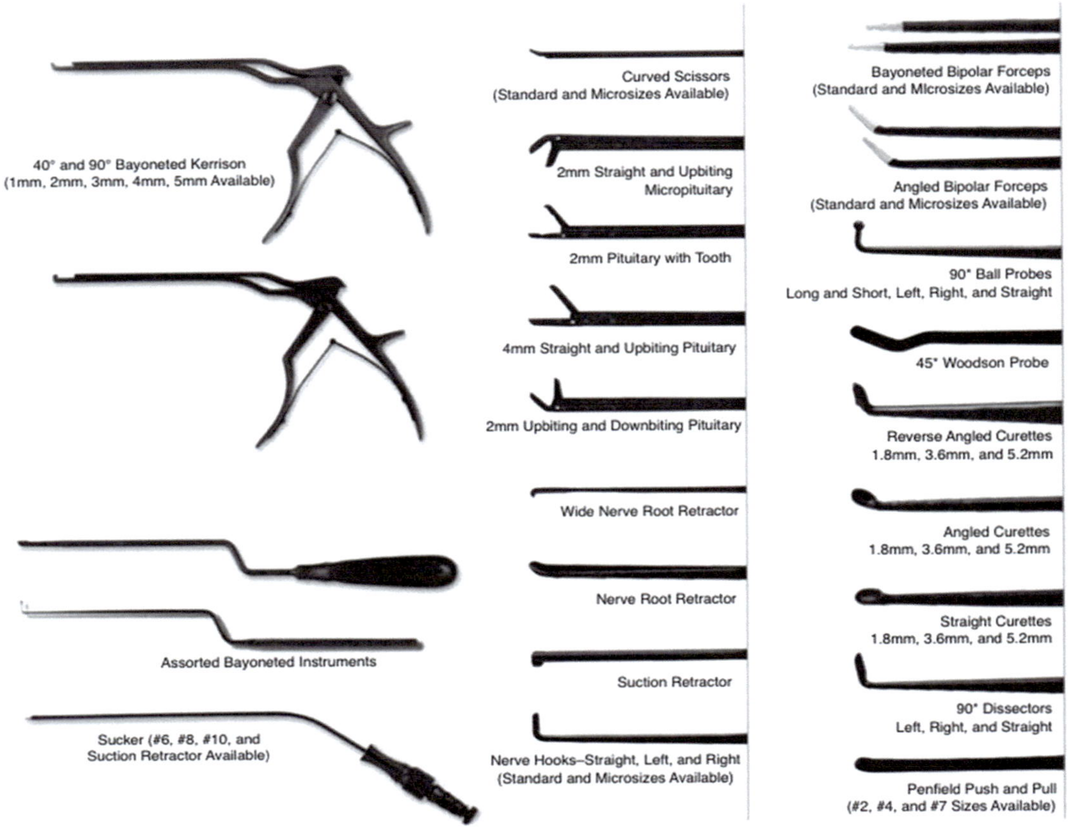

Fig. 11 METRx system part 2

pression, foraminal stenosis is approached in a same way as disc herniation—central stenosis can be approach through a unilateral laminectomy as shown by Weiner et al. [51]

The evolution of minimally invasive retractors, such as tubular or Mast Quadrant retractors (Fig. 12), along with the advancement of percutaneous minimally invasive spinal fixation, has facilitated the development of minimally invasive interbody fusion procedures. An accurate illustration is the evolution of the transforaminal lumbar interbody fusion (TLIF) since Harms' description in 1982. Indeed, in 2002 [36], Kevin Foley and Michael Lefkowitz introduced MIS-TLIF, a minimally invasive adaptation of the TLIF procedure. By utilizing two 1-inch paramedian incisions and a tubular or quadrant retractor to access the surgical site, this approach aimed at mitigating collateral damage in the traditional TLIF. By preserving soft tissue integrity, MIS-TLIF improved patient outcomes and reduced the risk of complications associated with open surgeries. The technique maintained the conceptual framework of TLIF while refining it to enhance safety and efficacy, and keep being improved today [52].

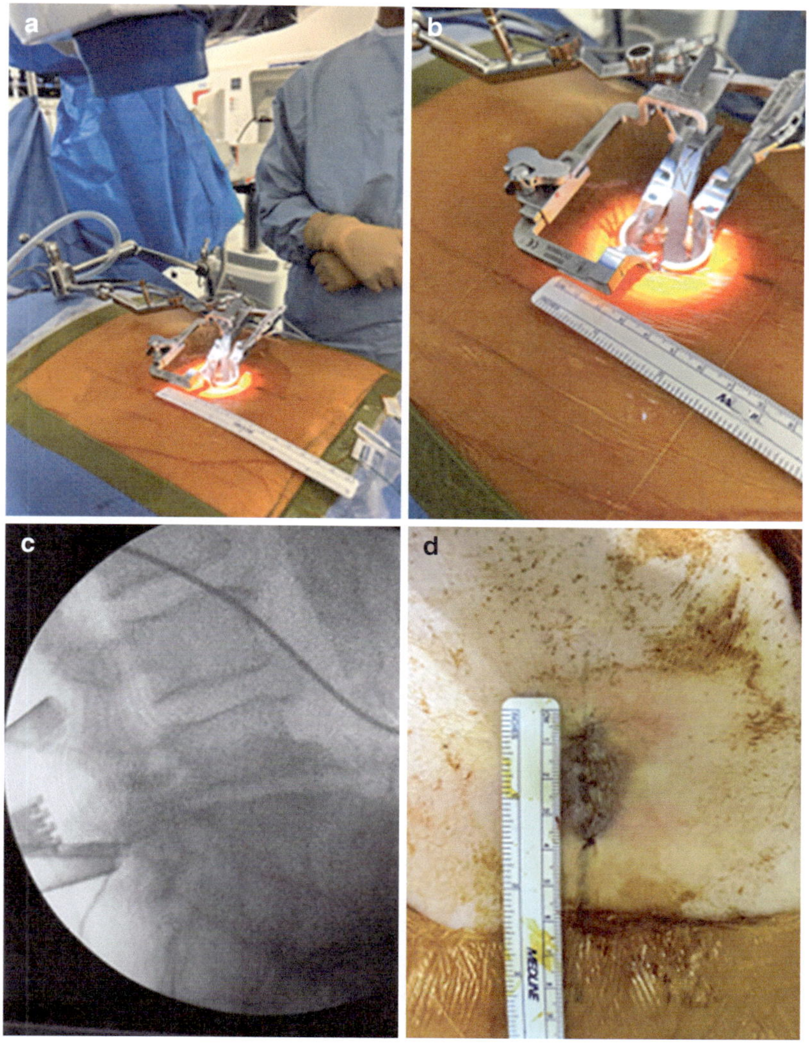

Fig. 12 Quadrant system enabling a two levels minimally invasive lumbar canal decompression through a 3 cm incision: (**a**) surgical view of the fixation system; (**b**) surgical view focused on the surgical field; (**c**) intraoperative lateral radiographs; (**d**) size of the incision

12 Uniportal Endoscopic Spine Surgery: An Overview

The first reported introduction of a modified arthroscope into the intervertebral disc space was in 1983 by Forst and Hausman [53]. In 1988, Kambin provided the first endoscopic views of a herniated nucleus pulposus through an endoscope, setting the stage for revolutionary developments [54, 55]. Two years later, in 1990, Kambin further described the anatomical transforaminal approach, defining the "Kambin's triangle" (Fig. 13), a milestone in full-endoscopic spine surgery [56]. The evolution continued with

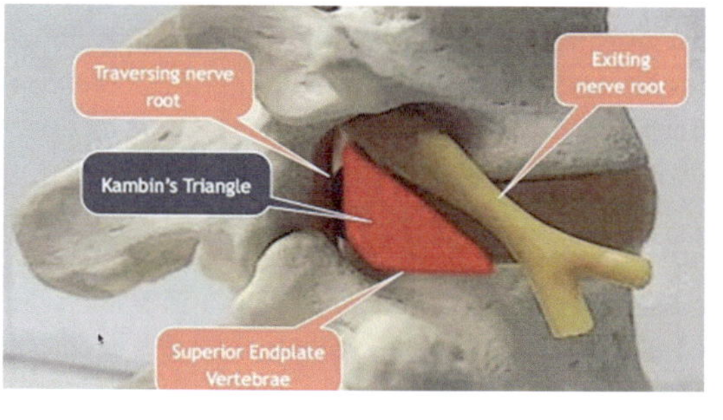

Fig. 13 Right side view of a spine with emphasis on the Kambin's triangle

Mayer's introduction of percutaneous endoscopic indirect lumbar disc resection in 1993 [57].

A significant leap came in 1999 with Anthony T. Yeung's Endoscopy Spine System (YESS) [58], replacing traditional indirect percutaneous endoscopic procedures. This multichannel endoscope had a working channel, an irrigation channel, and a video-recording system simultaneously. Initially, YESS had limited surgical indications, due to the poor instruments available and exposure, mainly an "inside-out" technique consisting in inserting a cannula inside the vertebral disc at the beginning of the procedure. This prompted Schubert and Hoogland with Joimax to introduce THESSYS (Thomas Hoogland Endoscopic spine system) between 1999 and 2002. Hoogland introduced a specialized reamer to expand the intervertebral foramen before disc removal. He described the epidural "outside-in" technique in 2005, broadening the scope of transforaminal approach [59]. Both the inside-out and the outside-in methods later became the most famous basics principles of TELD (transforaminal endoscopic lumbar diskectomy). In 2007, Lee et al. reported a "half-and-half" technique combining the advantages of both methods [60].

Following these emerging technologies, many surgeons worked to widen the range of indications for endoscopic microdiscectomy. In 2004, Ahn et al. emphasized the usefulness of TELD in the context of recurrent lumbar disc herniation [61], and in 2005 described the anterior endoscopic cervical discectomy [62]. In 2008, Choi et al. detailed a surgical method for cases of severely migrated disc herniation through endoscopic surgery [63]. He also reported the first transforaminal endoscopic thoracic discectomy in 2010.

Nevertheless, these innovations and improvements harbored limitations. Indeed, high iliac crest restrain from reaching Kambin's triangle, what is more, central or lateral recess stenosis are difficult to treat through these approaches. To address those limitations, another major breakthrough was achieved by Ruetten in 2006, who described the interlaminar approach, greatly enhancing the technology's versatility [64]. The focus transitioned from endoscopic discectomy to decompression, with advancements in high resolution endoscopic technology and cutting equipment facilitating the treatment of spinal stenosis, previously considered a contraindication. Noteworthy, Ruetten also described full-endoscopic posterior cervical foraminotomy [65, 66].

13 Unilateral Biportal Endoscopic Surgery: Basics and Principles

More recently, in 2013 and 2015, Soliman was the first to describe the surgical management of disc herniation and lumbar stenosis through the use of two separate portals, what will later be known as "UBE (Unilateral Biportal Endoscopic surgery)" [67, 68]. Then, particularly thanks to the dedication of the spine surgery community in Korea, UBE became recognized as the most important endoscopic surgical technique of the spine, taking part in every lumbar degenerative conditions (including fusion), and to some degree, for cervical and thoracic spine surgery.

First, one key basic about UBE is that it might stand as the least invasive technique so far. Indeed, UBE consists of two 1 cm skin and fascial incisions; after a serial muscle dilation, two landmarks are reached after an atraumatic dissection (a fat-free space between the lateral side of the multifidus muscle and the lamina, plus the interfascicular area in between the multifidus bundles). Finally, the 30% of ipsilateral facet joint resection advised in microscopic decompression surgery [69] are not mandatory in UBE surgery, thanks to the undercutting or inclinatory resection of facet joint area [70].

Second, UBE has a fluid-medium, continuous saline irrigation that maintain a clean operative field. This flow can induce an adjusted hydrostatic pressure, limiting epidural bleeding and tissue oozing. Also, it allows to peel off the dura from the lamina, making a safe working space in lumbar stenosis patients. Lastly, it is hypothesized that it may reduce infections risks and lower tissue inflammation. Hydrostatic pressure of 30 mmHg in the lumbar epidural area is thought to be safe [71]. If the outflow is not maintained fluently, epidural pressure might be elevated and cause complications such as headache, intraocular hemorrhages, delayed awakening from anesthesia, and seizures [72]. The temperature control of the saline fluid is also important to avoid hypothermia. UBE boast a magnification lens view, potentially enabling lesion removal through identification of normal and pathologic tissue.

One of the main obstacles to the wide adoption of endoscopic techniques is the stiff learning curve. As UBE uses partly microscopic surgical maneuvers, this technique tends to spread more easily among spine surgeons already familiar with tubular surgery.

4. Image-Guided Navigation, Robots, Augmented and Virtual Reality: New Intraoperative Tools, in the Era of the Augmented Surgeon

Intraoperative imaging has become increasingly widespread and serves as an invaluable tool during spine surgery. Since its inception, continuous improvements have aimed to address surgeons' limitations in vision and touch to achieve better surgical outcomes. Ultimately, this would reduce surgical complications for patients and mitigate the medicolegal stress faced by healthcare teams. Examples such as image-guided navigation (IGN) and robotics are integrated into intraoperative imaging, illustrating technological progress in surgical practice. We will critically evaluate each of these techniques, considering factors such as cost-effectiveness, learning curve, and their impact on patient care, based on the latest literature.

14 Image-Guided Navigation

IGN relies on stereotaxis, utilizing intraoperative 3D fluoroscopy (3DF) or mobile computed tomography (CT) to map the spine. An array sensor is attached to the patient's bone before image acquisition (typically from the spinous process or pelvic bone) and serve as a landmark during the procedure. Then, surgical instruments are registered via an optical tracking system, leading to a real-time stereotactic navigation through the spine. IGN finds applications in a variety of situations, both in open and percutaneous procedures, in elective or urgent surgeries, for nerve decompression or spinal fusion.

Two imaging settings can be used to implement IGN in the operating room (OR): 3D fluoroscopy and mobile computed tomography, each with its own set of advantages and limitations. While 3D fluoroscopy scanners offer faster imaging and maneuverability, they may lack in image quality and field of view compared to mobile CT. On the other hand, mobile CT provides superior image resolution and wider field of view, making it particularly beneficial for complex surgeries or patients with high BMI (body mass index). However, the mobility of mobile CT scanners is restricted by their size and specialized equipment, unlike the more versatile and easily deployable 3D fluoroscopy systems.

Various examples of 3D fluoroscopy and mobile CT systems offer distinct features and functionalities. Among available 3DF, systems such as the Ziehm RFD 3D CMOS, Siemens CIOS Spin, Medtronic O-arm II, and BrainLab LoopX (Figs. 14 and 15) provide different capabilities, such as compatibility with navigation platforms, improved image quality, and mobility. The latter, released in 2021 in the United States (2023 in France) has an enhanced workflow, providing both 2D and 3D imaging with a motorized design, and enable IGN with BrainLab software. On the other hand, two mobile 32 slice CT are available on the market (Fig. 16). First, the Mobius Airo has an integrated operating table, restraining its use to one OR; nevertheless, this CT can operate with BrainLab platform for IGN. Then, the Samsung BodyTom uses a detachable carbon fiber table, allowing to move it after surgery. This CT also requires a navigation software as BrainLab's one to benefit from IGN. Both CT can serve as diagnostic imaging in between operations. The choice of imaging setting will be determined by the intended usage in relation to the surgical team's activity and the possibility of mutualizing technical resources, with prices

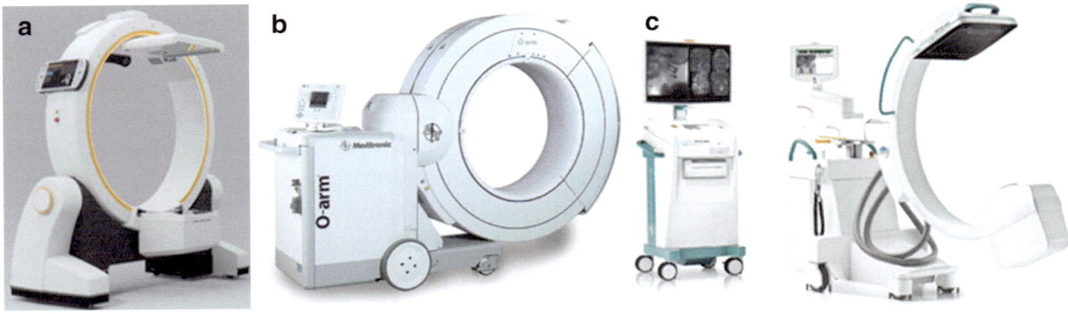

Fig. 14 Examples of 3D fluoroscopy: (**a**) BrainLab Loop-X; (**b**) Medtronic OARM II; (**c**) Ziehm RFD 3D

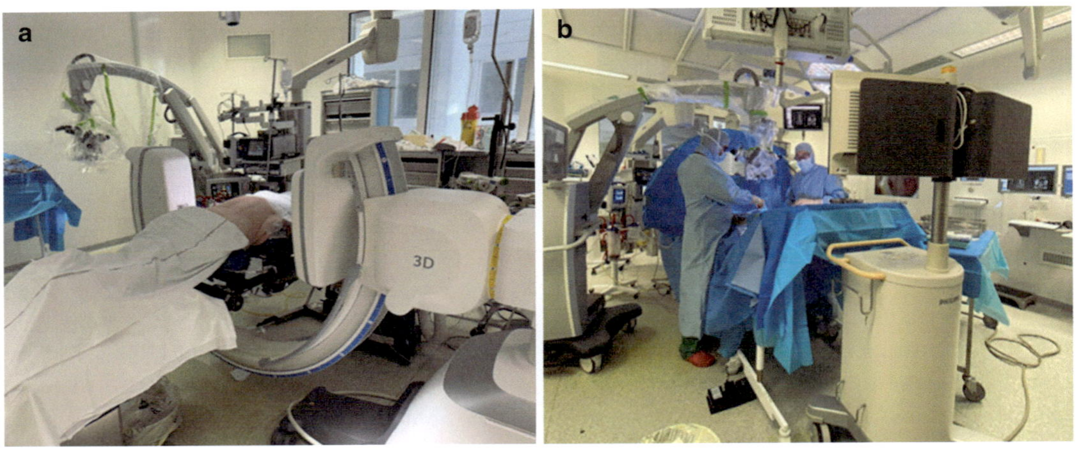

Fig. 15 Intraoperative view of fluoroscopy: (**a**) before surgical draping; (**b**) after surgical draping

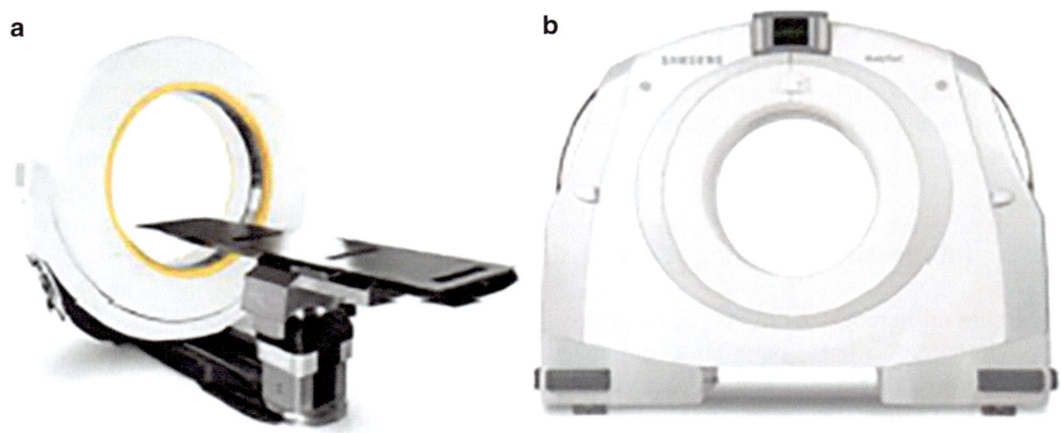

Fig. 16 Example of mobile 32 slice CT: (**a**) Stryker Airo

ranging from approximately €300,000 for a 3D fluoroscopy to over €one million for a 32-slice CT scanner in the operating room.

Systems, or platform or software and associated instrumentation necessary for IGN are getting increasingly standardized. Within the field of spine surgery, there exists a plethora of navigation platforms available on the market. Among the most widely used systems are Medtronic Stealth S8, BrainLab Curve Navigation, Stryker Navigation, 7D Surgical, Augmedics XVision, and NuVasive Pulse. The Medtronic Stealth S8 boasts comprehensive instrument options for spinal fusion outside of pedicle screws (e.g., interbody fusion navigated instruments, navigated high-speed burr) and provides seamless integration with Medtronic implants. BrainLab, an independent navigation company, offers compatibility with various imaging modalities and features surface matching for registration. Stryker Navigation stands out with its battery-powered instruments and innovative SpineMask technology (noninvasive array that does not require invasive bone attachment, stick on the skin instead). 7D surgical distinguishes itself with its flash optical tracking registration and rapid registration capabilities, ideal for long-construct surgeries. Augmedics XVision introduces augmented reality headsets for improved visualization, while NuVasive Pulse integrates surgical assistance technologies into a single system, optimizing floor space and enhancing surgical planning. These platforms represent advancements in technology tailored to meet the diverse needs of spine surgeons.

15 Robots in Spine Surgery

Robotics can refer to the addition of a mechanical arm that locks navigated instruments into a predetermined trajectory. They leverage navigated imaging particularly for tasks like pedicle screw placement. Operating on a shared-control principle, these tools merge surgeon input with automated execution. Theoretical advantages include heightened accuracy in comparison to free-hand methods, facilitated by precise trajectory planning; adoption of minimally invasive techniques, marked by smaller incisions, reduced tissue retraction, limited dissection, bleeding, and infection risks; decreased healthcare team radiation exposure compared to traditional fluoroscopic guidance methods; and unique robotic capabilities such as immunity to fatigue, tremor, and reproducibility. *The Da Vinci system is not included in this type of surgical robot and will be discussed in a separated section.*

Five notable robotic systems are MazorX (Medtronic), Excelsius GPS (Globus Medical), BrainLab Cirq (BrainLab), and the ROSA ONE (Zimmer Biomet) (Fig. 17). The MazorX Stealth Edition, developed by Medtronic, integrates Mazor Robotics technology with Stealth Navigation, offering automatic registration with

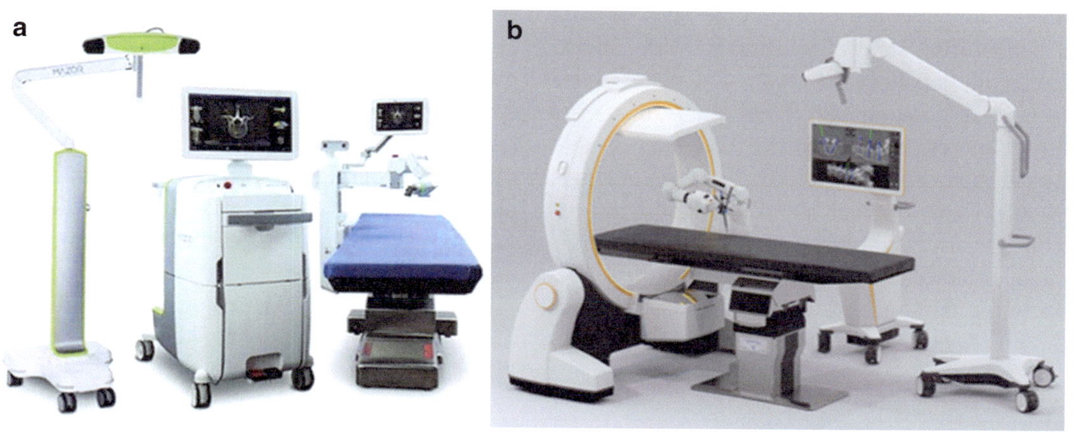

Fig. 17 Notable robotic systems: (**a**): MazorX Stealth edition; (**b**) Brainlab Robotic Suite

the O-arm II. This platform facilitates preoperative screw planning and enables percutaneous screw placement. Similarly, the Excelsius GPS robot from Globus Medical combines a robotic arm with navigated instrumentation, providing increased efficiency and navigation-assisted interbody work. The system is adaptable for both robotic and freehand navigation and automatically registers with the Excelsius 3D mobile 3D imaging platform. In contrast, the BrainLab Cirq functions as a surgical assistant, attaching to operative table rails and working in conjunction with BrainLab's Curve Navigation system. It offers trajectory guidance during drilling and K-wire placement, with options for both passive and active versions. Prices range from 200,000 euros to 1.000,000.

16 Safety and Efficiency of Robots and Image-Guided Navigation

Robots accurately align preoperative planning with postoperation imaging, confirming the screws are positioned as intended. Vardiman [73] showed a 97.5% accuracy rate for his series of 350 screws in the first 56 patients operated in his institution through this technic. He also showed a 93% accuracy in 75 thoracic screws from patients with thin pedicles [74]. The same excellent rates are found in the traumatic setting [75]. Compared to fluoroscopy-assisted free-hand screw placement, robots offer comparable or superior accuracy in screw placement with higher Gertzbein and Robbins grades [76–78] and less facet joint violation [79]. Additionally, they offer higher scores in quality of life (Oswestry disability index and EVA at last follow-up), lower length of stay, same to lower blood loss, and less revisions regardless of the robot model used [76, 80–83]. However, some studies point at higher operation duration. In the cervical spine, which present added difficulty due to the segment's mobility and the influence of patient's position, Zhan et al. demonstrated superior accuracy of robot compared to the traditional free-hand technique in a comparative study involving 26 patients treated with each method in the traumatic setting [84]. However, he shows higher operation duration with similar blood loss. In a patient with a C2 odontoid fracture, Farah et al. demonstrated the feasibility and accuracy of percutaneous posterior fixation of C1 and C2, utilizing the Cirq Robot to achieve precise screw placement [85]. Furthermore, it is noteworthy that while Cirq has FDA approval for use in cervical spine, The Mazor does not [86]. In oncology, robots prove beneficial for tasks such as augmented pedicle screw placement, guiding trajectories for en bloc osteotomies, targeting benign bone lesions, and facilitating minimally invasive removal of paraspinal thoracic and lumbosacral schwannomas and ganglioneuromas, particularly when utilizing the Da Vinci Robot (further discussed later) [87]. Meyer et al. demonstrated the safety and feasibility of using the Cirq Robot to assist in C1 lateral mass kyphoplasty, a surgical intervention to address painful osteolytic lesion of C1, pioneering use of robotic assistance in this procedure [88].

Two studies focused on the learning curve agreed that 25 cases are sufficient to reach a plateau [89, 90]. Furthermore, Lee et al., in their multicenter study spanning 5 years and involving seven surgeons, demonstrated a continuous improvement in the quality of care over time [91]. McDonnell focused on assessing a surgeon's proficiency in robotic surgery and compiled platforms that aid in learning and developing these skills [92]. Fiani conducted a review on the financial aspects of spinal surgery robots. He highlighted a lack of data and concluded that due to the shorter duration of hospital stays, this investment could prove beneficial in the long run [93].

Likewise, Sielatycki demonstrated comparable or superior accuracy in pedicle screw placement compared to the conventional fluoroscopy-assisted free-hand technique [94]. However, as for now, there is no compelling evidence indicating that image-guided screw placement is superior to conventional techniques in terms of clinical outcome. In his retrospective study conducted across two tertiary centers and two community hospitals, comparing single-level fusion for spondylolisthesis, Crawford found no significant difference between these two techniques in terms of 90-day adverse events and 3-year revision rates [95]. In a retrospective cohort study comparing robots and guided navigation, conducted by Shafi et al., involving 90 patients with robots and 120 with IGN, robots were found to be superior to IGN. They exhibited greater accuracy in screw placement, allowing for larger diameter screws, and had fewer breaches of the articular facet [96].

17 The Da Vinci Robot

The Da Vinci Robot (DVR) (Fig. 18) represents a pioneering advancement in medical technology, blending robotics with surgical precision. Developed by Intuitive Surgical, this robotic platform offers surgeons enhanced dexterity, control, and visualization during minimally invasive procedures across various surgical specialties. With its articulating arms and high-definition 3D camera, Da Vinci enables surgeons to perform complex maneuvers with unparalleled accuracy, leading to reduced patient trauma, faster recovery times, and superior clinical outcomes in various field of medicine. By combining human expertise with robotic assistance, the Da Vinci System continues to redefine the possibilities of modern surgery, ushering in a new era of precision and patient care. Compared to traditional robotic systems such as Mazor, Cirq, or ExcelsiusGPS, the Da Vinci Surgical System offers greater versatility, precision, and 3D visualization. Da Vinci's articulating arms and intuitive controls enable enhanced maneuverability in complex spinal surgeries, resulting in improved patient outcomes and reduced surgical trauma.

While a comprehensive scoping review spanning all applications of the Da Vinci robotic system has not been conducted, analysis of PubMed searches associating "Da Vinci Robot" with MeSH terms such as "urology," "gynecology," or "colorectal surgery" suggests higher attention given by these specialties to the Da Vinci Robot compared to spine surgery. This is due to the fact that the DVR was initially designed for soft tissue surgery.

Loniewski et al. published a DVR-assisted transperitoneal approach in oblique lumbar interbody fusion (OLIF) especially useful for obese patients [97]. The three dimensions view and the 360° instrument mobility provide a safer

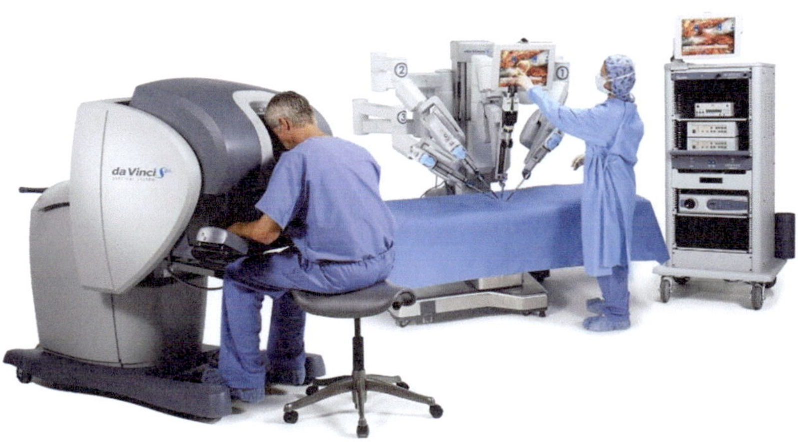

Fig. 18 Da Vinci Robot

approach in regard with neurovascular nearby structures as well as urologic or visceral organs. The DVR is involved into the surgical transperitoneal approach to reach and expose vertebral bodies and lumbar discs, then the surgeon performs the discectomy or the corporectomy [98]. Until the DVR is coupled with a surgical robot that operates on bones (as the ROSA, or SpineAssist) with navigation, this remains a hybrid procedure. Butler published the first anterior lumbar interbody fusion (ALIF) assisted by DVR through a transperitoneal approach [99]. Ye et al. described two case reports of pyogenic spondylodiscitis that required a DVR-assisted anterior retroperitoneal approach. In these complex cases, DVR enabled a safe exposition [100]. Lee reported the use of DVR for transoral odontoidectomy in case of basilar invagination [101]. Finally, DVR use in spine surgery have been reported for paraspinal tumor resection, such as schwannomas or ganglioneuroma, especially for patients with Neurofibromatosis 1 [87, 102, 103].

18 Autonomous Robots

Autonomous robotic surgery represents a pioneering field dedicated to the integration of robotic systems with varying degrees of autonomy for the execution of surgical procedures. This edging technology is enabled by paralleling breakthrough in artificial intelligence and machine learning. While most autonomous robotic systems remain in the experimental phase, a notable subset has successfully transitioned into clinical applications. Noteworthy procedures include venipuncture, intestinal anastomosis, total knee replacement, cochlear implant, among others [104]. In spine surgery, the literature is very limited to this day with two studies implementing autonomous robotic systems for transforaminal lumbar epidural injection [105, 106]. Li et al. shared a cadaveric study on an autonomous spine robot performing thoracolumbar laminectomy based on a preoperative planning [107]. Hao et al. explores new algorithms facilitating future autonomous robots to perform pedicle screw placement [108].

19 Augmented Reality and Virtual Reality

AR (Fig. 15) refers to virtual images that are projected over the actual physical field. It overlays digital information onto the real world, enhancing user perception. AR gear typically involves devices such as smart glasses or heads-up displays (HUDs), enabling users to see both physical surroundings and virtual elements simultaneously but can also display on tablets and phones with camera or in the surgical microscope. This technology consists of three components: tracking, display, and computation systems.

Virtual reality (VR) (Fig. 19) immerses users in simulated environments. VR equipment includes headsets that block out the real world and display computer-generated environments. These headsets often incorporate motion tracking and hand controllers for interactive experiences.

In McCloskey recent systematic review on AR and VR in spine surgery published in May 2023, 48 studies were included [109]. They found that AR and VR has multiple benefits to spine surgery. It enhances education and surgical training with reduced penetration rates and increased accuracy rates compared to lecture-based training [110]. VR use in preoperative planning can significantly impact surgical strategy [111], radiation exposure, operating duration, and estimated blood loss. AR was also found to improve accuracy in pedicle screw placement with three studies showing 95–100% accuracy rate (Gertzbein classification). AR/VR were also found useful in vertebroplasty, bone biopsy, rod bending, or tumor resections. Finally, four studies showed reduced radiation exposition in operations involving fluoroscopy [112].

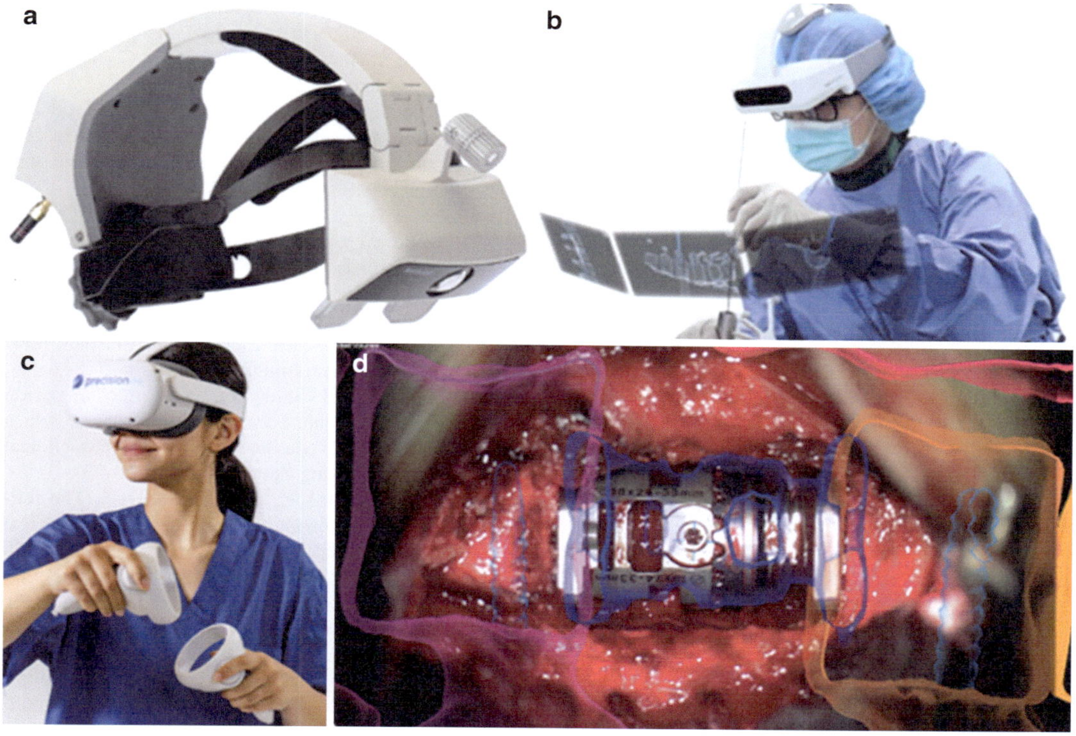

Fig. 19 Augmented reality and virtual reality examples: (**a**) XVision Spine system from Augmedics; (**b**) surgeon wearing the XVision gear (augmented reality); (**c**) surgical resident training on a virtual reality system; (**d**) example of what a surgeon wearing an augmented reality system may see during the surgery

20 Conclusion

In conclusion, spine surgery is undergoing rapid transformation driven by technological advancements, encompassing improvements in the surgical environment, techniques, and intelligent tools augmenting surgeon skills. Enhanced surgical tables and intraoperative imaging have led to the emergence of robotics and image-guided navigation, promising better accuracy, reduced complications, and shorter hospital stays. Intraoperative imaging technologies have also brought new surgical possibilities, approaches, and corridors, leading to the rise of minimally invasive spine surgery. The latter embodies the Ethos of "doing more with less," providing optimal outcome with less collateral damage. The benefits are as much for the patient as for the healthcare team with less exposition to operating radiation.

However, the initial costs and learning curves associated with these technologies necessitate cautious adoption. Looking ahead, emerging tools such as exoscopes and developments in artificial intelligence and autonomous robotics hold further promise for optimizing efficiency and patient outcomes. Adapting a critical mindset while embracing innovation will be crucial for maximizing the benefits of these advancements and advancing spine surgery.

Conflict of Interest and Disclosure of Funding Statement The authors certify that there is no conflict of interest with any financial organization regarding the material discussed in the manuscript. There is no disclosure of funding.

References

1. Essex-Lopresti M. Operating theatre design. Lancet. 1999;353:1007–10.
2. Habibi AA, et al. History, indications, and advantages of orthopaedic operating room tables: a review. Eur J Orthop Surg Traumatol. 2022;32:1207–13.
3. Shriver MF, et al. Lumbar spine surgery positioning complications: a systematic review. Neurosurg Focus. 2015;39:E16.
4. Cunha PD, et al. The ideal patient positioning in spine surgery: a preventive strategy. EFORT Open Rev. 2023;8:63–72.
5. Shen Y, Drum M, Roth S. The prevalence of perioperative visual loss in the United States: a 10-year study from 1996 to 2005 of spinal, orthopedic, cardiac, and general surgery. Anesth Analg. 2009;109:1534–45.
6. Joaquim AF, Makhni MC, Riew KD. Post-operative nerve injuries after cervical spine surgery. Int Orthop. 2019;43:791–5.
7. Uribe JS, et al. Brachial plexus injury following spinal surgery: a review. J Neurosurg Spine. 2010;13:552–8.
8. Nicol M, Sun Y, Craig N, Wardlaw D. Incidence of thromboembolic complications in lumbar spinal surgery in 1,111 patients. Eur Spine J. 2009;18:1548–52.
9. https://www.brainlab.com/surgery-products/overview-platform-products/robotics/.
10. Kato S, et al. Risk of infectious complications associated with blood transfusion in elective spinal surgery—a propensity score matched analysis. Spine J. 2016;16:55–60.
11. Janssen SJ, Braun Y, Wood KB, Cha TD, Schwab JH. Allogeneic blood transfusions and postoperative infections after lumbar spine surgery. Spine J. 2015;15:901–9.
12. Andersen K, Thastum M, Nørholt SE, Blomlöf J. Relative blood loss and operative time can predict length of stay following orthognathic surgery. Int J Oral Maxillofac Surg. 2016;45:1209–12.
13. Mikhail C, et al. Minimizing Blood Loss in Spine Surgery. Glob Spine J. 2020;10:71S–83S.
14. Willner D, et al. Spine surgery and blood loss: systematic review of clinical evidence. Anesth Analg. 2016;123:1307–15.
15. Sadrameli SS, Chan TM, Lee JJ, Desai VR, Holman PJ. Resection of spinal meningioma using ultrasonic BoneScalpel microshaver: cases, technique, and review of the literature. Oper Neurosurg. 2020;19:715–20.
16. Sanborn MR, et al. Safety and efficacy of a novel ultrasonic osteotome device in an ovine model. J Clin Neurosci. 2011;18:1528–33.
17. A, K., et al. Thoracic spine stenosis: does ultrasonic Osteotome improve outcome in comparison to conventional technique? Malays Orthop J. 2021;15:62–9.
18. Wu L, Wang S. Effect of ultrasonic Osteotome on therapeutic efficacy and safety of spinal surgery: A system review and meta-analysis. Comput Math Methods Med. 2022;2022:1–8.
19. Bartley CE, Bastrom TP, Newton PO. Blood loss reduction during surgical correction of adolescent idiopathic scoliosis utilizing an ultrasonic bone scalpel. Spine Deform. 2014;2:285–90.
20. Hazer DB, Yaşar B, Rosberg H-E, Akbaş A. Technical aspects on the use of ultrasonic bone shaver in spine surgery: experience in 307 patients. Biomed Res Int. 2016;2016:1–8.
21. Matsuoka H, et al. Recapping hemilaminoplasty for spinal surgical disorders using ultrasonic bone curette. Surg Neurol Int. 2012;3:70.
22. Bydon M, et al. Safety of spinal decompression using an ultrasonic bone curette compared with a high-speed drill: outcomes in 337 patients: clinical article. J Neurosurg Spine. 2013;18:627–33.
23. Onen MR, Yuvruk E, Akay S, Naderi S. The reliability of the ultrasonic bone scalpel in cervical Spondylotic myelopathy: a comparative study of 46 patients. World Neurosurg. 2015;84:1962–7.
24. Al-Mahfoudh R, et al. Applications of the ultrasonic bone cutter in spinal surgery—our preliminary experience. Br J Neurosurg. 2014;28:56–60.
25. Chen H-T, et al. Effects of combined use of ultrasonic bone scalpel and hemostatic matrix on perioperative blood loss and surgical duration in degenerative thoracolumbar spine surgery. Biomed Res Int. 2019;2019:1–7.
26. Rittipoldech C, Limsomwong P, Thamrongskulsiri N. Bisturi ósseo ultrassônico versus técnica convencional para descompressão espinhal torácica: Um teste controlado randomizado prospectivo. Rev Bras Ortop. 2023;58:e706–11.
27. Landi A, Gregori F, Marotta N, Delfini RE. Security, and manageability of Gelified hemostatic matrix in bleeding control during thoracic and lumbar spine surgery: FloSeal versus Surgiflo. J Neurol Surg Part Cent Eur Neurosurg. 2015;77:139–43.
28. FloSeal. Hemostatic matrix instructions for use. Baxter; 2014.
29. Surgiflo. Hemostatic matrix kit, technical report. Ethicon; 2012.
30. Price JS, Tackett S, Patel V. Observational evaluation of outcomes and resource utilization from hemostatic matrices in spine surgery. J Med Econ. 2015;18:777–86.
31. Renkens KL, et al. A multicenter, prospective, randomized trial evaluating a new hemostatic agent for spinal surgery. Spine. 2001;26:1645–50.
32. Magerl FP. Stabilization of the lower thoracic and lumbar spine with external skeletal fixation. Clin Orthop. 1984:125–41.
33. Ishii K, et al. The history and development of the percutaneous pedicle screw (PPS). System Medicina (Mex). 2022;58:1064.

34. Mathews H, Long B. Endoscopy assisted percutaneous anterior interbody fusion with subcutaneous suprafascial internal fixation: evolution, techniques, and surgical considerations. Orthop Int Ed. 1995;3:496–500.
35. Wiesner L, Kothe R, Rüther W. Anatomic evaluation of two different techniques for the percutaneous insertion of pedicle screws in the lumbar spine. Spine. 1999;24:1599.
36. Foley KT, Gupta SK, Justis JR, Sherman MC. Percutaneous pedicle screw fixation of the lumbar spine. Neurosurg Focus. 2001;10:1–9.
37. Galibert P, Deramond H, Rosat P, Le Gars D. Preliminary note on the treatment of vertebral angioma by percutaneous acrylic vertebroplasty. Neurochirurgie. 1987;33:166–8.
38. Kushchayev SV, et al. Percutaneous Vertebroplasty. Neuroimaging Clin N Am. 2019;29:481–94.
39. Jensen ME, Dion JE. Vertebroplasty relieves osteoporosis pain. Diagn Imaging. 1997;19(68):71–2.
40. Jasper LE, Deramond H, Mathis JM, Belkoff SM. The effect of monomer-to-powder ratio on the material properties of cranioplastic. Bone. 1999;25:27S–9S.
41. Mathis JM. Percutaneous vertebroplasty or kyphoplasty: which one do I choose? Skeletal Radiol. 2006;35:629–31.
42. https://www.forbes.com/2007/07/27/medtronic-kyphon-kyphoplasty-biz-sci-cx_mh_0727kyphon.html -7157e39c2831.
43. Avinens V, et al. Radiological analysis of minimally invasive treatment of type A thoracolumbar fractures based on a series of 135 fractures. Orthop Traumatol Surg Res. 2023;109:103486.
44. Prost S, Pesenti S, Fuentes S, Tropiano P, Blondel B. Treatment of osteoporotic vertebral fractures. Orthop Traumatol Surg Res. 2021;107:102779.
45. Meyer M, et al. Management of Spinal Metastasis by minimally invasive surgical techniques: surgical principles and indications—A literature review. J Clin Med. 2023;12:5165.
46. Stevens KJ, et al. Comparison of minimally invasive and conventional open posterolateral lumbar fusion using magnetic resonance imaging and retraction pressure studies. J Spinal Disord Tech. 2006;19:77–86.
47. Smith MM. Microendoscopic discectomy system: surgical technique and initial clinical results, vol. 99. Neurological Focus; 1997. p. S105.
48. Afathi M, et al. Minimally invasive transmuscular approach for the treatment of benign intradural extramedullary spinal cord tumours: technical note and results. Neurochirurgie. 2015;61:333–8.
49. Arts MP. Tubular Diskectomy vs conventional Microdiskectomy for sciatica: a randomized controlled trial. JAMA. 2009;302:149.
50. Ryang Y-M, Oertel MF, Mayfrank L, Gilsbach JM, Rohde V. Standard open microdiscectomy versus minimal access trocar microdiscectomy: results of a prospective randomized study. Neurosurgery. 2008;62:174–82.
51. Weiner BK, Walker M, Brower RS, McCulloch JA. Microdecompression for lumbar spinal canal stenosis. Spine. 1999;24:2268.
52. May AT, Farah K, Meyer M, Fuentes S. How I do it: mini invasive transforaminal lumbar interbody fusion. Acta Neurochir. 2021;163:289–93.
53. Forst R, Hausmann B. Nucleoscopy? A new examination technique. Arch Orthop Trauma Surg. 1983;101:219–21.
54. Kambin P, Nixon JE, Chait A, Schaffer JL. Annular protrusion: pathophysiology and roentgenographic appearance. Spine. 1988;13:671–5.
55. Kambin P, Sampson S. Posterolateral percutaneous suction-excision of herniated lumbar intervertebral discs. Report of interim results. Clin Orthop. 1986:37–43.
56. Kambin P. Arthroscopic microdiskectomy. Mt Sinai J Med N Y. 1991;58:159–64.
57. Mayer HM, Brock M. Percutaneous endoscopic lumbar discectomy (PELD). Neuro Surg Rev. 1993;16:115–20.
58. Yeung AT. Minimally invasive disc surgery with the Yeung endoscopic spine system (YESS). Surg Technol Int. 1999;8:267–77.
59. Schubert M, Hoogland T. Die transforaminale endoskopische Nukleotomie mit Foraminoplastik bei lumbalen Bandscheibenvorfällen. Oper Orthop Traumatol. 2005;17:641–61.
60. Lee S, et al. Percutaneous endoscopic lumbar discectomy for migrated disc herniation: classification of disc migration and surgical approaches. Eur Spine J. 2007;16:431–7.
61. Ahn Y, et al. Percutaneous endoscopic lumbar discectomy for recurrent disc herniation: surgical technique, outcome, and prognostic factors of 43 consecutive cases. Spine. 2004;29:E326–32.
62. Ahn Y, Lee S-H, Shin S-W. Percutaneous endoscopic cervical discectomy: clinical outcome and radiographic changes. Photomed Laser Surg. 2005;23:362–8.
63. Choi G, et al. Percutaneous endoscopic approach for highly migrated Intracanal disc Herniations by Foraminoplastic technique using rigid Working Channel endoscope. Spine. 2008;33:E508–15.
64. Ruetten S, Komp M, Godolias G. A new full-endoscopic technique for the Interlaminar operation of lumbar disc Herniations using 6-mm endoscopes: prospective 2-year results of 331 patients. Min – Minim Invasive Neurosurg. 2006;49:80–7.
65. Ruetten S, Komp M, Merk H, Godolias G. A new full-endoscopic technique for cervical posterior Foraminotomy in the treatment of lateral disc Herniations using 6.9-mm endoscopes: prospective 2-year results of 87 patients. Min - Minim Invasive Neurosurg. 2007;50:219–26.

66. Ahn Y, Park J-K, Park C-K. Core techniques of minimally invasive spine surgery. Singapore: Springer; 2023. https://doi.org/10.1007/978-981-19-9849-2.
67. Soliman HM. Irrigation endoscopic decompressive laminotomy. A new endoscopic approach for spinal stenosis decompression. Spine J. 2015;15:2282–9.
68. Soliman HM. Irrigation endoscopic discectomy: a novel percutaneous approach for lumbar disc prolapse. Eur Spine J. 2013;22:1037–44.
69. Guha D, Heary RF, Shamji MF. Iatrogenic spondylolisthesis following laminectomy for degenerative lumbar stenosis: systematic review and current concepts. Neurosurg Focus. 2015;39:E9.
70. Heo DH, Lee DC, Park CK. Comparative analysis of three types of minimally invasive decompressive surgery for lumbar central stenosis: biportal endoscopy, uniportal endoscopy, and microsurgery. Neurosurg Focus. 2019;46:E9.
71. Choi CM, Chung JT, Lee SJ, Choi DJ. How I do it? Biportal endoscopic spinal surgery (BESS) for treatment of lumbar spinal stenosis. Acta Neurochir. 2016;158:459–63.
72. Lin C-Y, et al. Seizure after percutaneous endoscopic surgery—incidence, risk factors, prevention, and management. World Neurosurg. 2020;138:411–7.
73. Vardiman AB, Wallace DJ, Booher GA, Toossi N, Bucklen BS. Decreasing the pedicle screw misplacement rate in the thoracic spine with robot-guided navigation. Clin Spine Surg Spine Publ. 2023;36:431–7.
74. Vardiman AB, et al. Pedicle screw accuracy in clinical utilization of minimally invasive navigated robot-assisted spine surgery. J Robot Surg. 2020;14:409–13.
75. Diaz-Aguilar LD, et al. The use of robot-assisted surgery for the unstable traumatic spine: a retrospective cohort study. North Am Spine Soc J NASSJ. 2023;15:100234.
76. Fan Y, et al. Accuracy of pedicle screw placement comparing robot-assisted technology and the free-hand with fluoroscopy-guided method in spine surgery: an updated meta-analysis. Medicine (Baltimore). 2018;97:e10970.
77. Li W, Li G, Chen W, Cong L. The safety and accuracy of robot-assisted pedicle screw internal fixation for spine disease: a meta-analysis. Bone Jt Res. 2020;9:653–66.
78. Fu W, et al. Robot-assisted technique vs conventional freehand technique in spine surgery: a meta-analysis. Int J Clin Pract. 2021;75:e13964.
79. Zhou L-P, Zhang R-J, Li H-M, Shen C-L. Comparison of cranial facet joint violation rate and four other clinical indexes between robot-assisted and freehand pedicle screw placement in spine surgery: a meta-analysis. Spine. 2020;45:E1532–40.
80. Li Y, et al. Comparison of short-term clinical outcomes between robot-assisted and freehand pedicle screw placement in spine surgery: a meta-analysis and systematic review. J Orthop Surg. 2023;18:359.
81. Peng Y-N, Tsai L-C, Hsu H-C, Kao C-H. Accuracy of robot-assisted versus conventional freehand pedicle screw placement in spine surgery: a systematic review and meta-analysis of randomized controlled trials. Ann Transl Med. 2020;8:824.
82. Romagna A, et al. Robot-assisted versus navigated transpedicular spine fusion: A comparative study. Int J Med Robot. 2023;19:e2500.
83. Li J, Fang Y, Jin Z, Wang Y, Yu M. The impact of robot-assisted spine surgeries on clinical outcomes: A systemic review and meta-analysis. Int J Med Robot. 2020;16:1–14.
84. Zhou L-P, et al. Clinical application of spinal robot in cervical spine surgery: safety and accuracy of posterior pedicle screw placement in comparison with conventional freehand methods. Neurosurg Rev. 2023;46:118.
85. Farah K, et al. Cirq® robotic assistance for minimally invasive C1-C2 posterior instrumentation: report on feasibility and safety. Oper Neurosurg. 2020;19:730–4.
86. Zhou L-P, et al. Robotics in cervical spine surgery: feasibility and safety of posterior screw placement. Neurospine. 2023;20:329–39.
87. Amin AG, Barzilai O, Bilsky MH. CT-based image-guided navigation and the DaVinci robot in spine oncology: changing surgical paradigms. HSS J® Musculoskelet J Hosp Spec Surg. 2021;17:294–301.
88. Meyer M, Farah K, Albader F, Fuentes S. Cirq® robotic assistance for percutaneous kyphoplasty of C1: report on feasibility. Acta Neurochir. 2023;165:3975–8.
89. Pennington Z, et al. Learning curves in robot-assisted spine surgery: a systematic review and proposal of application to residency curricula. Neurosurg Focus. 2022;52:E3.
90. Akazawa T, et al. Learning curves for robotic-assisted spine surgery: an analysis of the time taken for screw insertion, robot setting, registration, and fluoroscopy. Eur J Orthop Surg Traumatol. 2023;34:127–34.
91. Lee NJ, et al. A multicenter study of the 5-year trends in robot-assisted spine surgery outcomes and complications. J Spine Surg. 2022;8:9–20.
92. McDonnell JM, et al. Surgeon proficiency in robot-assisted spine surgery: a narrative review. Bone Jt J. 2020;102-B:568–72.
93. Fiani B, et al. Impact of robot-assisted spine surgery on health care quality and neurosurgical economics: A systemic review. Neurosurg Rev. 2020;43:17–25.
94. Sielatycki JA, Mitchell K, Leung E, Lehman RA. State of the art review of new technologies in spine deformity surgery–robotics and navigation. Spine Deform. 2022;10:5–17.
95. Crawford AM, et al. Intraoperative CT for lumbar fusion is not associated with improved short- or long-term complication profiles. Spine J. 2023;23:791–8.
96. Shafi KA, et al. Does robot-assisted navigation influence pedicle screw selection and accuracy in

minimally invasive spine surgery? Neurosurg Focus. 2022;52:E4.
97. Loniewski S, Farah K, Malikov S, Da Fuentes S. Vinci robotic-assisted anterolateral lumbar arthrodesis: operative technique. Acta Neurochir. 2023;165:2711–6.
98. Loniewski S, et al. Da Vinci robotic assistance for anterolateral lumbar arthrodesis: results of a French multicentric study. World Neurosurg. 2024;181:e685–93.
99. Beutler WJ, Peppelman WC, DiMarco LA. The da Vinci robotic surgical assisted anterior lumbar interbody fusion: technical development and case report. Spine. 2013;38:356–63.
100. Ye J, et al. Da Vinci robot-assisted laparoscopic retroperitoneal debridement for lumbar septic spondylodiscitis: A two-case report. Front Surg. 2022;9:930536.
101. Lee JYK, et al. Da Vinci robot-assisted Transoral Odontoidectomy for basilar invagination. ORL. 2010;72:91–5.
102. Perez-Cruet MJ, et al. Use of the da Vinci minimally invasive robotic system for resection of a complicated Paraspinal Schwannoma with thoracic extension: case report. Oper Neurosurg. 2012;71:onsE209–eE214.
103. Finley D, Sherman J, Avila E, Bilsky M. Thorascopic resection of an apical Paraspinal Schwannoma using the da Vinci surgical system. J Neurol Surg Part Cent Eur Neurosurg. 2013;75:058–63.
104. Rivero-Moreno Y, et al. Autonomous robotic surgery: has the future arrived? Cureus. 2024; https://doi.org/10.7759/cureus.52243.
105. Margalit A, et al. Autonomous spinal robotic system for Transforaminal lumbar epidural injections: a proof of concept of study. Glob Spine J. 2024;14:138–45.
106. Gao C, et al. Fluoroscopy-guided robotic system for Transforaminal lumbar epidural injections. IEEE Trans Med Robot Bionics. 2022;4:901–9.
107. Li Z, et al. Accuracy evaluation of a novel spinal robotic system for autonomous laminectomy in thoracic and lumbar vertebrae: A cadaveric study. J Bone Jt Surg. 2023;105:943–50.
108. Hao L, et al. An improved path planning algorithm based on artificial potential field and primal-dual neural network for surgical robot. Comput Methods Prog Biomed. 2022;227:107202.
109. McCloskey K, et al. Virtual and augmented reality in spine surgery: a systematic review. World Neurosurg. 2023;173:96–107.
110. Luca A, et al. Innovative educational pathways in spine surgery: advanced virtual reality–based training. World Neurosurg. 2020;140:674–80.
111. Zheng, C. et al. Development of a Virtual Reality Preoperative Planning System for Postlateral Endoscopic Lumbar Discectomy Surgery and Its Clinical Application. World Neurosurg. 2019;123:e1–e8.
112. Gasco, J. et al. Virtual reality spine surgery simulation: an empirical study of its usefulness. Neurol. Res. 2014;36:968–73.

MIX
Papier aus verantwortungsvollen Quellen
Paper from responsible sources
FSC® C105338

If you have any concerns about our products,
you can contact us on
ProductSafety@springernature.com

In case Publisher is established outside the EU,
the EU authorized representative is:
Springer Nature Customer Service Center GmbH
Europaplatz 3, 69115 Heidelberg, Germany

Printed by Libri Plureos GmbH
in Hamburg, Germany